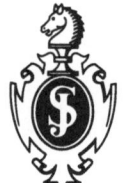

Christopher R. Chapple (Ed.)

Prostatic Obstruction

Pathogenesis and Treatment

With 67 Figures

Springer-Verlag
London Berlin Heidelberg New York
Paris Tokyo Hong Kong
Barcelona Budapest

Christopher R. Chapple BSc, MD, FRCS(Urol)
Consultant Urologist, Royal Hallamshire Hospital,
The Central Sheffield University Hospitals,
Glossop Road, Sheffield S10 2JF, UK

Cover illustration: cf. page 66

British Library Cataloguing in Publication Data
Prostatic Obstruction – Pathogenesis and Treatment
I. Chapple, Christopher R.
616.6

Library of Congress Cataloging-in-Publication Data
Prostatic Obstruction – Pathogenesis and Treatment/edited by
Christopher R. Chapple.
p. cm.
    Includes bibliographical references and index.
    ISBN-13: 978-1-4471-1868-8   e-ISBN-13: 978-1-4471-1866-4
    DOI: 10.1007/978-1-4471-1866-4

    1. Prostrate—Hypertrophy. 2. Prostrate—Surgery. 3. Bladder—
Obstruction. 4. Bladder Neck Obstruction—therapy. 5. Prostrate—
innervation. 6. Bladder—innervation. I. Chapple, Christopher R.
[DNLM: 1. Prostrate Diseases—physiopathology. 2. Prostatic Diseases—
therapy. 3. Bladder Neck Obstruction—physiopathology.
WJ 752 P2965 1993]   RC899.P34 1993   616.6'5—dc20
DNLM/DLC   93–17266

Typeset by The Electronic Book Factory Ltd, Fife, Scotland

28/3830–543210 Printed on acid-free paper

As men draw near the common goal,
Can anything be sadder
Than he who, master of his soul,
Is servant to his bladder.

Anonymous

Preface

The human prostate gland is of undoubted importance in reproductive physiology and is one of the commonest causes of clinical urological problems in the male patient. Despite the wealth of published literature relating to the prostate gland surprisingly little is understood about its neural innervation, the influence of pharmacological factors and its precise physiological functions.

Indeed, benign disorders of the prostate gland including benign prostatic hyperplasia, bladder neck dyssynergia and inflammatory disorders of the prostate (prostatitis, prostatodynia) although well recognised clinically, are as yet poorly characterised and understood. It was not until the late 1960s that the subject of urodynamics, which for the first time allowed scientific assessment of the function of the lower urinary tract, was introduced.

The first section of this book considers recent advances in our understanding of the innervation of the bladder and prostate gland and the changes in bladder function which accompany prostate mediated bladder outflow obstruction. The clinical consequence of benign prostatic hyperplasia in many patients is bladder outflow obstruction and although the traditional treatment of these conditions is by the use of ablative surgery, in recent years a number of new modalities have been investigated and are reviewed in the second section of the book.

Surgical prostatectomy is the most commonly used treatment for benign prostatic enlargement causing obstruction to the bladder outflow tract. Approximately 90% of patients will undergo a transurethral prostatectomy (Mebust, 1988) and this is the gold standard, against which other therapies need to be judged. This finding, coupled with the significant morbidity and indeed mortality associated with surgery, in particular via the transurethral route (Roos et al. 1989), recognition of the slow clinical progression of benign prostatic obstruction and increased public awareness recently of alternative non-surgical or minimally invasive treatment options, have raised a number of questions as to the ideal therapy in contemporary practice. The principles of pre-operative investigation and surgical intervention are discussed in Chapters 6 and 7. The condition of bladder neck dyssynergia is often unrecognised. Bladder neck dyssynergia and the condition of non-bacterial prostatitis (prostatodynia) are reviewed in Chapter 13. The controversy relating to the safety of prostatic surgery is reviewed in Chapter 8.

Alternative therapies to transurethral prostatectomy (TURP) are reviewed in depth. These are best considered under the headings pharmacological and mechanical.

Mechanical Therapy

Prostatic Stents

Of the many alternative treatments available for treating prostatic obstruction, only prostate stents relieve the obstruction to the same degree as prostatic surgery. These devices can broadly be considered as either temporary or permanent. The principal point of differentiation between these two categories is that the former are intraluminal in their position and hence will encrust with phosphatic debris if left long enough in contact with urine and are liable to become infected. The permanent stents are considerably more expensive than the temporary ones and are currently under investigation as a minimally invasive alternative to conventional surgical prostatectomy. This subject is reviewed in Chapter 9.

There seems to be no doubt that both permanent and temporary prostatic stents have a role in the contemporary management of prostatic obstruction. They are particularly suited to the elderly unfit patient where a major surgical procedure is contraindicated, providing a rapid treatment which can be carried out under local anaesthesia. Although considerably more expensive than the temporary stents, the permanent stents could potentially provide an alternative to surgical prostatectomy; provided that adequate stent placement can be achieved, thereby avoiding encrustation and the inevitable complications which will ensue from this in the long term.

Balloon Dilatation

The principle of prostatic dilatation is not new, the subject is very clearly and extensively reviewed in Chapter 11. A few more recent reports are worth noting. McLoughlin et al. (1991), studied 54 men using a 35 mm balloon, 46% of whom presented with acute urinary retention. Although they noted a marked improvement in patients with prostatic obstruction, very few of those in retention responded and the response in those who were obstructed appeared to be wearing off at 6 months follow-up. Lepor et al. (1991) in a single-blind comparison of balloon dilatation to cystoscopy reported there to be no apparent benefit accruing from the dilatation procedure. Others have reported an improvement in 67% of patients with benign prostatic hyperplasia lasting for up to 12 months following cystoscopy (Pollack, 1991). Indeed, it must be remembered that all treatments have a placebo effect which may be as high as 50% in a condition such as BPH where the progress of the disease is very slow with marked spontaneous fluctuations in the severity of symptoms.

Although it may be of particular benefit to the younger male, where the reduced likelihood of retrograde ejaculation and hence preservation of fertility is particularly important, it is now becoming increasingly clear that balloon dilatation is not a technique which is likely to replace transurethral resection of the prostate. Its mechanism of action remains unknown, the actual technique is not yet standardised in terms of size of balloon and duration of dilatation and the duration of action of treatment appears to be short-lived. Furthermore in the current economic climate it must be remembered that although balloon dilatation can be used in a day-case setting it has been calculated that the actual cost of the procedure may be as high as 50% of that of a transurethral prostatectomy (McCullough, 1990).

Prostatic Hyperthermia

Recent interest has centred upon the possibility of reducing outflow obstruction by microwave hyperthermia of the prostate (Chapter 10). Objective assessment of the results of this therapy is hampered by the variety of different devices which have been developed, using either transrectal or transurethral probes, different treatment regimens and the ethical and practical problems associated with randomised placebo-controlled studies. Although a number of hypotheses have been advanced for the mechanism of action of this therapy, it still remains unknown.

Microwave therapy offers the potential of a well-tolerated, safe, outpatient alternative to surgery. Whilst in the flurry of current enthusiasm new devices are being continually introduced, it must be borne in mind that contemporary microwave therapy, in particular, via the transurethral route is expensive. Furthermore, the improvements in voiding parameters do not appear to be as marked as those to be expected following surgical prostatectomy. As yet, the existing evidence is too incomplete for a definitive statement to be made as to the efficacy and long-term place of this therapy in the management of benign prostatic obstruction.

Other Minimally Invasive Techniques

Alternative therapies are continuously being evaluated and developed. Transurethral ultrasound-guided laser-induced prostatectomy (TULIP) (Roth et al. 1991; Wishnow et al. 1991) has been evaluated in an animal model and found to be a potentially effective therapy for the future. Laser photo-irradiation of the prostate is a technique which is currently under investigation, initial pilot studies have produced interesting results which warrant further investigation (Costello et al. 1991; Watson et al. 1991). High-energy shock waves (HESW) have been tested in an animal model and demonstrated to provide high-volume ablation of the prostate without injury to adjacent tissues (Foster et al. 1991). A preliminary clinical study in 21 patients using HESW from an ultrasound generator demonstrated a 111% improvement in flow rate at a mean follow-up of 6 months, with a marked improvement in symptoms and no significant side effects (Lobel et al. 1991).

Pharmacological Therapy

Whilst the pathogenesis of benign prostatic hypertrophy (BPH) is poorly understood it seems clear that hormonal factors are important in its pathogenesis, since it does not occur in patients who have been castrated before the age of 40 years (Moore, 1944). Although there are no significant differences in androgen levels in age-matched men with and without BPH (Bartsch et al. 1979), it seems likely that androgens provide a hormonal milieu that is essential to the development of BPH. A number of theories exist as to the mechanism of development of BPH (Geller, 1989). It is theoretically possible for hormonal therapy acting on the prostate to be targeted at many levels; the evidence for the clinical efficacy of existing therapy is discussed in Chapter 12.

Following on from the initial work of Caine and associates (Caine et al. 1976), pharmacological and ligand-binding studies by a number of workers have demonstrated the functional and ultrastructural pre-eminence of α_1 over α_2 receptors within the stromal compartment of the prostate (Chapple et al. 1989); thereby providing a scientific basis for the use of specific α_1 blockade in the non-surgical management of benign prostatic hyperplasia. The clinical studies relating to the use of α blockers are reviewed in Chapter 12.

Existing pharmacotherapy has a limited clinical role but is not comparable in terms of efficacy to surgical prostatectomy. The concurrent use of selective α_1-adrenergic blockade to relax prostatic smooth muscle combined with prostate selective hormonal blockade (e.g. 5α-reductase inhibitors) to shrink the glandular tissue, may provide additional therapeutic benefits in the future.

References

Bartsch, G., Muller, H.R., Oberholzer, M., Rohr, H.P. (1979). Light microscopic stereological analysis of the normal human prostate and of benign prostatic hyperplasia. J. Urol. 122:487

Caine, M., Pfau, A., Perlberg, S. (1976). The use of alpha-adrenoceptor blockers in benign prostatic obstruction. Br. J. Urol. 48:255–263

Chapple, C.R., Aubry, M.L., James, S., et al. (1989). Characterisation of human prostatic adrenoceptors using pharmacology, receptor binding and localisation. Br. J. Urol. 63:487–496

Costello, A.J., Johnson, D.E., Bolton, D.M., Bowsher, W.G. (1991). Nd:YAG laser ablation of the prostate as a treatment for benign prostatic hypertrophy. Presented at the annual meeting of the British Association of Urological Surgeons, 1991

Foster, R.S., Bihrle, R., Sanghvi, N.T., et al. (1991). Non-invasive ultrasound produced volume lesion in prostate. J. Urol. 145:396A

Geller. (1989). Pathogenesis and medical treatment of benign prostatic hyperplasia. Prostate (suppl) 2:95–104

Lepor, H., Sypherd, D., Derus, J., Machi, G. (1991). A randomised double-blind study comparing the efficacy of cystoscopy versus balloon dilatation of the prostate in males with symptomatic benign prostatic hyperplasia. J. Urol. 145:362A

Lobel, B., Gille, F., Cipolla, B., et al. (1991). High-energy shock waves for the treatment of benign prostatic hypertrophy. J. Urol. 145:396A

McCullough, D.L. (1990). Editorial comment. J. Urol. 144:88–89

McLoughlin, J., Keane, P.F., Jager, R., Gill, K.P., Machann, L., Williams, G. (1991). Dilatation of the prostatic urethra with a 35 mm balloon. Br. J. Urol. 67:177–181

Mebust, W.K. (1988). Surgical management of benign prostatic obstruction. Urology 32:12

Moore, R.A. (1944). Benign hypertrophy and carcinoma of the prostate: occurrence and experimental production in animals. Surgery 16:152–167

Pollack, H.M. (1991). Balloon dilatation of the prostate: effective treatment or dilatory tactic? Radiology 178:331–333.

Roos, N.P., Wennberg, J.E., Malenka D.J., et al. (1989). Mortality and re-operation after open and transurethral resection of the prostate for benign prostatic hyperplasia. N. Engl. J. Med. 320:1120–1123

Roth, R.A., Babayan, R., Aretz, T. (1991). TULIP: Transurethral ultrasound-guided laser-induced prostatectomy. J. Urol. 145:390A

Watson, G., Perlmutter, A., Shah, T. (1991). A laser balloon for prostatic outflow obstruction. Presented at the annual meeting of the British Association of Urological Surgeons, 1991

Wishnow, K.I., Newman, C.T., Croomens, D.E., Price R.E., von Eschenbach, A.C. (1991). Safety of transurethral laser treatment of the prostate. J. Urol. 145:267A

Acknowledgements

I would like to thank my colleagues for all their support in producing this book, the Medical Illustration Unit at the Middlesex Hospital for help with illustrations and Springer-Verlag London Ltd for all the editorial help which they have provided.

Contents

Contributors

Christopher R. Chapple, BSc, MD, FRCS(Urol)
Consultant Urological Surgeon,
The Royal Hallamshire Hospital,
Glossop Road,
Sheffield S10 2JF, UK

Timothy J. Christmas, MD, FRCS(Urol)
Consultant Urological Surgeon,
Department of Urology,
Charing Cross Hospital,
Fulham Palace Road,
London W6 8RF, UK

J. W. Hugh Evans, MS, FRCS
Senior Registrar in Urology,
St. Thomas' Hospital,
Lambeth Palace Road,
London S61 7EH, UK

Karl J. Kreder, MD, FACS
Department of Urology,
University of Iowa,
Hospital and Clinics,
Iowa City,
Iowa 52242, USA

N. MacCartney, FFARCS
Anaesthetic Registrar,
Department of Anaesthetics,
The Middlesex Hospital,
Mortimer Street,
London W1N 8AA, UK

Ian R. Marshall, BSc, PhD
Senior Lecturer in Pharmacology,
Department of Pharmacology,
University College,
Gower Street,
London WC1E 6BT, UK

Euan J.G. Milroy, FRCS
Consultant Urological Surgeon,
The Middlesex Hospital,
Mortimer Street,
London W1N 8AA, UK

Jeremy G. Noble, FRCS
Registrar,
Department of Urology,
Battle Hospital,
Oxford Road,
Reading RG3 1AG, UK

J. Brantley Thrasher, MD
Staff Urologist,
Madigan Army Medical Center,
Tacoma,
Washington, USA

Richard Turner-Warwick, CBE, DSc, FRCS, FACS
Honorary Senior Lecturer and Consultant Urological Surgeon,
The Institute of Urology and St Peter's Group of Hospitals,
The Middlesex Hospital,
Mortimer Street,
London W1N 8AA, UK

The Importance of Neural Factors in the Presentation and Treatment of Prostatic Obstruction

Chapter 1

Introduction: The Clinical Problem

C.R. Chapple

Historical Review

Male bladder outflow obstruction has presented a clinical problem throughout medical history. Catheters were used by the ancient Egyptians and Chinese as treatment for acute retention (Murphy, 1972). Jean Riolan the younger (1577–1657) is credited with being amongst the first to suggest that prostatic enlargement could result in mechanical obstruction to the bladder outflow tract (Shelley, 1965).

Morgagni (1769) reported that "the swelling of the prostate is most common in the decline of life". John Hunter in his "treatise on venereal disease" (1786) first recognised the structural and functional implications of lower urinary tract obstruction. He described the necessity for hormonal factors derived from the testis to the normal structure and function of the prostate and noted the asymmetric nature of prostatic enlargement. He presented such a clear synopsis of the functional problem that it is worth quoting it in its entirety: "the lateral width of the urethra gives such a resistance to the force or power of the bladder in expelling the urine as is easily overcome by the natural action of the bladder; but when the canal is lessened, either by stricture, spasm, swelled prostate gland or any other means, this proportion is lost, by which means the bladder finds greater difficulty than normal and is of course thrown into an increased action to overcome the resistance, which becomes a cause of the irritability and increased strength of this viscus in such diseases . . . the disease of the bladder arising from obstruction alone is increased irritability and its consequences, by which the bladder admits of little distension, becomes quick in its action and thick and strong in its coats". Despite providing this marked insight into the clinical problem such ideas were not followed up by other workers (cf Thompson, 1882) for nearly two centuries.

Urodynamic Investigation

The introduction of technology enabling measurement of intravesical pressure during filling (Dubois, 1876) and voiding (Mosso and Pellacani, 1882) laid the foundations for the development of techniques to study both

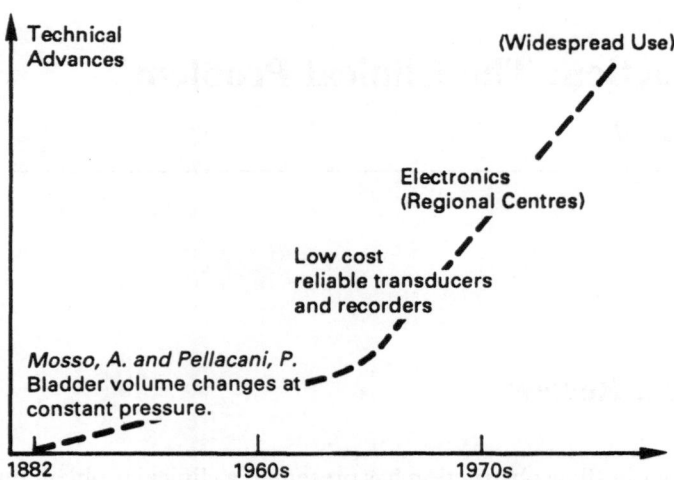

Fig. 1.1. Diagrammatic representation of the time scale underlying the development and distribution of urodynamic technology.

normal and disordered bladder function (Fig. 1.1). Rose (1932) reported an increased intravesical pressure during filling cystometry in patients with prostatic obstruction. However, the ability to measure pressure and flow parameters awaited the development of strain gauge transducers (Von Garrelts, 1956; Smith 1968; Claridge, 1966). Smith (1968) clearly defined the pressure/flow relationship in obstruction and suggested a mathematical relationship (maximum voiding detrusor pressure/ maximum flow rate) for the calculation of urethral resistance. Claridge (1966) suggested that many of the symptoms of obstruction were due to changes in the detrusor; he noted that the intravesical pressure at rest prior to micturition was higher in obstructed patients and concluded that frequency and urgency were related to this increased pressure. Hodgkinson et al. (1963) had previously reported similar bladder over-activity in a group of women presenting with urge incontinence and noted the ability of a normal subject to inhibit such bladder contractions. In both groups of patients there were no demonstrable associated urological abnormalities, an important consideration since other workers had suggested that detrusor over-activity could be attributed solely to an underlying urological abnormality (Miller et al. 1965).

Bates (1971; Bates et al. 1970; Bates and Corney, 1971) defined the role of clinical urodynamics and from the unit at The Middlesex Hospital described the technique of synchronous cine/flow/cystourethrography (videocystometrography). He stressed the importance of measuring the *true* detrusor pressure (total bladder pressure minus abdominal pressure) and of carrying out such studies in both standing and lying positions in order to unmask any underlying abnormality (vide infra). In addition he clearly showed that if the bladder was filled at a rate of 100 ml/minute in "normal subjects" who were specifically asked to hold their urine, then there was little rise in detrusor pressure during filling, even when the patient felt uncomfortably full; the so-called stable detrusor.

This group of workers applied the term "unstable" bladder (detrusor instability) to the over-active detrusor behaviour previously recognised by Hodgkinson in 1963. In the absence of a demonstrable neurological abnormality they noted its occurrence in a number of groups of patients; including up to 10% of the general population and as a secondary phenomenon in over 50% of those with proximal urethral outflow obstruction (Turner-Warwick et al. 1973). Based on this work urodynamics has now received widespread international acceptance. The techniques and terminology used in urodynamic investigation are monitored and standardised by the International Continence Society (Abrams et al. 1988). Initial experience suggested that an involuntary detrusor pressure rise in excess of 15 cm H_2O was pathognomonic of detrusor instability. Subsequent work has suggested that an absolute value of this nature should be avoided and that the pattern of the pressure rise is more important (see Fig. 1.2).

Controversy remains concerning the differentiation of marginal or "steep" instability from "low compliance" (Abrams et al. 1988); and indeed whether they might not represent the same phenomenon (see Fig. 1.2). Compliance is defined as the change in volume for a given change in pressure. During normal bladder filling there is little or no pressure change, although the mural tension increases as the bladder fills (Smith, 1976). This phenomenon can be attributed to the physiological property of smooth muscle known as receptive relaxation; this is not nerve mediated, but rather reflects the physiological and physical properties of the bladder wall (Tang and Ruch, 1955).

Unfortunately, a barrier to resolution of the debate over the distinction between low compliance and detrusor instability is raised both by our lack of understanding of the pathogenesis of detrusor instability and our limited knowledge of the mechanisms underlying the normal function and, in particular, neural control of human detrusor smooth muscle. Therefore the majority of cases of detrusor instability remain idiopathic.

Further progress in our understanding of detrusor instability has awaited the development of a suitable model in which an identifiable factor can be related to the subsequent onset of secondary detrusor instability. Investigation of prostatic bladder outflow obstruction provides this opportunity.

Prostate Obstruction and Detrusor Instability

A review of the literature (see Table 1.1) reveals that detrusor instability occurs in between 52% and 80% of men with bladder outlet obstruction due to benign prostatic hyperplasia. Conversely, surgical relief of bladder outflow obstruction results in a recovery of normal detrusor behaviour in the majority of patients (Table 1.2). Such observations lend support to the hypothesis that there is a causal link between the two conditions.

The scientific investigation of prostate obstruction using urodynamic principles has allowed the recognition of two main groups of symptoms:

1. *Obstructive*: hesitancy, poor stream, feeling of incomplete bladder emptying.

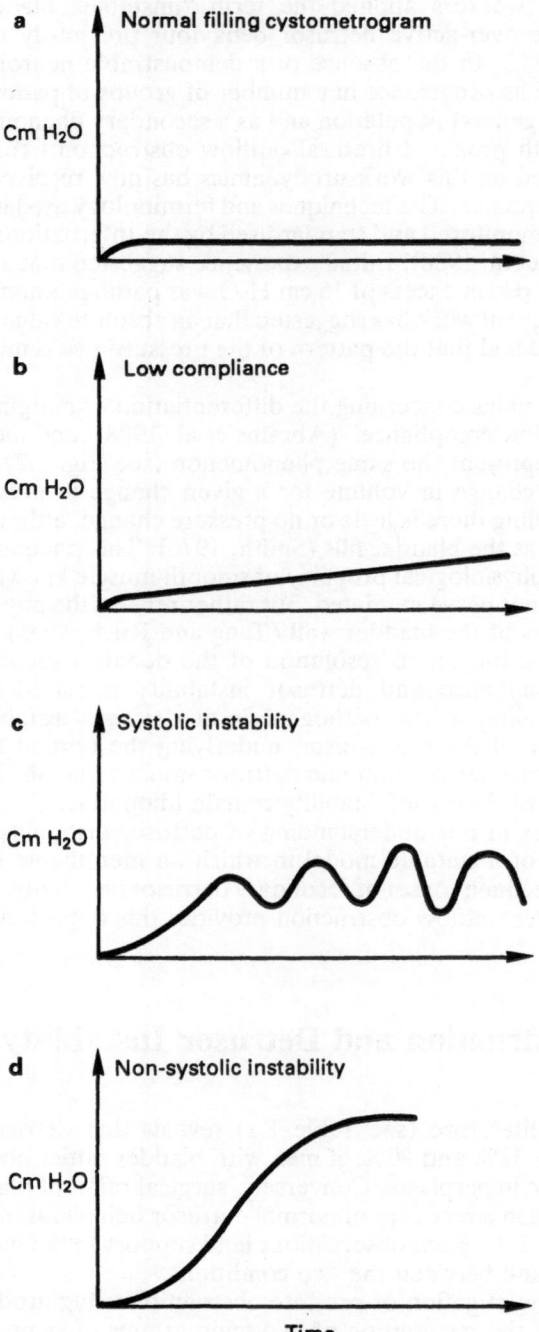

Fig. 1.2. Stylised filling cystometry traces to demonstrate **a** normal, **b** low compliance, **c** systolic instability, **d** non-systolic instability.

Table 1.1. The prevalence of detrusor instability demonstrated urodynamically in patients with prostate obstruction (after Abrams 1985)

Reference	No. of patients	% detrusor instability	Text refers to:
Leppanen 1962[a]	43	56	"Hypertonic"
Makrigiannis and Gaca 1972[a]	50	56	Detrusor instability
Andersen 1982	93	49	"Hyperreflexia"
Abrams 1977[a]	203	63	Detrusor instability
Price et al. 1980	40	72	Detrusor instability
Meyhoff et al. 1984	60	80	Detrusor instability
Coolsaet et al. 1984	139	52	Detrusor instability
Frimodt-Moller et al.1984[a]	84	65	Detrusor instability

[a] These series may contain unobstructed patients as no definition of obstruction in relation to instability was presented.

2. *Irritative*: daytime frequency, nocturia, urgency, and urge incontinence.

The normal male voids to completion at a maximum pressure of 40–50 cmH$_2$O and a free flow rate in excess of 25 ml/sec. In the initial stages of bladder outflow obstruction an increase in the maximum micturition pressure compensates for the increased outflow resistance and there is often no reduction in the free flow rate until a later stage when the classical picture of high pressure/low flow is seen.

Irritative symptoms could arise from either motor or sensory dysfunction (Bates and Corney, 1971), but are usually the symptomatic manifestation of secondary detrusor instability. Indeed symptoms associated with detrusor instability are often the most troublesome to the patient and usually provide the stimulus prompting medical referral. Although effective relief of bladder outflow obstruction usually leads to complete resolution of associated detrusor instability within 6 months, such symptoms may persist for up to 1 year following relief of obstruction. When detrusor instability persists following surgery it commonly results in troublesome symptoms. Studies of patients with post-prostatectomy incontinence reveal a significant association with persisting detrusor instability. Fitzpatrick et al. (1979) studied 68 patients: 45 had persisting instability associated with post-prostatectomy incontinence, 37 had no urodynamic evidence of residual obstruction.

The causal association between instability and prostatic obstruction has recently been challenged by Abrams (1985), who notes that other types of outflow obstruction are not associated with a similar predisposition to detrusor instability. In addition, the incidence of detrusor instability increases with advancing age in the population, even in unobstructed patients. Andersen

Table 1.2. The incidence of detrusor instability before and after prostatectomy (after Abrams 1985)

Reference	Pre-operative %	Post-operative %
Leppanen	80 after RPP	0
1962	35 after TURP	22
Makrigiannis and Gaca	34 after RPP	0
1972	50 after TURP	25
Andersen	49	31
1982		
Abrams	56	23
1977		
Price et al.	72	28
1980		
Meyhoff et al.	81 after RPP	55
1984	79 after TURP	44
Frimodt-	65	22
Moller et al. 1984		

TURP, transurethral resection of the prostate; RPP, retropubic prostatectomy.

(1982) showed detrusor hyperreflexia in 53% of 17 asymptomatic elderly males aged 60–75 and in addition, he confirmed the poor correlation between detrusor instability and "severity of obstruction" as judged by urodynamic parameters, which had previously been reported by Arnold (1973).

Although the possibility of a causal link between detrusor instability and outflow obstruction is contentious, it is clear from animal studies that bladder outflow obstruction does lead to important functional changes within the bladder (Sibley, 1987). The resultant reversible changes in detrusor function appear to provide a good model for the secondary detrusor instability seen in the human. The literature on this subject is reviewed in detail in Chapter 4.

It is therefore evident that there is an association between bladder outlet obstruction and detrusor instability which resolves in up to two thirds of patients following surgery, and is an important cause of troublesome symptoms. There have been few reported studies of the combined morphological and physiological changes which occur in the bladder in response to obstruction and which may contribute to disordered detrusor function. The logical solution is to investigate this matter further using a combination of histochemical and pharmacological techniques to study the effect of outflow obstruction on the innervation and function of the human detrusor.

The Neural Control of the Human Prostate: Neural Influences and Benign Prostatic Hyperplasia

Benign prostatic hyperplasia is an almost universal finding in men with normal gonadal function, from the 5th decade of life. Prostatic enlargement causes urethral compression and results in an increased resistance to the bladder outflow tract. The incidence of prostatic obstruction increases with age from the 6th decade of life onwards; but the onset of symptoms is gradual and usually only slowly progressive (Ball et al. 1981). However, it has been estimated that a 40-year-old man has a 29% risk of undergoing a prostatectomy during his lifetime (Glynn et al. 1985).

The traditional view of the pathogenesis of prostatic obstruction regards simple mechanical urethral compression, resulting from an increase in prostatic bulk, as being the major component. In recent years this view has been challenged. It is now well recognised that the degree of prostatic enlargement as assessed clinically correlates poorly with the severity of outflow obstruction (Turner-Warwick et al. 1973). Whilst this can be attributed solely to the asymmetric nature of prostatic enlargement (Hunter, 1786) an additional factor which has been increasingly recognised in recent years is the important contribution provided by the neural control of the prostate to the genesis of bladder outflow obstruction (Donker et al. 1972; Furuya et al. 1982).

A substantial body of evidence now exists to support the hypothesis that the sympathetic nervous system controls the contraction of the prostatic musculature via the release of noradrenaline which binds onto adrenoceptors within prostatic muscle. This has allowed the development of non-surgical pharmacological treatment of benign prostatic outflow obstruction using sympathetic α-adrenoceptor blockade (Caine 1986 a,b).

Despite the undoubted importance of the prostate gland in both health and disease, surprisingly little information is available relating to the ultrastructure of its innervation. Recent reports have suggested that sensory nerve stimulation within the prostate gland may be important in the aetiology of the associated secondary detrusor instability (Chalfin and Bradley, 1982). However, few previous studies have documented the motor innervation and only one has described the sensory innervation of the human prostate (Crowe et al 1991).

References

Abrams, P.H. 1977. The investigation of bladder outflow obstruction in the male. MD thesis, University of Bristol

Abrams, P.H. 1985. Detrusor instability in bladder outlet obstruction. Neurourol. Urodynamics 4:317–328

Abrams, P.H., Blaivas, J.G., Stanton, S.L., Andersen, J.T. 1988. The standardisation of terminology of lower urinary tract function. Scand. J. Urol. Nephrol. (suppl.) 114:5–19

Andersen, J.T. 1982. Prostatism. III. Detrusor hyperreflexia and residual urine. Clinical and urodynamic aspects and the influence of surgery on the prostate. Scand. J. Urol. Nephrol. 16:25–30

Arnold, E.P. 1973. A urodynamic analysis of detrusor dysfunction. PhD thesis, University of London

Ball, A.J., Feneley, R.C.L., Abrams, P.H. 1981. The natural history of untreated "prostatism". Br. J. Urol. 53:613–616

Bates, C.P., Whiteside, C.G., Turner-Warwick, R.T. 1970. Synchronous cine/pressure/flow/cysto-urethrography with special reference to stress and urge incontinence. Br. J. Urol. 42:714–723

Bates, C.P. 1971. Continence and incontinence. A clinical study of the dynamics of voiding and of the sphincter mechanism. Ann. R. Coll. Surg. Engl. 49:18–35

Bates, C.P., Corney, C.E. 1971. Synchronous cine/pressure/flow cystourethrography: a method of routine urodynamic assessment. Br. J. Radiol. 44:44–50

Caine, M. 1986a. Clinical experience with α-adrenoceptor antagonists in benign prostatic hypertrophy. Fed. Proc. 45:2604–2608

Caine, M. 1986b. The present role of α-adrenergic blockers in the treatment of benign prostatic hypertrophy. J. Urol. 136:1–4

Chalfin, S.A., Bradley, W.E. 1982. The aetiology of detrusor hyperreflexia in patients with infravesical obstruction. J. Urol. 127:938–942

Claridge, M. 1966. Analyses of obstructed micturition. Ann. R. Coll. Surg. 39:30–53

Coolsaet, B.L.R.A., Van Venroois, G.E.P.M., Blok, C. 1984. Prostatism: rationalisation of urodynamic testing. World J. Urol. 2:216–221

Crowe, R., Chapple, C.R., Burnstock, G. 1991. The human prostate gland: a histochemical and immunohistochemical study of neuropeptides, serotonin, dopamine β-hydroxylase and acetylcholinesterase in autonomic nerves and ganglia. Br. J. Urol. 68:53–61

Donker, P.J., Ivanovici, F., Noach, E.L. 1972. Analyses of the urethral pressure profile by means of electromyography and the administration of drugs. Br. J. Urol. 44:180–193

Dubois, P. 1876. Ueber den Druck in der Harnblase. Dtsch. Arch. Klin. Med. 17:148–163

Fitzpatrick, J.M., Gardiner, R.A., Worth, P.H.L. 1979. The evaluation of 68 patients with post-prostatectomy incontinence. Br. J. Urol. 51:552–555

Frimodt-Moller, P.C., Jensen, K.M.E., Iversen, P., Madsen, P.O., Bruskewitz, R.C. 1984. Analysis of presenting symptoms in prostatism. J. Urol. 132:272–276

Furuya, S., Kumamoto, Y., Yokoyama, E., Tsukamoto, T., Izumi, T., Abiko, Y. 1982. Alpha-adrenergic activity and urethral pressure profilometry in prostatic zone in benign prostatic hypertrophy. J. Urol. 128:836–839

Glynn, R.J., Campion, E.W., Bouchard, G.R., Silbert, J.E. 1985. The development of benign prostatic hyperplasia among volunteers in the normative aging study. Am. J. Epidemiol. 121:78–90

Hodgkinson, C.P., Ayers, M.A., Drukker, B.H. 1963. Dyssynergic detrusor dysfunction in the apparently normal female. Am. J. Obstet. Gynecol. 87:717–730

Hunter, J. 1786. Treatise on venereal disease. In: The works of John Hunter FRS. Vol 11. Palmer, J.F., ed. Paternoster Row, London, Longman Rees Orme Brown Green and Longman, 1835, p 284

Lepannen, M.K. 1962. A cystometric study of the function of the urinary bladder in prostatic patients. Urol. Int. 14:226–238

Makrigiannis, D., Gaca, A. 1972. Cystometric studies of detrusor function after prostatectomy and transurethral electrosurgery. Int. Urol. Nephrol. 4:175–178

Meyhoff, H.H., Nordling, J., Hald, T. 1984. Urodynamic evaluation of transurethral versus transvesical prostatectomy. Scand. J. Urol. 18:27–35

Miller, H.G., Simpson, C.A., Yeates, W.K. 1965. Bladder dysfunction in multiple sclerosis. Br. Med. J. i:1265–1269

Morgagni, G. 1769. The seats and causes of disease. In: Investigated by Anatomy. Book 3. Miller, A., Cadell, T., eds. London, Johnson and Payne, pp 46–462

Mosso, A., Pellacani, P. 1882. Sur les fonctions de la vessie. Arch. Ital. Biol. 1:97–128, 291–324

Murphy, L.J.T. 1972. The history of urology. Springfield, Illinois, C.C. Thomas

Price, D.A., Ramsden, P.D., Stobbart, D. 1980. The unstable bladder and prostatectomy. Br. J. Urol. 52:529–531

Rose, D.K. 1932. Changes in the wall of the bladder secondary to prostatic obstruction. Arch. Surg. 25:783–795

Shelley, H.S. 1965. The enlarged prostate, a brief history of its treatment. J. Hist. Med. 20:452–473

Sibley, G.N.A. 1987. The physiological response of the detrusor muscle to experimental bladder outflow obstruction in the pig. Br. J. Urol. 60:332–336

Smith, J.C. 1968. Urethral resistance to micturition. Br. J. Urol. 40:125–156

Smith, J.C. 1976. The function of the bladder. In: Urology Vol 2. Blandy, J., ed. Oxford, Blackwell, pp 672–686

Tang, P.C., Ruch, T.C. 1955. Non-neurogenic basis of bladder tonus. Am. J. Physiol. 181:249–257

Thompson, H. 1882. The diseases of the prostate; their pathology and treatment. London, J. and A. Churchill, pp 1–152

Turner-Warwick, R.T., Whiteside, C.G., Arnold, E.P., et al. 1973. A urodynamic view of prostate obstruction and the results of prostatectomy. Br. J. Urol. 45:632–645

Von Garrelts, B. 1956. Analysis of micturition. A new method of recording the voiding of the bladder. Acta Chir. Scand. 112:326–340

Chapter 2

The Anatomy and Innervation of the Bladder

C.R. Chapple

Introduction

The urinary tract provides a highly sophisticated system of conduits, which allows the conversion of a continuous and involuntary production of urine by the kidneys into the intermittent, consciously controlled voiding of urine (micturition) in appropriate circumstances. It is also designed to protect the nephrons of the kidney from damage by the retrograde transmission of pressure or infection from the bladder.

The urinary bladder has two main functions: the collection and low–pressure storage of urine and its subsequent expulsion at an appropriate time and place. Disruption of the normal action of the bladder usually produces significant clinical symptoms. Such symptoms may be the consequence of either local pathological conditions affecting the bladder and its outflow tract or disordered neural control of detrusor muscle. In order to understand the clinical consequences of disordered bladder function, it is necessary first to appreciate the structure of the bladder, its innervation and neurophysiological control.

Historical Aspects

The first recorded reference to the human bladder is to be found in the ancient Indian literature: in the "Susmata Samhita" (Mettler, 1947). Fallopius is accredited with being the first to recognise that the bladder is not an inert reservoir, but is emptied by active contraction of its muscle coat. A later account attributable to Galen (second century AD) described the walls of this organ to be comprised of fibres arranged in discrete functional layers (Hald, 1969). This concept was considered to be correct until the early part of this century (McCrea, 1926). Although Spiegel initially coined the term musculus detrusor urinae (detrudare = to drive out), and applied it to the longitudinal muscle coat alone (Griffiths, 1891), more recent studies have demonstrated that individual muscle fibres traverse all layers of the bladder wall (Hunter, 1954; Woodburne, 1960).

Anatomy

The human urinary bladder is an organ of variable size and shape as dictated by the volume of fluid present within its lumen. It has three distinct histological layers: an outer adventitial connective tissue layer, a middle smooth muscle coat and an innermost mucous membrane of transitional cell epithelium. This mucous membrane is supported by lamina propria and muscularis mucosa (Dixon et al. 1983) and provides an elastic lining which is impervious to urine.

The mammalian bladder can be subdivided into three distinct regions on the basis of embryological, histological and functional criteria:

- bladder body
- trigone
- bladder neck

The detrusor muscle is responsible for the normal motor function of the bladder and although it can be further subdivided into three concentric ill-defined layers it is best considered as a single unit comprising interlocking muscle fibres which combine to form a functional syncytium. The detrusor muscle is under the control of the autonomic nervous system and receives a rich innervation comprising three main groups of nerves which form dense plexuses amongst the smooth muscle cells. Within the bladder, nerves pursue a tortuous course, which provides slack that can be taken up during bladder distension (Fletcher and Bradley, 1969).

In the male there are two important sphincteric mechanisms, a proximal "bladder neck mechanism" and a urethral sphincteric mechanism lying at the apex of the prostate (the "distal sphincter mechanism").

The male bladder neck subserves two functions. It is a powerful urinary sphincter and its contraction during ejaculation is essential to the prevention of the retrograde transmission of semen into the bladder. In addition, there is a more distal urethral sphincteric mechanism lying at the apex of the prostate. This distal sphincteric mechanism is extremely powerful as evidenced by its ability to maintain continence even when the bladder neck has been rendered totally incompetent by bladder neck incision or prostatectomy. The urethral sphincter mechanism is comprised of intrinsic urethral smooth muscle and extrinsic striated muscle components.

Although bladder neck and urethral smooth muscle receive a dual autonomic innervation, the sympathetic nervous system is thought to be of principal importance in the male. The efferent innervation of the striated muscle (the extrinsic component of the urethral sphincter), arises predominantly from cell bodies lying in a specific area of the sacral anterior horn known as Onufs nucleus (Onufrowicz, 1900). A number of aspects of the innervation of this sphincter are controversial, for example, whether the somatic nerve fibres pass via the pudendal nerve (Vodusek and Light, 1983) or the pelvic splanchnic nerves (Gosling et al. 1983) and whether there is a significant autonomic innervation.

The trigone is a triangular area framed by the ureteric orifices above and the internal urethral meatus below. The majority of the muscle cells comprising the trigonal detrusor muscle are histologically indistinguishable from their counterparts in the remainder of the bladder. A thin superficial muscle layer is thickened superiorly to form a prominent slightly curved ridge known as the superficial trigonal muscle. This is comprised of small-diameter muscle cells which are morphologically distinct from the detrusor muscle (Gosling et al. 1983); they arise from mesodermal structures and hence have a different embryological origin from the bladder. Despite its rather insignificant mass, it is suggested that by contracting during micturition, this muscle occludes the ureteric orifices to prevent vesicoureteric reflux (Hutch, 1963, Tanagho and Pugh, 1963).

Innervation

In mammalian species the urinary bladder receives an innervation from the parasympathetic and sympathetic divisions of the autonomic nervous system which traditionally contain the neurotransmitters acetylcholine and noradrenaline respectively (Langley and Anderson, 1895; Elliott, 1907), although recently, a number of non-adrenergic, non-cholinergic (NANC) neurotransmitters have been identified (Ambache and Aboo Zar, 1970). In the human bladder, parasympathetic stimulation initiates bladder contraction (Learmonth, 1931) via the release of the transmitter acetylcholine. At present, the role of adrenergic sympathetic neurons and NANC sensorimotor nerves containing putative peptidergic, amine and purinergic neurotransmitters is still the subject of debate. The remainder of this chapter reviews the anatomy and ultrastructure of bladder innervation and its potential neurophysiological role.

Mobley and co-workers (1966) were the first to report that the body and the base of the human bladder have a dual parasympathetic and sympathetic innervation which is distributed both in company with and separately from blood vessels. However it has been recognised for a long time that there is a dual autonomic innervation to the bladder in most mammalian species (Langley and Anderson, 1895; Elliott, 1907). The subsequent literature contains a number of conflicting observations, which can be related to the extreme heterogeneity of the material studied by different authors, occasioned by the difficulties inherent in obtaining "normal" human tissue. A review of the literature reveals the following as being the principal sources of error:

1. Differences in the age and sex of the subjects studied
2. The coexistence of unrecognised disease
3. Difficulties in standardising the site and type of tissue samples collected
4. The diversity and limitations of the investigative techniques used.

Motor Innervation

Parasympathetic Neurons

Considerable methodological problems are associated with the specific histo-chemical localisation of peripheral acetylcholine-containing neurons. Current techniques rely on the relatively non-specific technique first described by Koelle and Friendenwald (1949), which demonstrates the presence of the ubiquitous enzyme acetylcholinesterase (AChE). Indeed, it has been suggested that much of the AChE activity which can be demonstrated in detrusor muscle is related to non-specific staining of the muscle cell membrane (Raezer et al. 1973). A more specific technique for the histochemical demonstration of acetylcholine-containing nerve fibres depends upon the visualisation of ChAT (choline acetyl transferase), the acetylcholine synthesising enzyme (Burt and Silver, 1973). This technique is unfortunately not suitable for use in the demonstration of peripheral nerves, since it only stains neuronal cell bodies and not terminals (Alm, 1978). Despite the problems outlined above it is now generally considered that AChE staining does provide reliable visualisation of peripheral cholinergic neurons (Elbadawi, 1982), although it must be remembered that it will also non-specifically stain nerves containing a variety of other neurotransmitters.

Cholinergic nerves identified by their AChE content (Gosling et al. 1983) are the principal neuronal population within the detrusor body. These AChE-positive neurons form a net-like plexus in all areas of the bladder body with large AChE-positive nerve trunks clearly identifiable in the basal layers of smooth muscle cells (Ek et al. 1977). Electron microscopy has shown these neurons to lie in close apposition to muscle cells (Taira, 1972), where they are likely to mediate the motor control of detrusor smooth muscle via the release of acetylcholine.

Sympathetic Neurons

Techniques specifically to identify noradrenergic nerves demonstrate that in contrast to the rich parasympathetic nervous supply the sympathetic supply to the bladder body is sparse and non-uniformly distributed. In the normal bladder adrenergic terminals can be identified predominantly in association with blood vessels rather than smooth muscle and are thought to be important in the control of vasculature (Elbadawi and Schenk, 1966; Sundin et al. 1977).

The trigone can be subdivided anatomically into two areas as noted above, each of which has a distinctive neural innervation. The deep layer is identical in terms of structure and innervation to the main detrusor muscle: the trigonal detrusor muscle. In contrast, the superficial layer of the trigone possesses few AChE-positive nerves but a predominance of noradrenergic sympathetic neurons (Gosling et al. 1983; Ek et al. 1977).

Benson et al. (1979) demonstrated adrenergic nerve terminals using a fluorescent glyoxylic acid technique; the distribution was patchy within muscle bundles, but there was an association between these nerve fibres and blood vessels. No sex-related difference in the innervation of the bladder wall was evident, but they described an age-related decline in adrenergic innervation, a similar phenomenon to that which had previously been noted in human sympathetic ganglia (Hervonen et al. 1978). Nordling (1983) reported a sparse distribution of noradrenergic nerve terminals both within the detrusor and the trigonal smooth muscle.

The differences reported by various investigators in the morphology and distribution of adrenergic nerves within the human bladder may be more apparent than real. Catecholamines are labile and histochemical results are notoriously subject to methodological errors arising from the collection of tissue and its subsequent handling.

Electron microscopy (vide infra) confirms that in the bladder dome the majority of nerve fibres are likely to be cholinergic whilst, in the trigone, adrenergic endings still represent only a small proportion of the total (Dixon and Gosling, 1987). Such work confirms the results of light microscopy studies and in particular supports the use of the non-specific AChE technique. As elsewhere in the body, it is likely that the sympathetic and parasympathetic nerve supplies to the bladder have opposing actions. Clearly, in view of the sparse distribution of innervation, sympathetically mediated inhibition of bladder smooth muscle activity is unlikely to depend upon a direct action on detrusor musculature.

Sympathetic/Parasympathetic Interaction

Evidence from animal studies suggests that detrusor inhibition is mediated by sympathetic neurons acting via α_1 receptors located upon parasympathetic cell bodies within perivesical or pelvic plexuses and acting via the presynaptic inhibition of acetylcholine release (De Groat and Booth, 1980). A plausible hypothesis is that vesical ganglia act as filters on the efferent pathways to the bladder, functioning as blocks when preganglionic firing is low, but conversely facilitating neurotransmission when activity is increased. Although numerous ganglia each containing up to 20 neuronal cell bodies can be identified within the human bladder wall, these appear to contain cholinergic neurons with no evidence of noradrenergic terminals within them. In view of the absence of associated adrenergic nerve terminals it therefore seems unlikely that there is a significant interaction between cholinergic parasympathetic and sympathetic autonomic neurons at the level of the bladder ganglia (Dixon et al. 1983; Gilpin et al. 1983). However, in both the perivesical and pelvic plexuses there are numerous synaptic contacts between the constituent sympathetic and parasympathetic neurons (Dixon et al. 1983).

Non-adrenergic, Non-cholinergic Innervation

A third population of neurons found within the bladder comprises the so-called non-adrenergic, non-cholinergic (NANC) sensorimotor nerves (Mundy,

1984). These nerves contain a number of putative neurotransmitters, which can be identified by the use of immunofluorescence techniques (Ambache and Aboo Zar, 1970). The existence of peripheral nerves that conformed to neither of the traditional autonomic groups was first suggested in the 1960s (Burnstock, 1969). The original reason for the interest in this third group of NANC nerves was to find an explanation for the so-called atropine resistance found in studies of the animal bladder (Ambache and Aboo Zar, 1970).

In electron microscopy studies, differentiation between cholinergic and adrenergic nerve terminals depends on identification of the type of transmitter vesicles present. Presumptive cholinergic terminals contain small agranular vesicles whilst adrenergic endings contain small dense-core vesicles. In both neural populations large granular vesicles which are thought to contain peptides may also be found (Larsson et al. 1977). More recently, a precise correlation between morphological appearance and the contents of vesicles has been challenged (Daniel et al. 1983). Nevertheless, in recent years a considerable body of histochemical and biochemical evidence has accumulated which indicates that peptide neurotransmitters are widely distributed in structures involved in the regulation of bladder and urethral function by both central and peripheral nervous systems (Maggi and Meli, 1986; De Groat and Kawatani, 1985).

Unfortunately, despite the abundance of research there have been few attempts to integrate structural and functional observations. An important contributory factor in the case of the human bladder is the paucity of physiological and pharmacological data on the functional role of these putative neurotransmitters. If the classical criteria required to identify a putative neurotransmitter are strictly applied, few if any of these putative peptide neurotransmitters would have an established role.

Criteria for Classical Neurotransmitters.

1. Synthesis and storage in nerve terminals
2. Calcium-dependent release on nerve stimulation
3. Occupation of specific receptors on the post-junctional cell leading to changes in its activity
4. Inactivation by enzyme and/or by uptake
5. Drugs producing parallel block (or potentiation) of the responses to neural stimulation and the exogenously applied substance.

In an attempt to integrate and explain the role of these NANC substances it has been suggested that some neurons may store and release more than one transmitter. This hypothesis is based on the work of Burn and Rand (1965) and comparative studies of the evolution of the autonomic nervous system (Burnstock, 1969). There is now considerable support for the intraneuronal coexistence of peptides and purine nucleotides with classical neurotransmitters such as acetylcholine and noradrenaline outside the urinary tract (Hokfelt et al. 1980; Burnstock, 1986 a,b; Gu et al. 1984). Although the functional interaction of these putative peptide neurotransmitters within the classical autonomic innervation remains to be established, possible roles include: co-transmission, neuromodulation and a trophic function.

In the early 1970s a large number of compounds (including peptides, purines, monoamines and amino acids) were screened for a potential role as NANC neurotransmitters within the bladder. A substance that satisfied the classical criteria (see above) was the purine nucleotide adenosine 5-triphosphate (ATP). Nerves containing this were termed "purinergic" (Burnstock, 1972). Histological attempts to identify purinergic nerves have so far been disappointing, but on electron microscopy it has been reported that purinergic nerve terminals contain granulated vesicles larger than those within cholinergic or adrenergic endings, so-called "large opaque vesicles" (Burnstock, 1972). There is well documented evidence of an important functional role for purinergic nerves in non-primate mammals, in particular the guinea pig (Burnstock et al. 1978; Mackenzie and Burnstock, 1984); but this subject is still the matter of some debate (Ambache et al. 1977; Levin et al. 1986). Recently a number of peptides including vasoactive intestinal polypeptide (VIP), neuropeptide Y (NPY), substance P (SP), somatostatin, calcitonin gene-related peptide (CGRP) and enkephalin have been identified in the bladder innervation in experimental animals and have been ascribed a neurotransmitter or neuromodulatory role (Maggi and Meli, 1986). Very little histochemical work on the human bladder has been reported, but the presence of VIP, NPY, substance P and somatostatin has been confirmed (Gu et al. 1984).

The role of the NANC neurotransmitters in the human bladder is as yet poorly understood. Although substance P and CGRP are thought to be involved in afferent nerve pathways (Maggi and Meli, 1986; Mundy, 1984), VIP is the only peptide transmitter for which any defined physiological role has been identified. In the cat 10%–15% of bladder ganglia exhibit VIP immunoreactivity (Kawatani et al. 1985). VIP has also been detected in intramural ganglia of the human urinary bladder and in nerve fibres which are particularly densely distributed beneath the epithelium, around blood vessels and in the muscle layers. VIP is present in higher concentration in the trigone than in the dome of the bladder (Polak and Bloom, 1984; Gu et al. 1984).

It has been reported that VIP tissue levels are markedly reduced in the bladder of patients with idiopathic detrusor instability (Gu et al. 1983). The myogenic (tetrodotoxin-resistant) contractile activity of the human detrusor, which is inhibited by exogenous VIP, is greater than normal in detrusor hyperreflexia as contrasted to that of urodynamically normal bladders (Kinder and Mundy, 1985). A plausible hypothesis which explains these observations is that detrusor instability results from a disorder of intrinsic inhibitory mechanisms, involving endogenous VIP-ergic fibres within the detrusor.

Sensory Innervation

Whilst there are still marked gaps in our knowledge of the efferent (motor) innervation of the lower urinary tract, even less is understood about afferent innervation. A major factor which has hindered further understanding of this aspect of bladder innervation is the difficulty in correlating structure and in vitro pharmacological results with in vivo sensory function. When considering sensation within the lower urinary tract it is important to regard the bladder, posterior urethra and trigone as a combined functional complex.

Although complex sensory nerve endings (Kleyntjens and Langworthy, 1937) and identifiable Pacinian corpuscles (Fletcher and Bradley, 1970; Feher et al. 1982) have been identified in animal bladders, no distinct anatomical sensory receptors have yet been identified in man. It seems probable that sensory information arises from stretch receptors in the detrusor muscle (Iggo, 1955), and it appears that in the cat the majority of bladder afferents respond to tension changes within detrusor musculature (Winter, 1971). In man, stimulating the mucosa of the urinary bladder with a needle (Moore, 1924) or using electrodes (Frimodt-Moller, 1972) does produce pain.

A fine plexus of acetylcholinesterase-positive nerve fibres can be demonstrated within the lamina propria of the urethra and bladder. This is especially dense beneath the epithelial lining and these nerves are particularly prominent at the base of the bladder, around the trigone and bladder neck (George and Dixon, 1986). It has been suggested that these acetylcholinesterase-positive nerves which contain numerous agranular synaptic-type vesicles are visceral afferent nerve endings (Gosling et al. 1974). The principal basis for this hypothesis is a lack of recognisable target sites with no apparent correlation of innervation with a demonstrable effector role. This hypothesis has been supported by observations in patients with cholinergic dysautonomia (Kirby, 1987); it was noted that despite a quantifiable reduction in the density of cholinergic nerves in the bladder muscle with a corresponding motor deficit, the subepithelial plexus was unaffected and bladder sensation was preserved. These conclusions are however challenged on the basis of animal studies, for example, observation of neuronal degeneration following surgical ablation of spinal ganglia documented that there was a degeneration rate of less than 1% for submucosal axons with agranular synaptic vesicles (Uemura et al. 1975). In recent years substance P-like immunoreactivity has been reported to occur within isolated nerve fibres in the lamina propria and subepithelial nerves (Gu et al. 1984; Alm et al. 1979). This peptide had previously been proposed as a sensory neurotransmitter (Nicoll et al. 1980). More recently CGRP has been shown to coexist within the same group of neurons (Yokokawa et al. 1986).

The density of innervation observed on ultrastructural study is supported by clinical experience, stimuli affecting the base of the bladder and trigone producing the most marked symptoms (e.g. strangury). Conversely, inflamed mucosa around the bladder dome is usually experienced by the patient as a dull suprapubic ache. It has been suggested that sensory perception within the bladder depends upon both extroceptive and proprioceptive receptors (Hald, 1969), indeed, proprioceptive receptors discharge at a rate dependent on the speed of bladder filling (Klevmark, 1974).

Frimodt-Moller (1972) reported a method of evaluating bladder sensation: the technique of mucosal electrosensitivity. A stimulator delivered a constant square wave impulse via a silver wire, the amplitude of which could be altered, the lowest amplitude producing a sensation recorded as the electrical perception threshold. Subsequent modifications have been made (Kiesswetter, 1977; Powell and Feneley, 1980), but this technique remains crude and of limited usefulness.

Summary

Morphological evidence indicates that the human bladder receives a dense AChE-positive innervation predominantly comprised of acetylcholine-containing parasympathetic neurons. There is limited evidence for a significant adrenergic sympathetic innervation to all except the base of the bladder (trigone, bladder neck). A number of nerves containing putative neurotransmitters have been identified, but their role in the human bladder is at present poorly substantiated. Ultrastructural studies have defined the occurrence and distribution of different neuronal populations, characterised by their content of neurotransmitter granules. Overall these results contribute little in isolation and their functional significance must be evaluated by the concurrent use of physiological and pharmacological studies. The central nervous system control of bladder innervation and its associated pharmacological mechanisms are reviewed in Chapter 3.

References

Alm, P. 1978. Cholinergic innervation of the human urethra and urinary bladder, a histochemical study and review of methodology. Acta Pharmacol. Toxicol. 43:56–62

Alm, P., Alumets, K., Ek, A. Sundler, F. 1979. Peptidergic (VIP) nerves in the human urinary tract. Proc. Ninth Int. Cont. Soc. Meeting, Rome, p 147

Ambache, N., Aboo Zar, M.A. 1970. Non-cholinergic transmission by post-ganglionic motor neurones in the mammalian bladder. J. Physiol. (Lond) 210:761–783

Ambache, N., Kilick, S.W., Woodley, J.P. 1977. Evidence against purinergic motor transmissions in guinea pig urinary bladder. Br. J. Pharmacol. 61:464

Benson, G.S., McConnell, J.A., Wood, J.G. 1979. Adrenergic innervation of the human bladder body. J. Urol. 122:189–191

Burn, J.H., Rand, M.J. 1965. Acetylcholine in adrenergic transmission. Ann. Rev. Pharmacol. 5:163–182

Burnstock, G. 1969. Evolution of the autonomic innervation of visceral and cardiovascular systems in vertebrates. Pharmacol. Rev. 21:247–324

Burnstock, G. 1972. Purinergic nerves. Pharmacol.Rev. 24:509–581

Burnstock, G. 1986a. The changing face of autonomic neurotransmission. Acta Physiol. Scand. 126:67–91

Burnstock, G. 1986b. Autonomic neuromuscular junctions: current developments and future directions. J. Anat. 146:1–30

Burt, A.M., Silver, A. 1973. Histochemistry of choline acetyl transferase: a critical analysis. Brain. Res. 62:509–516

De Groat, W.C., Booth, A.M. 1980. Inhibition and facilitation in parasympathetic ganglia of the urinary bladder. Fed. Proc. 39:2990–2996

De Groat, W.C., Kawatani, M. 1985. Neural control of the urinary bladder: possible relationship between peptidergic inhibitory mechanisms and detrusor instability. Neurourol. Urodynamics 4:285–300

Dixon, J.S., Gilpin, S.A., Gilpin, C.G., Gosling, J.A. 1983. Intramural ganglia of the human urinary bladder. Br. J. Urol. 55:195–198

Dixon, J.S., Gosling, J.A. 1983. Histology and fine structure of the muscularis mucosae of the human urinary bladder. J. Anat. 136:265–271

Dixon, J.S., Gosling, J.A. 1987. Structure and innervation in the human. In: Physiology in the lower urinary tract. Torrens, M., Morrison, J.F.B., eds. Berlin, Heidelberg, New York, Springer, pp 3–22

Ek, A., Alm, P., Andersson, K.E., Persson, C.G.A. 1977. Adrenergic and cholinergic nerves of the human urethra and urinary bladder. A histochemical study. Acta Physiol. Scand. 99:345–352

Elbadawi, A., Schenk, E.A. 1966. Dual innervation of the mammalian urinary bladder. A histochemical study of the distribution of cholinergic and adrenergic nerves. Am. J. Anat. 119:405–416

Elbadawi, A. 1982. Neuromorphologic basis of vesico-urethral function. I. Histochemistry, ultrastructure and function of intrinsic nerves of the bladder and urethra. Neurourol. Urodynamics 1:3–50

Elliott, T.R. 1907. The innervation of the bladder and urethra. J. Physiol. (Lond) 25:367–445

Feher, E., Hosszu, E., Vajda, J. 1982. Distribution of primary sensory nerve terminals in the cat urinary bladder wall. Acta Morph. Acad. Sci. Hung. 30:223–232

Fletcher, T.F., Bradley, W.E. 1969. Comparative morphological features of urinary bladder innervation. Am. J. Vet. Res. 30:1655–1662

Fletcher, T.F., Bradley, W.E. 1970. Afferent nerve endings in the urinary bladder of the cat. Am. J. Anat. 128:147–158

Frimodt-Moller, C. 1972. A new method for quantitative evaluation of bladder sensibility. Scand. J. Urol. Nephrol. 6 (suppl. 15):135–142

George, M.J.R., Dixon, J.S. 1986. In: George, N.J.R., Gosling, J.A., (eds.) Sensory disorders of the bladder and urethra. Springer, Berlin, Heidelberg, New York

Gilpin, C.J., Dixon, J.S., Gilpin, S.A., Gosling, J.A. 1983. The fine structure of autonomic neurones in the wall of the human urinary bladder. J. Anat. 137:705–713

Gosling, J.A., Dixon, J.S., Humpherson, J.R. 1983. Functional anatomy of the urinary tract. Edinburgh, Churchill Livingstone.

Griffiths, J. 1891. Observations on the urinary bladder and urethra. J. Anat. Physiol. 25:535–549

Gu, J., Restorick, J.M., Blank, M.A., et al. 1983. Vasoactive intestinal polypeptide in the normal and unstable bladder. Br. J. Urol. 55:645–647

Gu, J., Blank, M.A., Huang, W.M., et al. 1984. Peptide containing nerves in human urinary bladder. Urology 24:353–357

Hald, T. 1969. Neurogenic dysfunction of the urinary bladder. Thesis, University of Copenhagen

Hervonen, A., Vaalasti, A., Partanen, M., Kanerva, L., Hervonen, H. 1978. Effects of ageing on the histochemically demonstrable catecholamines and acetylcholinesterase neurones of human sympathetic ganglia. J. Neurocytol. 7:11–23

Hokfelt, T., Johansson, O., Ljungdahl, A., Lundberg, J.M., Schultzberg, M. 1980. Peptidergic neurones. Nature 284:515–521

Hunter, D.T. 1954. A new concept of urinary bladder musculature. J. Urol. 71:695–704

Hutch, J.A. 1963. Ureteric advancement operation: anatomy technique and early results. J. Urol. 89:180–184

Iggo, A. 1955. Tension receptors in the stomach and the urinary bladder. J. Physiol. 128:593–607

Kawatani, M., Rutigliano, M., De Groat, W.C. 1985. Selective facilitatory effect of vasoactive intestinal polypeptide (VIP) on muscarinic firing in vesical ganglia of the cat. Brain Res. 336:223–234

Kiesswetter, H. 1977. Mucosal sensory threshold of the urinary bladder and urethra measured electrically. Urol. Int. 32:437–448

Kinder, R.B., Mundy, A.R. 1985. Inhibition of spontaneous contractile activity in isolated human detrusor muscle strips by vasoactive intestinal polypeptide. Br. J. Urol. 57:20–23

Kirby, R.S. 1987. MD Thesis, University of Cambridge

Klevmark, B. 1974. Motility of the urinary bladder in cats during filling at physiological rates. I. Intravesical pressure patterns studied by a new method of cystometry. Acta Physiol. Scand. 90:565–577

Kleyntjens, F., Langworthy, O. 1937. Sensory nerve endings on the smooth muscle of the urinary bladder. J. Comp. Neurol. 67:367–380

Koelle, B.G., Friedenwald, J.S. 1949. A histochemical method for localising cholinesterase activity. Proc. Soc. Exp. Biol. 70:617–622

Langley, J.N., Anderson, H.K. 1895. The innervation of the pelvic and adjoining viscera. Part 2. The bladder. J. Physiol. (Lond) 19:85–139

Larsson, L.I., Fahrenkrug, J., Schaffalitzkyde de Muckadell, O.B. 1977. Occurrence of nerves containing VIP-immunoreactivity in the male genital tract. Life Sciences 21:503–508

Learmonth, J.R. 1931. A contribution to the neurophysiology of the urinary bladder in man. Brain 54:147–176

Levin, R.M., Ruggieri, M.R., Wein, A.J. 1986. Functional effects of the purinergic innervation of the rabbit urinary bladder. J. Pharmacol. Exp. Ther. 236:452–457

Mackenzie, I., Burnstock, G. 1984. Neuropeptide action on the guinea pig bladder. A comparison with the effects of field stimulation and ATP. Eur. J. Pharmacol. 105:85–94

Maggi, C.A., Meli, A. 1986. The role of neuropeptides in the regulation of the micturition cycle. J. Autonom. Pharmacol. 6:133–162

McCrea, E.D. 1926. The musculature of the bladder. Proc. R. Soc. Med. 19:35–43

Mettler, C.C. 1947. History of Medicine. Mettler, F.A., ed. New York, Blakiston Company.

Mobley, T.L., Elbadawi, A., McDonald, D.F., Schenk, E.A. 1966. Innervation of the human urinary bladder. Surg. Forum 27:505–506

Moore, T.D. 1924. Bladder sensibility. Arch. Surg. 9:176–187

Mundy, A.R. 1984. Neuropeptides in lower urinary tract function. World J. Urol. 2:211–215

Nicoll, R.A., Schenker, C., Leeman, S.E. 1980. Substance P as a transmitter candidate. Am. Rev. Neurol. Sci. 3:227–268

Nordling, J. 1983. Influence of the sympathetic nervous system on lower urinary tract in man. Neurourol. Urodynamics 2:3–26

Onufrowicz, B. 1900. On the arrangements and function of the cell groups of the sacral region of the spinal cord in man. Arch. Neurol. Psychopathol. 3:387–412

Polak, J.M., Bloom, S.R. 1984. Localisation and measurement of VIP in the genitourinary system of man and animals. Peptides 5:225–230

Powell, P.H., Fenely, R.C.L. 1980. The role of urethral sensation in clinical urology. Br. J. Urol. 52:539–541

Raezer, D.M., Wein, J., Jacobwitz, D., Corriere, J.N.J. 1973. Autonomic innervation of canine urinary bladder. Cholinergic and adrenergic contributions and interaction of sympathetic and parasympathetic nervous systems in bladder function. Urology 2:211–214

Sundin, T., Dahlstrom, A., Norlen, L., Svedmyr, N. 1977. The sympathetic innervation and adrenoceptor function of the human lower urinary tract in the normal state and after parasympathetic denervation. Invest. Urol. 14:328–332

Taira, N. 1972. The autonomic pharmacology of the bladder. Ann. Rev. Pharmacol. 12:197–208

Tanagho, E.A., Pugh, R.C.B. 1963. The anatomy and function of the ureterovesical junction. J. Urol. 35:151–165

Uemura, E., Fletcher, T.F., Bradley, W.E. 1975. Distribution of lumbar and sacral afferent axons in submucosa of cat urinary bladder. Anat. Rec. 183:579–588

Vodusek, D.B., Light, J.K. 1983. The motor nerve supply of the external urethral sphincter muscles; an electrophysiological study. Neurourol. Urodynamics 2:193–200

Winter, D.L. 1971. Receptor characteristics and conduction velocities in bladder afferents. J. Psychiatr. Res. 8:225–235

Woodburne, R.T. 1960. Structure and function of the urinary bladder. J. Urol. 84:79–85

Yokokawa, K.M., Tohuama, M., Shiosaka, S., et al. 1986. Distribution of calcitonin gene-related peptide containing fibres in the urinary bladder of the rat and their origin. Cell Tissue Res. 244:271–278

Chapter 3

The Physiology of Micturition

C.R. Chapple

Before considering the investigation of disorders of micturition it is first essential to analyse the neural mechanisms which control bladder function. Bladder function can be subdivided into two interrelated yet distinct phases, *urine storage* and its controlled *voiding* at an appropriate time and place. Most contemporary knowledge is based on studies with experimental animals. Although it can be difficult and is often misleading to relate findings from animal models to man, such information is essential since human data on the central nervous control of the bladder can only be derived from clearly defined clinical syndromes and isolated spinal cord lesions.

Neurophysiological Control of the Bladder

Local Neural Pathways

The spinal segments S2–S4 acting via efferent parasympathetic cholinergic neurons are responsible for the initiation and maintenance of detrusor contraction. Damage to these spinal segments results in abolition of the micturition reflex in man (Denny-Brown and Robertson, 1933b). After leaving the sacral foramina the pelvic splanchnic nerves, containing the parasympathetic innervation to the bladder and possibly some efferent somatic neurons to the intrinsic component of the urethral sphincter, pass lateral to the rectum to enter the inferior hypogastric or pelvic plexus. They are joined by the hypogastric nerve containing efferent sympathetic nerve fibres originating from the lower three thoracic and upper two lumbar segments of the spinal cord (Warwick and Williams, 1973). When combined they form a plexus lying at the base of the bladder. The limited knowledge available suggests that the pudendal nerve transmits urethral mucosal sensation (Nathan, 1956) and it has long been suggested that the afferent pathway of the micturition reflex is carried via the pelvic nerves (Learmonth, 1931). Additional afferent information is likely to be transmitted from the trigone via sympathetic neuronal pathways in the hypogastric nerves (Winter, 1971). From observation of patients undergoing anterolateral cordotomy Nathan and Smith (1951) concluded that some bladder and urethral sensation in the afferent limb of the micturition reflex passed proximally via the spinothalamic tracts.

Reflexes Governing Micturition

Barrington initially described five reflexes associated with micturition in the cat (1914), and added a further two on the basis of further study (1931, 1941). Two of these reflexes had their reflex centres in supraspinal sites (medulla and pons) and caused strong and sustained contractions. He considered these as essential for normal micturition, since bladder contraction and urethral relaxation were not coordinated after experimentally produced high spinal transection. The remaining five reflexes appeared confined to the spinal cord.

Although it is tempting to relate these findings to man, Denny-Brown and Robertson, (1933a) failed to detect either initiation of micturition or vesical contraction resulting from distension of the posterior urethra in man and concluded that micturition was a reflex act resulting from bladder distension and mediated by a centre in the sacral cord (Denny-Brown and Robertson 1933b). More recently, Kuru (1965) has proposed that many interrelated reflexes act upon the sacral micturition centre, exerting both excitatory and inhibitory effects.

Urine Storage

During bladder filling, afferent activity from stretch receptors increases and passes via the posterior roots of the sacral cord and the lateral spinothalamic tracts to the brain, thereby mediating the desire to void. Activity within the striated component of the urethral sphincter is increased, and local spinal reflex activity in turn stimulates the pudendal motor neurons of the nucleus of Onufrowicz, which enhances the activity within striated muscles of the pelvic floor and sphincter.

Local factors are important during bladder filling and these include not only receptive relaxation (Tang and Ruch, 1955), but also the passive viscoelastic properties of the bladder wall. Both abnormal bladder morphology resulting from collagenous infiltration, hypertrophy or altered muscle structure (e.g. obstructed bladder) and abnormal detrusor smooth muscle behaviour, either primary or secondary to neural dysfunction, could contribute to the genesis of poor bladder compliance and detrusor instability.

Initiation of Micturition

Once a threshold level of filling has been achieved, which will depend on circumstances and vary considerably between individuals, the increasing afferent activity impinges upon consciousness, and the subject becomes aware that the bladder is filling. Except during infancy, the normal human has complete volitional control over these reflex pathways.

When micturition is initiated by the cerebral cortex a complex series of bladder/brain stem reflexes are involved (Kuru, 1965). Urethral relaxation precedes detrusor contraction (Tanagho and Miller, 1970), there is a simultaneous relaxation of the pelvic floor muscles (Porter, 1962) and these events are accompanied by funnelling of the bladder neck (Lund et al. 1957). The inhibitory activity of the higher centres on the sacral centres is lifted, allowing parasympathetically controlled detrusor contraction to occur with a corresponding relaxation of the urethra/prostate/bladder neck complex resulting from reciprocal sympathetic nerve inhibition. In addition to these primary actions, other important secondary events include contraction of the diaphragm and anterior abdominal wall muscles, and the specific behavioural changes associated with voiding.

At the end of voiding the proximal urethra is closed in a retrograde fashion, the "milkback" seen at videocystometry. Once these events are completed inhibition is reapplied to the sacral centres by the cortex and the next filling cycle starts.

Pharmacological Responses of the Bladder

Animal experimentation has been helpful in clarifying the complex local neural interactions which participate in the control of lower urinary tract function. It is, however, important to take care in interpreting such data and extrapolating results from animals to man, since there are important inherent species differences. The following examples demonstrate this: physiological adaptations to encompass behavioural characteristics such as territorial marking; pharmacological differences with a high proportion of non-adrenergic, non-cholinergic neurotransmission in the control of detrusor function in rodents; anatomical differences, in particular, the upright position of the human and the extra-peritoneal position of the bladder base and urethra which completely change the influence of supporting tissues.

The traditional approach has been to subdivide the autonomic nervous system into two divisions, sympathetic and parasympathetic, based on the two neurotransmitter substances, noradrenaline and acetylcholine respectively. Bearing in mind the caveat expressed above it must be remembered that most of our knowledge of human bladder neurophysiology is derived from animal studies. Furthermore, in recent years, the recognition of new putative transmitter substances has complicated an already controversial area. It is the intention of this chapter to summarise the current literature on this subject.

The Role of the Parasympathetic Nervous System

Coordinated contraction of the urinary bladder at the time of micturition is initiated and maintained by parasympathetic nervous stimulation via the pelvic nerves in all mammalian species studied (Andersson and Sjogren, 1982). The early recognition of cholinergic transmission at many synapses resulted in acceptance of acetylcholine as the post-ganglionic transmitter in the bladder and formulation of the theory of cholinergic transmission (Dale, 1933). This hypothesis is in accordance with the histological evidence of a dense uniform network of cholinergic (acetylcholinesterase-positive) fibres and the corollary that all parts of the bladder, including the trigone and proximal urethra, contract when exposed to acetylcholine, an effect inhibited by atropine (Todd and Mack, 1969; Nergardh, 1975).

Further evidence in support of acetylcholine being an excitatory neuro-transmitter is provided by the work of Carpenter and Rand (1965) who studied whole bladder preparations from the rat and assayed the bath medium for acetylcholine both at rest and during nerve-mediated electrical stimulation. Acetylcholine output was increased 150-fold during electrical stimulation. These observations are supported by in vivo studies in both rhesus monkeys (Craggs and Stephenson, 1985) and humans (Cullumbine et al. 1955).

Work utilising receptor binding techniques with 1-quinuclidinyl (phenyl 4-^{3}H) benzilate (^{3}HQNB) to visualise cholinergic muscarinic receptor binding sites confirms that the human detrusor muscle contains a number of such receptors (Levin et al. 1982). Ligand binding data using the agonist carbachol suggest that there is more than one class of these muscarinic receptors (Nilvebrant et al. 1985), leading to the tempting speculation that in the future it might be possible to develop drugs with precise selectivity for muscarinic receptors in the human bladder.

Partial atropine resistance of bladder contractions was first noted by Langley and Anderson (1895a,b) during electrical stimulation of the parasympathetic nerve supply to the human bladder. Refractoriness to atropine was also documented by Henderson and Roepke (1934, 1935), in experiments using pelvic nerve stimulation in dogs. Despite further confirmation of this phenomenon in the cat bladder (Edge, 1955) and several other parasympathetically innervated organs, "the nature of parasympathetic post-ganglionic neurons in the bladder remain(ed) unsolved" (Ambache, 1955).

Vanov (1965) reported that atropine resistance noted during his experiments on the rat bladder was counteracted by a disruption of acetylcholine synthesis using hemicholinium; on this basis it was suggested that the phenomenon of atropine resistance was produced by a local build up of endogenous acetylcholine around the post-synaptic membrane, sufficient to antagonise receptor blockade by atropine. Other explanations which have been suggested to explain the presence of non-cholinergic transmission have included: (a) that muscarinic acetylcholine receptors in the detrusor muscle behave anomalously towards atropine; and (b) that neurogenic acetylcholine is released in close proximity to receptors and hence beyond the atropine barrier (Dale and Gaddum, 1930). Contemporary knowledge finds little evidence to support these hypotheses and in particular, the Dale and Gaddum hypothesis has further been discredited by Dumsday (1971) who calculated that the synaptic volume was sufficient to allow access of atropine to receptors.

Ambache and Aboo Zar (1970) taking note of these suggestions used much lower strength electrical stimulation to avoid flooding the receptors with neurotransmitter and provided clear evidence in animal studies, predominantly on guinea pigs but also in cats and rabbits, that atropine-resistant neurotransmission was a definite entity and appeared to be mediated via a truly non-cholinergic mechanism. They suggested that adrenergic nerves were unlikely to be implicated in non-cholinergic neurotransmission in the guinea pig, since administration of noradrenaline produced detrusor relaxation and neural stimulation was unaffected by both α- and β-adrenoceptor blockade. This has been confirmed by work showing that depletion of catecholamines from the bladder with reserpine was without effect (Dean and Downie, 1978).

The concept of non-adrenergic, non-cholinergic neurotransmission (NANC) is now widely accepted (Taira, 1972; Andersson and Sjogren, 1982) and the presence of marked interspecies variation in NANC bladder control is well recognised. The nature and indeed role of NANC neurotransmission is still the subject of debate, a situation further complicated by the likelihood that there are a number of different neurotransmitter substances involved (Burnstock, 1986a,b).

Hindmarsh et al. (1977) reported that electrically induced contraction of human detrusor muscle strips was only partially sensitive to atropine, thus lending support to the view that there might be a NANC component. Eaton and Bates (1982), reporting an in vitro pharmacological study investigating samples of both normal and unstable obstructed detrusor, noted only "partial inhibition" by atropine in both groups.

Cowan and Daniel (1983) in a study of normal female human detrusor suggested that there might be a tetrodotoxin (TTX)-resistant NANC excitatory system, representing approximately 50% of the contractile response to short-pulse electrical field stimulation. These findings are controversial, since their interpretation relies upon the postulate that there is stimulation of a TTX- resistant non-muscle site, where these nerves do not release mediator by the standard mechanism involving sodium conductance.

In contrast, Sjogren and his co-workers (1982) found that detrusor strips from 33 patients deemed to have normal bladders (although urodynamic investigation had not been carried out), invariably demonstrated a response to transmural electrical stimulation which was almost completely inhibited by atropine (95%). Interestingly, in the same study muscle strips from patients with prostatic outflow obstruction exhibited atropine resistance of up to 50%.

Kinder and Mundy (1985b), reported a study of 23 detrusor muscle strips obtained from 13 urodynamically normal patients and documented a 92.7% inhibition by atropine of the response to nerve-mediated stimulation.

Similarly, Sibley (1984a) concluded that nerve-mediated activity in normal human bladder is exclusively cholinergic, as contrasted to a significant atropine-resistant component in the rabbit (58%) and pig (22%). In the same comparative study bladder strips from patients undergoing prostatectomy were also studied, and although an atropine-resistant component of 20% was recorded, this was also TTX resistant and therefore unlikely to be nerve mediated.

The apparent conflict of data which exists in the literature can be explained by heterogeneity of the tissue investigated and variation in experimental procedures. It has to be concluded that since the normal human detrusor does not possess significant atropine resistance, the NANC component is under normal circumstances of little physiological importance. However, it is probable that the structural changes which occur in the obstructed bladder result in significant changes in the physiological response of detrusor muscle (Sibley, 1984b) and its pharmacological profile (Sjogren et al. 1982) which may indeed be related to the altered behaviour of the obstructed detrusor.

The Role of the Sympathetic Nervous System

Langley and Anderson (1895a,b) in their investigation of the innervation of the cat bladder reported that stimulation of the sympathetic neural innervation to the bladder via the hypogastric nerves resulted in a biphasic response, namely, a brief detrusor contraction followed by relaxation, the former being most pronounced in the region of the trigone.

Elliott (1907) reviewed a number of species and concluded that the hypogastric nerves contained both motor and inhibitory fibres, and that there were marked inter-species variations and also striking differences between the sexes within a species. He suggested that the sympathetic nervous system diminished in importance in higher mammals. Subsequently, it has been recognised that much of the confusion relating to the effect of sympathetic innervation in the cat is attributable to differing responses related to the depth of anaesthesia (Macdonald and McCrea, 1930).

Later work has clearly confirmed the presence of a typical biphasic response to sympathetic stimulation, comprising a short contraction followed by a marked relaxation of the urinary bladder, in the cat (Ingersoll et al. 1954; Edvardsen 1968a; Norlen, 1977) and dog (Ingersoll and Jones, 1958), but not the rhesus monkey (Ingersoll and Jones, 1962).

Most animal studies have been carried out in dogs and cats, where an abundant sympathetic innervation of the bladder base and proximal urethra has been reported, with a definite but sparse adrenergic innervation of the bladder body (Raezer et al. 1973; Sundin and Dahlstrom, 1973). It has been suggested by some workers that sympathetic fibres exert a tonic inhibitory influence on the bladder, hence the decrease in end-filling volume and increase in bladder tone produced by sympathectomy (Edvardsen 1968b; Wein et al. 1974). Although Klevmark (1977) could not reproduce these findings Nishizawa et al. (1985), in a study of the dog bladder, found that hypogastric nerve transection resulted in a small but significant reduction in bladder end-filling volume and pressure and in initial voiding pressure, with an increase in bladder compliance but with no effect on urodynamic voiding parameters. Nevertheless, in a cat model, increased activity has been demonstrated in the sympathetic neurons to the bladder during filling (Edvardsen, 1968a).

Following the functional classification of sympathetic nervous system receptors into α- and β-adrenoceptor subtypes (Ahlquist, 1948), attention has been directed towards determining their distribution and the correlation of this with pharmacological responses. In vitro studies have confirmed that there is a very pronounced regional variation in response to agonist.

In studies conducted in the dog, noradrenaline produced contraction of muscle strips from the bladder trigone and relaxation of tissue from the bladder dome (Rohner et al. 1971). To explain this, it has been suggested that at the trigone there is a functional predominance of α receptors which mediate contractile responses and in the bladder body of β receptors (Edvardsen and Setekleiv, 1968) which produce relaxation. Further characterisation studies have confirmed that α receptors predominate at the bladder base and β receptors in the detrusor muscle of the bladder dome (Awad et al. 1974; Wein and Levin, 1979).

The pioneering work of Learmonth (1931) confirmed that there was a similar situation in man. He reported that faradic stimulation of sympathetic nerves produced a contraction of the ureteric orifices, increased tonus in the trigone and contraction of the bladder neck, prostatic musculature and musculature of the seminal vesicles and ejaculatory ducts; but produced no observable effect on the musculature of the bladder walls and dome. Conversely, following division of the sympathetic nerves to the bladder, the ureteric orifices, trigone and bladder neck relaxed, but after three weeks appeared to regain their tone.

Subsequent detailed analyses of adrenoceptor subtypes in the human bladder has resulted in some debate as to their distribution. Some authors maintain that there are no α receptors detectable in the normal human detrusor (Sundin et al. 1977; Nergardh and Boreus, 1972). In contrast, Awad et al. (1974) noted that there are both α and β receptors within normal detrusor; a finding corroborated by the functional studies of Todd and Mack (1969) who reported contractile responses to α-stimulation and relaxation with β-stimulation in the normal human detrusor. Functional characterisation of β-adrenoceptors in the human bladder has suggested that they have neither β_1 nor β_2 characteristics (Nergardh et al. 1977; Larsen, 1979).

Learmonth (1931) reported, in an experiment conducted on himself, that the intravenous injection of noradrenaline produced bladder relaxation. Several investigators have demonstrated a relaxation response attributable to β-adrenoceptors in isolated human detrusor (Cowan and Daniel, 1983; Todd and Mack, 1969; Awad et al. 1974; Nergardh et al. 1977; Larsen, 1979). Cowan and Daniel (1983) correlated these findings with the sparse sympathetic innervation to the bladder, and suggested that such responses could result in vivo from the stimulation of adrenoceptors by circulating catecholamines.

Review of the literature reveals that in clinical trials, β-adrenoceptor stimulation and blockade has little effect on the normal detrusor. Beta-adrenoceptor agonists (terbutaline, isoprenaline) have been reported to produce a small increase in bladder capacity (Norlen et al. 1978). In another study, propranolol decreased rather than increased intravesical pressure in normal man and had no influence on bladder capacity (Jensen, 1981).

In isometric muscle strip experiments carried out on the human bladder body, α-adrenoceptor agonists appear to be without significant effect (Sundin et al. 1977; Awad et al. 1974). Furthermore, contraction induced by transmural stimulation is little affected by α-adrenoceptor blockade with phentolamine (Cowan and Daniel, 1983). In normal men, α-adrenoceptor stimulation with phenylpropanolamine did not result in an alteration of either intravesical pressure or capacity and α-blockade (phentolamine/thymoxamine) had little effect (Jensen, 1981).

On the basis of available evidence, the most plausible hypothesis is that bladder filling is influenced by β- rather than α-adrenoceptors. However, the minor and rather variable effects of α and β agonists and antagonists documented in experimental studies make the importance of such a role uncertain in the normal detrusor.

An important alternative physiological pathway is that provided by neuronal interaction within the autonomic nervous system. Although synaptic contacts between adrenergic and cholinergic neurons at axonal and axon terminal levels have *not* been described in man, ultrastructural evidence to support such neuronal interaction is provided by the juxtaposition of adrenergic and cholinergic neurons within extra-vesical ganglia. It is of interest that recent work reported by Mattiason and colleagues (1987), documented that nerve-mediated release of noradrenaline in normal detrusor muscle strip preparations was decreased by the cholinergic agonist carbachol.

It must therefore be concluded that although the basic mechanism of sympathetic neuromuscular coupling within the human detrusor is well documented, there remains considerable debate as to the precise neurophysiological role of the sympathetic nervous system in the control of the normal bladder and the importance of neural interaction with the parasympathetic and NANC sensorimotor nerves within the autonomic nervous system.

The Role of Non-adrenergic, Non-cholinergic Neurotransmission

In recent years a considerable body of anatomical, biochemical and pharmacological evidence (as outlined above) has demonstrated that NANC neurotransmitters are widely distributed within the body and may play an important role alongside the classical neurotransmitters. Much of the information currently available is rather fragmentary and its derivation from a number of animal species does raise doubts as to the advisability and indeed validity of cross-relating these results. The current knowledge on the neuropharmacological actions of many of these compounds with particular reference to the bladder will now be considered.

Primary afferent neurons contain a number of regulatory peptides (Gibbins et al. 1987) which include substance P, calcitonin gene-related peptide (CGRP), somatostatin (Som), vasoactive intestinal polypeptide (VIP) and neurokinin A (NKA) (Jancso et al. 1977; Sundler et al. 1985). The submucosal population of peptide-containing nerves demonstrated in the animal bladder is thought to be associated with sensory innervation. Many of the putative neurotransmitters have also been demonstrated to produce motor effects. In the following section the current knowledge on each putative neurotransmitter as relating to the bladder will be reviewed.

Adenosine Triphosphate (ATP)

Scanty evidence is available to substantiate the role of this agent in the human bladder. Husted and co-workers (1983) reported from an in vitro study of muscle from the human bladder dome that ATP produced three types of contractile response, the maximal response being approximately one third of that achieved by acetylcholine. ATP and adenine nucleotides initially potentiated, then subsequently reduced nerve-mediated stimulation and reduced acetylcholine-mediated contraction. Since TTX did not influence the responses in any way they concluded that ATP produced this action by a direct effect on bladder smooth muscle cells.

At present it must be concluded that although the role of purinergic neurotransmission is well established in the animal bladder its potential role in man remains undetermined.

Gamma-Aminobutyric Acid (GABA)

Gamma-aminobutyric acid (GABA), although well recognised as an inhibitory neurotransmitter in the central nervous system, has in recent years been identified in peripheral tissues and has been noted to have inhibitory effects on animal bladder both in vivo and in vitro (Maggi et al. 1983, 1985).

5-hydroxytryptamine (5-HT)

5-hydroxytryptamine (5-HT) has been ascribed a neurotransmitter role in the human and animal bladder. Holt et al. (1985) and Klarskov and Horby-Petersen (1986) demonstrated that 5-HT evoked a dose-dependent and reversible contractile response in the human detrusor and produced dose-dependent relaxation of trigone, bladder neck and urethral smooth muscle. It has been postulated that 5-HT derived from blood platelets may act as a neuromodulator within detrusor muscle (Holt et al. 1985).

Histamine

Histamine is known to produce contraction of smooth muscle in a number of sites within the body. Evidence from animal studies suggests that there are H_1 receptors which mediate histamine-induced contraction of the guinea pig bladder whilst H_2 receptors mediate inhibition of non-cholinergic contraction (Kondo et al. 1985). No evidence for a functional role for this agent in human detrusor has so far been reported.

Vasoactive Intestinal Polypeptide (VIP)

Vasoactive intestinal polypeptide (VIP), a 28-amino acid compound, was isolated from the gut (Said and Mutt, 1970) and has since been demonstrated in the bladder, prostate and urethra of a number of species (Alm et al. 1977, 1980).

A role for VIP in mediating bladder muscle contractility, possibly by an action on post-ganglionic excitatory neurotransmission, has been suggested. Work with guinea pig isolated bladder strips, where VIP produces small contractions and potentiates nerve-mediated responses (Johns, 1979), supports this suggestion. In other species VIP inhibits the motility of isolated vesicourethral preparations (Maggi and Meli, 1986) and in in vitro animal studies VIP produces relaxation of detrusor smooth muscle (Levin and Wein,

1981). The distribution of VIP-immunoreactive nerves suggests that they may participate in regulating local blood flow and epithelial function (Alm et al. 1980).

VIP may have an important role in the control of human detrusor motor function. Gu et al. (1983a) reported a dramatic reduction of VIP immunoreactivity in the detrusor muscle of unstable human bladder as compared to control. Subsequent in vitro muscle strip studies have demonstrated that the application of VIP produced a significant reduction in muscle strip basal tension and the amplitude and frequency of spontaneous contractions in the normal and hyperreflexic human detrusor (Kinder and Mundy, 1985a; Kinder et al. 1985). Klarskov et al. (1984a) reported that VIP exerted a concentration-dependent relaxation of human detrusor which did not appear to be acting via neuromodulation of neural pathways and was likely to be producing its effects via a direct action on smooth muscle cells. In support of this, the muscular relaxation occurred at a slower rate than that which had been observed following NANC responses resulting from electrical field stimulation (Andersson et al. 1983; Klarskov et al. 1983). In contrast, studies of VIP from other anatomical sites suggest that it may act by modulation of neural pathways. For example, in the cat submandibular gland VIP possibly potentiates the action of acetylcholine by increasing the affinity of acetylcholine binding to muscarinic receptors (Lundberg, 1981). No evidence to support such a role in man was found by Sjogren and co-workers (1985) in an in vitro study of human bladder strips where effects on neither acetylcholine-induced responses nor contractions induced by electrical field stimulation were evident.

Few in vivo studies of the action of VIP on the bladder have been reported. Andersson et al. (1987) noted in the anaesthetised cat that stimulation of parasympathetic nerves induced a marked increase in VIP output accompanied by a much smaller relative increase in blood flow; they suggested that this discrepancy could be explained by an additional action on bladder musculature. The intravenous infusion of VIP into male and female volunteers (Klarskov 1984b, Klaksov et al.1987) has failed to confirm these expectations, with no demonstrable change in urodynamic parameters of bladder function.

Neuropeptide Y (NPY)

Neuropeptide Y (NPY) is a 36-amino acid peptide, widely distributed in both the peripheral and central nervous systems. It is the peptide present in the highest concentration in the mammalian brain. NPY may be released in conjunction with noradrenaline upon stimulation of sympathetic nerves in man, with apparent pre-and post-junctional effects on the sympathetic control of blood vessels (Lundberg et al. 1985). Recent work using denervation studies in the rat bladder have revealed that there may be a non-adrenergic population of NPY fibres originating from cell bodies in the pelvic ganglia (Mattiasson et al. 1985).

NPY has potent biological actions which include the inhibition of nerve-mediated muscular contraction (mouse vas deferens) and vasoconstriction

(Adrian et al. 1984). NPY occurs in high concentration in the male genital tract and may play a role in erectile function.

To date few pharmacological studies have been carried out on the human bladder; this is an important oversight, since NPY is the neuropeptide present in greatest concentration in the human detrusor.

Calcitonin Gene-Related Peptide (CGRP) and Substance P (SP)

Calcitonin gene-related peptide (CGRP) is a 37-amino acid peptide encoded in the calcitonin gene. Calcitonin gene-related peptide often coexists with substance P within cholinergic neurons in the spinal cord. It has been shown to both stimulate and relax smooth muscle in vitro and via potent effects on blood vessels produces vasodilatation. In the central nervous system it potentiates the action of substance P (Goodman and Iverson, 1986). CGRP and substance P seem to be localised to sensory nerve fibres and CGRP has been reported to be a potent inhibitor of substance P degradation (Le Greves et al. 1985). CGRP has been localised within the rat and guinea pig bladder (Gibbins et al. 1985; Mulderry et al. 1985), but not so far in the human.

Substance P was first isolated from extracts of brain and intestine by von Euler and Gaddum in 1931. It was found to cause contraction of intestinal smooth muscle and to lower blood pressure, actions not influenced by atropine blockade. Substance P was proposed as a sensory transmitter by Lembeck (1953) and certainly fulfils the principal criteria; it is present in sensory neurons, is released on neural stimulation and exerts appropriate effects on post-synaptic cells in the spinal cord.

CGRP and SP have been shown to coexist in the same nerves in the rat urinary bladder (Sundler et al. 1985). Capsaicin, a substance derived from Hungarian red peppers, is known to selectively affect primary unmyelinated sensory nerve fibres (C-fibres) (Szolesanyi, 1977). Neonatal treatment with capsaicin leads to a complete degeneration of C-fibres, whereas treatment of the adult animal leads to a depletion of the neural content of both SP and CGRP and a desensitisation to further capsaicin (Maggi et al. 1984; Jancso et al. 1985). Cystometric investigation during anaesthesia has shown that rats subjected to neonatal treatment with capsaicin have an increased bladder capacity compared to control rats (Maggi and Meli, 1986) and resultant urinary retention has also been reported (Sharkey et al. 1983).

A preliminary study of the intravesical instillation of capsaicin into 6 patients has reported that it produces a concentration-related reduction in the first desire to void, bladder capacity and detrusor pressure at the onset of micturition. Of particular interest was the finding that all 5 patients with hypersensitivity disorders of the lower urinary tract reported either disappearance or marked attenuation of their symptoms for a few days after capsaicin instillation (Maggi et al. 1989).

Recent observations in the rat bladder have suggested that capsaicin treatment may lead to the development of a selective supersensitivity of muscarinic receptors, albeit with no demonstrable cystometric changes (Malmgren, 1989, personal communication). Further data indicate that the administration of SP releases acetylcholine from the rat urinary bladder (Andersson, 1989, personal communication).

In recent years it has been recognised that a number of compounds belonging to a group of compounds related to SP – the tachykinins (Erspamer et al. 1981) – also occur in the mammalian bladder (Maggi and Meli, 1986). Albeit both SP and other neurokinins can produce contraction of the rat (Maggi et al. 1983) or the human urinary bladder (Kalbfleisch and Daniel, 1987; Dion et al. 1988; Erspamer et al. 1981). It has been suggested that SP is unlikely to function as a NANC motor neurotransmitter because selective SP tachyphylaxis is common and the use of a substance P inhibitor failed to reduce NANC responses to field stimulation (Kalbfleisch and Daniel, 1987).

The physiological consequences of a sensory neurotransmitter having motor effects remain hypothetical and the contractile effects of SP may represent pharmacological rather than physiological responses. Nevertheless, an attractive hypothesis is that when SP is released in response to afferent stimuli it aids muscle contraction not only by a direct effect but also indirectly via a local action on parasympathetic pathways (a possible explanation for the observation that SP releases acetylcholine in an animal model). This would augment the effects of increased activity within local spinal reflexes, thereby increasing the efficiency of detrusor contraction at the time of voiding.

Met- and Leu-Enkephalin (m-Enk and l-Enk)

Methionine-enkephalin (m-Enk) and leucine-enkephalin (l-Enk) are closely related pentapeptides (Beaumont, 1983). The two peptides are localised to synaptic vesicles in nerve terminals within the central nervous system and in peripheral autonomic nerves (La Motte and de Lanerolle, 1981; Miller, 1981). M-Enk and l-Enk have been reported to occur in different nerve populations (Larsson et al. 1979). Enkephalin-immunoreactive nerves have been demonstrated in the lower urinary tract smooth muscle and within ganglia of the cat urinary bladder. It has been suggested that urinary bladder motility is depressed by enkephalin-like substances via a direct action on vesical ganglia (Booth et al. 1981; Simonds et al. 1983) and by intrathecal administration (Hisamitsu et al. 1982). Both m-Enk and l-Enk seem to be implicated in the neural control of micturition (De Groat and Kawatani, 1985), but little evidence is currently available to support a substantive role for these agents in the local control of bladder function (Maggi and Meli, 1986).

In an in vitro study of pig lower urinary tract muscle and human detrusor, enkephalins did not influence the basal tension or spontaneous contraction of muscle strips, or of contractions evoked pharmacologically. However, both m-Enk and l-Enk significantly inhibited electrically evoked contractions particularly at low stimulation frequencies, m-Enk being 1.4 times more potent than l-Enk (Klarskov, 1987a), and it was concluded that there was a presynaptic inhibition of detrusor muscle contraction. In this study up to 30% of the control of muscular contraction appeared to be NANC mediated. A major criticism of this work is that TTX was not used to quantify the component due to direct muscle stimulation; hence the results obtained could partly be due to a direct depressant effect of enkephalins on detrusor muscle contractile activity. Furthermore, a long pulse duration was used (1 msec) for electrical stimulation, which could produce significant direct muscle stimulation (Sibley, 1984a).

Summary

It is evident from this brief review that our current knowledge of neuropeptide substances and the amine 5-HT is fragmentary and based on observations taken from a number of species. In view of the ubiquitous distribution of these substances it is to be presumed that they do have a functional role in the nervous system. Nevertheless, surprisingly little information is available as to the distribution of NANC neurotransmitters in the human bladder or prostate in either health or disease.

References

Adrian, T.E., Gu, J., Allen, J.M., Tatemoto, K., Polak, J.M., Bloom, S.R. 1984. Neuropeptide Y in the human male genital tract. Life Sci. 35:2643–2648

Ahlquist, R.P. 1948. A study of the adrenotropic receptors. Am. J. Physiol. 53:586–600

Alm, P., Alumets, J., Hakanson, R., Sundler, F. 1977. Peptidergic (vasoactive intestinal polypeptide) nerves in the genitourinary tract. Neuroscience 2:751–754

Alm, P., Alumets, J., Hakanson, R., et al. 1980. Origin and distribution of vasoactive intestinal polypeptide (VIP) nerves in the genito-urinary tract. Cell Tissue Res. 205:337–347

Ambache, N. 1955. The use and limitations of atropine for pharmacological studies on autonomic effectors. Pharmacol. Rev. 7:467–494

Ambache, N., Aboo Zar, M.A. 1970. Non-cholinergic transmission by post-ganglionic motor neurones in the mammalian bladder. J. Physiol. (Lond) 210:761–783

Andersson, K.E., Sjogren, C. 1982. Aspects on the physiology and pharmacology of the bladder and urethra. Progr. Neurobiol. 19:71–89

Andersson, K.E., Mattiasson, A., Sjogren, C. 1983. Electrically induced relaxation of the noradrenaline contracted isolated urethra from rabbit and man. J. Urol. 129:210–213

Andersson P.O., Bloom, S.R., Mattiasson, A., Uvelius, B. 1987. Bladder vasodilatation and release of vasoactive intestinal polypetide from the urinary bladder of the cat in response to pelvic nerve stimulation. J. Urol. 138:671–673

Awad, A.A., Bruce, G., Carrocampi, J.W., Lin, M., Marks, G.S. 1974. Distribution of α- and β-adrenoceptors in human urinary bladder. Br. J. Pharmacol. 50:525–529

Barrington, F.J.F. 1914. The nervous mechanism of micturition. Q. J. Exp. Physiol. 8:33–71

Barrington, F.J.F. 1931. The component reflexes of micturition in the cat. Parts 1 & 2. Brain 54:177–188

Barrington, F.J.F. 1941. The component reflexes of micturition in the cat. Part 3. Brain 64:239–243

Beaumont, A. 1983. Putative peptide neurotransmitters. The opioid peptides. Int. Rev. Exp. Pathol. 25:279–305

Booth, A.M., Ostrowski, N., McLinden, S., Lowe, I., De Groat, W.C. 1981. An analysis of the inhibitory effects of leucine enkephalin on transmission in vesical parasympathetic ganglia of the cat. Soc. Neurosci. Symposia Abstract 8:214

Burnstock, G. 1986a. The changing face of autonomic neurotransmission. Acta Physiol. Scand. 126:67–91

Burnstock, G. 1986b. Autonomic neuromuscular junctions: current developments and future directions. J. Anat. 146:1–30

Carpenter, F.G., Rand, S.A. 1965. Relation of acetylcholine release to responses of the rat urinary bladder. J. Physiol. (Lond) 180:371–382

Cowan, W.D., Daniel, E.E. 1983. Human female bladder and its non-cholinergic contractile function. Can. J. Physiol. Pharmacol. 61:1236–1246

Craggs, M.D., Stephenson, J.D. 1985. Bladder electromyograms and function in monkeys after atropine. Br. J. Urol. 57:341–345

Cullumbine, H., McKee, W.H.E., Creasey, N.H. 1955. The effects of atropine sulphate upon healthy male subjects. Q. J. Exp. Physiol. 30:309–319

Dale, H.H. 1933. Nomenclature of fibres in the autonomic system and their effects. J. Physiol. (Lond) 80:10–11

Dale, H.H., Gaddum, J.H. 1930. Reactions of denervated voluntary muscle and their bearing on the mode of action of parasympathetic and related nerves. J. Physiol. (Lond) 70:109–144

Dean, D.M., Downie, J.W. 1978. Contribution of adrenergic and "purinergic" neurotransmission to contraction in rabbit detrusor. J. Pharmacol. Exp. Ther. 207:431–445

De Groat, W.C., Kawatani, M. 1985. Neural control of the urinary bladder: possible relationship between peptidergic inhibitory mechanisms and detrusor instability. Neurourol. Urodynamics 4:285–300

Denny-Brown, D, Robertson, E.G. 1933a. On the physiology of micturition. Brain 56:149–190

Denny-Brown, D., Robertson, E.G. 1933b. The state of the bladder and its sphincters in complete transverse lesions of the spinal cord and cauda equina. Brain 56:397–462

Dion, S., Corcos, J., Carmel, M., Drapeau, G., Regoli, D. 1988. Substance P and neurokinins as stimulants of the human isolated urinary bladder. Neuropeptides 11:83–87

Dumsday, B. 1971. Atropine resistance of the urinary bladder innervation. J. Pharm. Pharmacol. 23:222–225

Eaton, A.C., Bates, C.P. 1982. An in vitro physiological study of normal and unstable human detrusor muscle. Br. J. Urol. 54:653–657

Edge, N.D. 1955. A contribution to the innervation of the urinary bladder of the cat. J. Physiol. (Lond) 127:54–68

Edvardsen, P. 1968a. Nervous control of urinary bladder in cats. 1. The collecting phase. Acta Physiol. Scand. 72:157–171

Edvardsen, P. 1968b. Nervous control of urinary bladder in cats. III. Effects of autonomic blocking agents in the intact animal. Acta Physiol. Scand. 99:345–352

Edvardsen, P., Setekleiv, J. 1968. Distribution of adrenergic receptors in the urinary bladder of cats, rabbits and guinea pigs. Acta Pharmacol. Toxicol. 26:437–445

Elliott, T.R. 1907. The innervation of the bladder and urethra. J. Physiol. (Lond) 25:367–445

Erspamer, V., Ronzoni, G., Falconieri-Erspamer, G. 1981. Effects of active peptides on the isolated muscle of the human urinary bladder. Invest. Urol. 18:302–304

Gibbins, I.L., Furness, J.B., Costa, M. 1985. Pathway-specific patterns of the co-existence of substance P, calcitonin gene-related peptide, cholecystokinin and dynorphin in neurones of the dorsal root ganglia of the guinea pig. Cell Tissue Res. 248:417–437

Goodman, E.C., Iverson, L.L. 1986. Calcitonin gene-related peptide: novel neuropeptide. Life Sci. 38:2169–2178

Gu, J., Restorick, J.M., Blank, M.A., et al. 1983a. Vasoactive intestinal polypeptide in the normal and unstable bladder. Br. J. Urol. 55:645–647

Gu, J., Polak, J.M., Polak, P.L. 1983b. Peptidergic innvervation of the human genital tract. J. Urol. 130:386–391

Henderson, V.E., Roepke, M.H. 1934. The role of acetylcholine in bladder contractile mechanisms and in parasympathetic ganglia. J. Pharmacol. Exp. Ther. 51:97–111

Henderson, V.E., Roepke, M.H. 1935. The urinary bladder mechanisms. J. Pharmacol. Exp. Ther. 54:408–414

Hindmarsh, J.R., Idowu, A.O., Yeates, W.W., Aboo Zar, M.A. 1977. Pharmacology of electrically evoked contraction of the bladder. Br. J. Pharmacol. 61:115P

Hisamitsu, T., Roques, B.P., De Groat, W.C. 1982. The role of enkephalins in the sacral parasympathetic reflex pathways to the urinary bladder of the cat. Soc. Neurosci. Symposia Abstract 8:227

Holt, S.E., Cooper, M., Wyllie, J.H. 1985. Evidence for purinergic transmission in mouse bladder and for modulation of responses to electrical stimulation by 5-hydroxytryptamine. Eur. J. Pharmacol. 116:105–111

Husted, S., Sjogren, C., Andersson, K.E. 1983. Direct effects of adenosine and adenine nucleotides on isolated human urinary bladder and their influence on electrically induced contractions. J. Urol. 130:392–398

Ingersoll, E.H., Jones, L.L., Hegre, E.S. 1954. Urinary bladder response to unilateral stimulation of hypogastric nerves. J. Urol. 72:178–190

Ingersoll, E.H., Jones, L.L. 1958. Effect upon the urinary bladder of unilateral stimulation of hypogastric nerves in the dog. Anat. Rec. 130:605–615

Ingersoll, E.H., Jones, L.L. 1962. Effect of stimulation of autonomic outflow to urinary bladder of rhesus monkey. Proc. Soc. Exp. Biol. Med. 110:858–861

Jancso, G., Kiraly, E., Jancso-Gabor, A. 1977. Pharmacologically induced selective degeneration of chemo-sensitive primary sensory neurons. Nature 270:741–742

Jancso, G., Kiraly, E., Joo, F., Such, G., Nagy, A. 1985. Selective degeneration of a subpopulation of primary sensory neurones in the adult rat. Neurosci. Lett. 59:209–214

Jensen, D. 1981. Pharmacological studies of the uninhibited neurogenic bladder. Acta Neurol. Scand. 64:175–195

Johns, A. 1979. The effect of VIP on the urinary bladder and taenia coli of the guinea-pig. Can. J. Physiol. Pharmacol. 57:106–108

Kalbfleisch, R.E., Daniel, E.E. 1987. The role of substance P in the human urinary bladder. Arch. Int. Pharmacodyn. 285:238–248

Kinder, R.B., Mundy, A.R. 1985a. Inhibition of spontaneous contractile activity in isolated human detrusor muscle strips by vasoactive intestinal polypeptide. Br. J. Urol. 57:20–23

Kinder, R.B., Mundy, A.R. 1985b. Atropine blockade of nerve-mediated stimulation of the human detrusor. Br. J. Urol. 57:418–421

Kinder, R.B., Restorick, J.M., Mundy, A.R. 1985. Vasoactive intestinal polypeptide in the hyperreflexic neuropathic bladder. Br. J. Urol. 57:289–291

Klarskov, P., Gerstenberg, T., Ramirez, D., Hald, T. 1983. Non-cholinergic, non-adrenergic nerve mediated relaxation in trigone, bladder neck and urethral smooth muscle in vitro. J. Urol. 129:848–850

Klarskov, P., Gerstenberg, T., Hald, T. 1984a. Vasoactive intestinal polypeptide influence on lower urinary tract smooth muscle from human and pig. J. Urol. 131:1000–1004

Klarskov, P., Fahrenkrug, J., Holm-Bentzen, M., et al. 1984b. Vasoactive intestinal polypeptide (VIP) concentration in bladder neck, smooth muscle and VIP influence on urodynamic parameters. Proc. 14th Meeting of the Int. Cont. Soc., pp 228–230

Klarskov, P., Horby-Petersen, J. 1986. The influence of serotonin on lower urinary tract smooth muscle in vitro. Br. J. Urol. 58:507–513

Klarskov, P. 1987a. Enkephalin inhibits presynaptically the contractility of urinary tract smooth muscle. Br. J. Urol. 59:31–35

Klarskov, P. 1987b. Non-cholinergic non-adrenergic nerve mediated relaxation of pig and human detrusor muscle in vitro. Br. J. Urol. 59:414–419

Klarskov, P. 1987c. Non-cholinergic non-adrenergic inhibitory nerve responses of bladder outlet smooth muscle in vitro. Br. J. Urol. 60:337–342

Klarskov, P., Holm-Bentzen, M., Norgaard, T., Ottesen, B., Walter, S., Hald, T. 1987. Vasoactive intestinal polypeptide concentration in human bladder neck smooth muscle and its influence on urodynamic parameters. Br. J. Urol. 60:113–118

Klevmark, B. 1977. Motility of the urinary bladder in cats during filling at physiological rates. II. Effects of extrinsic bladder denervation on intravesical pressure patterns. Acta Physiol. Scand. 101:176–184

Kondo, M., Taniyama, K., Tanaka, C. 1985. Histamine H^1-receptors in the guinea-pig urinary bladder. Eur. J. Pharmacol. 114:89–92

Kuru, M. 1965. Nervous control of micturition. Physiol. Rev. 45:425–494

LaMotte, C.C., de Lanerolle, N.C. 1981. Human spinal neurons innervation by both substance P and enkephalin. Neuroscience 6:713–723

Langley, J.N., Anderson, H.K. 1895a. The innervation of the pelvic and adjoining viscera. Part 2. The bladder. J. Physiol. (Lond) 19:85–139

Langley, J.N., Anderson, H.K. 1895b. The innervation of the pelvic and adjoining viscera. Part 1. J. Physiol. (Lond) 19:71–84

Larsen, J.J. 1979. α- and β-adrenoceptors in the detrusor muscle and bladder base of the pig and β-adrenoceptors in the detrusor muscle of man. Br. J. Pharmacol. 65:215–222

Larsson, L.I., Childers, S., Synder, S.H. 1979. Met- and leu-enkephalin immunoreactivity in seperate neurones. Nature 282:407–410

Learmonth, J.R. 1931. A contribution to the neurophysiology of the urinary bladder in man. Brain 54:147–176

Le Greves, P., Nyberg, F., Terenius, L., Hokfelt, T. 1985. Calcitonin gene-related peptide is a potent inhibitor of substance P degradation. Eur. J. Pharmacol. 115:309–311

Lembeck, F. 1953. Zur Frage der zentralen Übertragung afferenter impulse. III. Das vorkommen und die Bedeutung der Substanz p in den dorsalen Wurzeln des Ruckenmarks. Naunyn Schmiedebergs Arch. Pharmakol. 219:197–213

Levin, R.M., Wein, A.J. 1981. Effect of vasoactive intestinal polypeptide on the contractility of the rabbit urinary bladder. Urol. Res. 9:217–218

Levin, R.M., Staskin, D.R., Wein, A.J. 1982. The muscarinic cholinergic binding kinetics of the human urinary bladder. Neurourol. Urodynamics 1:221–226

Lund, C.J., Benjamin, J.A., Tristan, T.A., Fullerton, R.E., Ramsey, G.H., Watson, J.S. 1957. Cinefluorographic studies of the bladder and urethra in women. I. Urethrovesical relationships in voluntary and involuntary urination. Am. J. Obstet. Gynecol. 74:896–908

Lundberg, J.M. 1981. Evidence for coexistence of vasoactive intestinal polypeptide (VIP) and acetylcholine in neurons of cat exocrine glands. Morphological, biochemical and functional studies. Acta Physiol. Scand. (suppl.) 496:1–57

Lundberg, J.M., Torssell, L., Sollevi, A., et al. 1985. Neuropeptide Y sympathetic vascular control in man. Regul. Pept. 13:41–52

Macdonald, A.D., McCrea, E.D. 1930. Observations on the control of the bladder. The effects of nervous stimulation and of drugs. Q. J. Exp. Physiol. 20:379–391

Maggi, C.A., Santicioli, P., Grimaldi, G., Meli, A. 1983. The effect of peripherally administered GABA on spontaneous contractions of rat urinary bladder in vivo. Gen. Pharmacol. 14:455–458

Maggi, C.A., Santicioli, P., Meli, A. 1984. The effect of capsaicin on micturition reflex in urethrane anaesthetised rats. Proc. Int. Continence Soc. pp 217–218

Maggi, C.A., Santicioli, P., Meli, A. 1985. GABAa and GABAb receptors in detrusor strips from guinea-pig bladder dome. J. Autonom. Pharmacol. 5:55–64

Maggi, C.A., Meli, A. 1986. The role of neuropeptides in the regulation of the micturition cycle. J. Autonom. Pharmacol. 6:133–162

Maggi, C.A., Barbanti, G., Santicioli, P., et al. 1989. Cystometric evidence that capsaicin-sensitive nerves modulate the afferent branch of micturition reflex in humans. J. Urol. 142:150–154

Mattiasson, A., Ekblad, E., Sundler, R.F., Uvelius, B. 1985. Origin and distribution of neuropeptide Y, vasoactive intestinal polypeptide and substance P containing nerve fibres in the urinary bladder of the rat. Cell Tissue Res. 239:141–146

Mattiasson, A., Andersson, K.E., Elbadawi, A., Morgan, E., Sjogren, C. 1987. Interaction between adrenergic and cholinergic nerve terminals in the urinary bladder of rabbit, cat and man. J. Urol. 137:1017–1019

Miller, R.J. 1981. Peptides as neurotransmitters focus on the enkephalins and endorphins. Pharmacol. Ther. 12:73–108

Mulderry, P.K., Ghatei, M.A., Rodrigo, J., et al. 1985. CGRP in cardiovascular tissues of the rat. Neuroscience 14:947–954

Nathan, P.W., Smith, M.C. 1951. The centripetal pathway from the bladder and urethra within the spinal cord. J. Neurol. Neurosurg. Psychiatr. 14:262–280

Nathan, P.W. 1956. Sensations associated with micturition. Br. J. Urol. 28:126–131

Nergardh, A., Boreus, L.O. 1972. Autonomic receptor function in the lower urinary tract of man and cat. Scand. J. Urol. Nephrol. 6:32–36

Nergardh, A. 1975. Autonomic receptor functions in the lower urinary tract: a survey of recent experimental results. J. Urol. 113:180–185

Nergardh, A., Boreus, L.O., Naglo, A.S. 1977. Characterisation of the adrenergic β receptor in the urinary bladder of man and cat. Acta Pharmacol. Toxicol. 40:14–21

Nilvebrant, L., Andersson, K.E., Mattiasson, A. 1985. Characterisation of the muscarinic cholinoceptors in the human detrusor. J. Urol. 134:418–423

Nishizawa, O., Fukuda, T., Matsuzaki, A., Moriya, I., Harada, T., Tsuchida, S. 1985. The role of the sympathetic nerves in bladder and urethral sphincter function during the micturition cycle in the dog evaluated by pressure flow EMG study. J. Urol. 134:1259–1261

Norlen, L. 1977. Efects on the urinary bladder and urethra of different pharmacological treatments. An in vitro study in normal and parasympathetically denervated cats. Scand. J. Urol. Nephrol. 11:7–16

Norlen, L., Sundin, T., Waagstein, F. 1978, β-adrenoceptor stimulation of the human urinary bladder in vitro. Acta Pharmacol. Toxicol. (suppl.) 43:26–30

Porter, N.H. 1962. A physiological study of the pelvic floor in rectal prolapse. Ann. R. Coll. Surg. 31:379–404

Raezer, D.M., Wein, J., Jacobwitz, D., Corriere, J.N.J. 1973. Autonomic innervation of canine urinary bladder. Cholinergic and adrenergic contributions and interaction of sympathetic and parasympathetic nervous systems in bladder function. Urology 2:211–214

Rohner, T.J., Hannigan, J.D., Sanford, E.J. 1971. Altered in vitro adrenergic responses of dog detrusor muscle after chronic bladder outlet obstruction. Urology 11:357–361

Said, S.I., Mutt, V. 1970. Polypeptide with broad biological activity. Isolation from small intestine. Science 169:1217–1218

Sharkey, K.A., Williams, R.G., Schultzberg, M., Dockray, G. 1983. Sensory substance P innervation of the urinary bladder possible site of action of capsaicin in causing urinary retention in rats. Neuroscience 10:861–868

Sibley, G.N.A. 1984a. A comparison of spontaneous and nerve-mediated activity in bladder muscle from man, pig and rabbit. J. Physiol. (Lond) 354:431–443

Sibley, G.N.A. 1984b. The response of the bladder to lower urinary tract obstruction. DM Thesis, University of Oxford

Simonds, W.F., Booth, A.M., Thor, K.B., Ostrowski, N.L., Nagel, J.R., De Groat, W.C. 1983. Parasympathetic ganglia naloxone antagonises inhibition by leucine-enkephalin and GABA. Brain Res. 271:365–370

Sjogren, C., Andersson, K.E., Husted, S., Mattiasson, A., Moller-Madsen, B. 1982. Atropine resistance of transmurally stimulated isolated human bladder muscle. J. Urol. 128:1368–1371

Sjogren, C., Andersson, K.E., Mattiasson, A. 1985. Effects of vasoactive intestinal polypeptide on isolated urethral and urinary bladder smooth muscle from rabbit and man. J. Urol. 133:136–140

Sundin, T., Dahlstrom, A. 1973. The sympathetic innervation of the urinary bladder in the normal state and after parasympathetic denervation at the spinal root level. Scand. J. Urol. Nephrol. 7:131–149

Sundin, T., Dahlstrom, A., Norlen, L., Svedmyr, N. 1977. The sympathetic innervation and adrenoceptor function of the human lower urinary tract in the normal state and after parasympathetic denervation. Invest. Urol. 14:332–328

Sundler, F., Brodin, E., Ekblad, E., Hakansson, R., Uddman, R. 1985. Sensory nerve fibres distribution of substance P, neurokinin A and calcitonin gene-related peptide. In: Tachykinin antagonists. Hakansson, R., Sundler, F., eds. Amsterdam, Elsevier, pp 3–14

Szolesanyi, J. 1977. A pharmacological approach to elucidation of the role of different nerve fibres and receptor endings in mediation of pain. J. Physiol. 73:251–259

Taira, N. 1972. The autonomic pharmacology of the bladder. Ann. Rev. Pharmacol. 12:197–208

Tanagho, E.A., Miller, E.R. 1970. Initiation of voiding. Br. J. Urol. 42:175–183

Tang, P.C., Ruch, T.C. 1955. Non-neurogenic basis of bladder tonus. Am. J. Physiol. 181:249–257

Todd, J.K., Mack, A.J. 1969. A study of human bladder detrusor muscle. Br. J. Urol. 41:448–454

Vanov, S. 1965. Responses of the rat urinary bladder in situ to drugs and nerve stimulation Br. J. Pharmacol. 24:591–600

Von Euler, U.S., Gaddum, J.H. 1931. An unidentified depressor substance in certain tissue extracts. J. Physiol. (Lond) 72:74–87

Warwick, R. Williams, P.L. 1973. Neurology plexuses of the autonomic nervous system. In: Gray's anatomy. Warwick, R., Williams, P.L., eds. Edinburgh, Longman, pp 1079–1081

Wein, A.J., Gregory, J.G., Cromie, W.J., Corriere, J.N.J., Jacobwitz, D. 1974. Sympathetic innervation and chemical sympathectomy of canine bladder. Urology 9:27–31

Wein, A.J., Levin, R.M. 1979. Comparison of adrenergic receptor density in urinary bladder in man, dog and rabbit. Surg. Forum 30:576–578

Winter, D.L. 1971. Receptor characteristics and conduction velocities in bladder afferents. J. Psychiatr. Res. 8:225–235

Chapter 4

Pathophysiological Changes in the Obstructed Bladder

C.R. Chapple

A Review of Previous Experimental Animal Studies

The first reported studies concentrated on the effects of acute bladder outlet obstruction produced by urethral ligation in dogs and rabbits (Guyon and Albarron, 1890; Shigematsu, 1928; Creevy, 1934). This produced a non-physiological situation which resulted in marked vesical distension accompanied by acute vesical haemorrhage and mural necrosis. In an attempt to mimic the clinical course produced by prostatic obstruction, Duncan and Goodwin (1949) produced gradual obstruction to the urethra by implanting cellophane bands in dogs, thus stimulating an intense fibrotic response around the proximal urethra. However, this technique was unsatisfactory in that the obstruction was so marked that 4 out of the 7 animals so treated died within 6 months.

Subsequently, there have been a number of experimental studies on the morphological, contractile and functional effects of partial bladder outlet obstruction. Mayo and Hinman (1976) studied the functional and structural changes within the rabbit bladder at 6 months following bladder neck obstruction. They noted marked structural changes with collagenous infiltration of muscle and disruption of intracellular junctions. Brent and Stephens (1975), also using a rabbit model, recorded the sequential changes associated with obstruction; with an initial collagenous infiltration followed by an increased muscle cell mass due to hyperplasia (threefold increase in cell number) and hypertrophy (fivefold increase in cell volume). Uvelius et al. (1984) reported that in the initial stages following experimentally induced bladder outflow obstruction in the rat there was pronounced smooth muscle hypertrophy and hyperplasia with an approximately tenfold increase in the total bladder muscle mass by 6 weeks following obstruction. These changes occurred with marked rapidity with a significant increase in DNA content being evident after just 3 days. Levin et al. (1984) confirmed the rapidity of the bladder's response to chronic partial obstruction with a ninefold increase in bladder mass as a consequence of hypertrophy after just 1 week of obstruction.

These reports demonstrate that the bladder's response to obstruction involves both a collagenous infiltration and muscular hypertrophy and hyperplasia. Variation in results is evident between the different studies which may either be due to methodological differences or inter-species variation. The importance of study design is emphasised by two separate reports on the ultrastructural changes following short-term bladder distension. Gosling et al. (1977) reported transient oedema and haemorrhage following a 3-hour balloon distension of the rabbit bladder with no evidence of significant structural changes on either light or electron microscopy at up to 18 weeks following the procedure. Sehn (1978), using a similar technique in rats and rabbits, documented no changes following 2 hours of distension but demonstrated evidence of external injury in over half of the neuronal axons present within the bladder by 2 weeks after a 6-hour distension.

Despite extensive work, the mechanisms of functional disruption underlying these documented ultrastructural changes remain obscure. Mayo and Hinman (1976) noted that bladder neck obstruction in the rabbit did not appear to alter bladder contractility to pelvic nerve stimulation. Mattiasson and Uvelius (1982) observed that pelvic nerve stimulation resulted in obstructed rat bladders achieving a similar maximum force per unit cross-sectional area as controls but at a considerably greater volume. They concluded that hypertrophic rat detrusor therefore exhibited a decreased ability to generate pressures at smaller bladder volumes as compared to control bladder.

Ghoneim et al. (1986) studied rings of rabbit detrusor after 3 months of partial bladder outlet obstruction, using muscle strip techniques and concluded that the detrusor response varied with the degree of obstruction. These conclusions were based on the observations that the muscle length at which maximum contractility was exerted increased in moderate obstruction and decreased in severe obstruction, where hyperplasia and collagen infiltration were more evident.

Levin et al. (1984) reported that after 1 week of bladder outlet obstruction produced by the application of a ligature around the bladder neck, there resulted a 50% reduction in in vitro isometric contractile responses to bethanecol and electrical field stimulation and parallel reductions in muscarinic receptor density (77%) and intracellular ATP levels (71%). Using an in vitro whole bladder preparation, obstructed bladders had an increased capacity (threefold), but exhibited a 72% reduction in the ability of the bladder to empty its contents as compared to control. Although the contractile and metabolic dysfunction appeared reversible and the functional ability of the isolated bladder returned to 80% of control activity by 2 weeks following relief of obstruction, the residual functional deficit had not resolved after 4 weeks (Levin et al. 1985). Following on from this work Levin and co-workers (1986) in an acute study using a whole bladder preparation have shown that the obstructed bladder requires an increased intraluminal pressure to empty and does so at a slower rate than controls. In addition, the obstructed bladder is more prone to fatigue after repetitive stimulation. More recent work using an obstructed rat model has suggested that in the hypertrophic muscle the force per area had decreased (Uvelius et al. 1988). Subsequent biochemical study of the muscular proteins actin and myosin in the obstructed rat and human bladder demonstrated an increased actin/myosin ratio which appeared to correlate with this decrease in the maximal active force in hypertrophic bladder (Uvelius et al. 1989).

Detrusor instability is a complex functional disorder, which results from the interaction of a number of interrelated ultrastructural and pharmacological changes under the influence of an intact reflex arc. All of the experimental animal studies so far reported are difficult to relate directly to man, not only because of species differences but also in view of the limitations of the in vitro experimental techniques which are available. The importance of inter-species variation in pharmacological responses has been demonstrated by a recent comparative study contrasting rabbit, pig and man (Sibley, 1984a). In recent years, a great deal of attention has been directed to the development of a satisfactory animal model to reproduce the clinical picture seen in man and thereby allow in vivo physiological studies using urodynamics in combination with the application of ultrastructural and in vitro pharmacological techniques.

The first comprehensive validated model was developed by Sibley (1985) and utilised the pig. Previous workers had suggested that the pig lower urinary tract exhibited a number of similarities to man (Melick et al. 1978). It is of note that Jorgensen et al. (1983) had previously produced a situation akin to detrusor instability in 6 out of 7 female pigs at 10 weeks following proximal urethral obstruction. Similarly, Sibley produced a situation mimicking detrusor instability, albeit the cystometric pattern produced cannot be said to be unequivocal detrusor instability as this requires full subject cooperation. The pattern suggestive of detrusor instability occurred in nearly two thirds of the animals obstructed in Sibley's study (9/14), two pigs developed low compliant bladders, one pig a picture suggestive of chronic retention and two pigs remained stable. Following relief of the chronic obstruction in 6 pigs (4 of whom had developed instability), reassessment at 3 months demonstrated that two pigs reverted to stable detrusor function and two remained with abnormal filling cystometrograms. There was no evidence to suggest that this detrusor instability was related to the severity of the bladder outflow obstruction produced. Pharmacological studies on muscle strips obtained from these animals after 3–5 months of obstruction demonstrated appearances consistent with post-junctional supersensitivity, with exaggerated responses to agonists such as acetylcholine and potassium and a reciprocal reduction in the responses observed to nerve-mediated stimulation of the bladder (Sibley, 1987).

The dynamic nature of the pathophysiological changes accompanying bladder outlet obstruction must not be forgotten. For instance Ekstrom et al. (1986), from work on the obstructed rat urinary bladder, postulated that supersensitivity initially occurred as a consequence of a dilution of the density of intramuscular nerve fibres by muscle hypertrophy which was subsequently compensated for by an increase in the field of innervation of individual nerve fibres. Conversely, Sibley postulated that this supersensitivity was not due to an increase in muscle bulk consequent upon hypertrophy or hyperplasia, but represented a true partial denervation of the obstructed detrusor muscle and confirmed this with preliminary non-quantitative ultrastructural studies (Sibley, 1984b).

Further support for this denervation hypothesis follows from in vitro experimental studies in the rat, where an almost direct relationship was noted between the fraction of motor nerves left intact in the bladder and electrically induced contractile effects (Carpenter and Rubin, 1967), work which has been confirmed in vivo in the rat (Elmer, 1974), and in vitro in the cat (Mattiasson et al. 1983) and dog bladder (Raz, 1983).

Speakman et al. (1987) have extended the work with the pig model up to 18 months. Thirty pigs were studied (8 control and 22 obstructed); 17/22 (77%) of the obstructed pigs developed detrusor instability. This work again suggested a post-junctional supersensitivity. Concomitant objective quantitative studies using light and electron microscopy to count AChE-positive and total nerve profiles respectively, revealed a significant negative correlation between the nerve profile count per mm^2 detrusor muscle and the duration of obstruction. It is of particular note that these workers failed to demonstrate any significant physiological or morphological differences between animals with obstructed and stable bladders and those with obstruction and detrusor instability.

Malmgren and co-workers (1987) have subsequently developed a similar model using the rat. Sprague-Dawley rats had their urethras partially obstructed using ligatures and concurrently had intravesical pressure lines inserted which allowed the measurement of cystometric parameters in conscious animals. After 6 weeks' obstruction, isometric muscle strip experiments demonstrated increased spontaneous activity in the bladder of most obstructed rats (83%), again reminiscent of detrusor instability, with significant increases in bladder capacity (25-fold), bladder compliance, micturition pressure and residual volumes. Further studies using this model (Andersson et al. 1988) have demonstrated a decreased concentration of substance P and increased concentrations of VIP in obstructed as compared to control bladder. Furthermore, obstructed bladder exhibited a reduced response to neural stimulation, with little corresponding change in response to carbachol. Although VIP could not be demonstrated to produce any pharmacological effect, substance P produced contractions of reduced amplitude in obstructed bladder as compared to control. Two weeks following the relief of 6 weeks of bladder outlet obstruction, Malmgren et al. (1988) documented that strips from these rat bladders exhibited an apparent supersensitivity to carbachol and electrical field stimulation, the latter response being reduced below control and obstructed response levels by scopolamine. The previous reduction in contractile response to substance P was reversed towards control levels. They suggested that instability in this model was not related to cholinergic neurons but rather represented increased myogenic reactivity of smooth muscle cells.

Steers and De Groat (1988) carried out partial urethral ligation in female rats which reproduced the previously described changes in urodynamic variables. They examined changes in the central control of the bladder related to obstruction and noted that experimentally induced bladder distension produced no obvious differences in afferent and efferent nerve activity. In contrast, electrical stimulation of the pelvic nerve afferents evoked two distinct reflexes, a supraspinal and a spinal component. Whilst the supraspinal reflex was unchanged, the spinal reflex was present in a significantly greater percentage of obstructed (100%) than sham operated controls (35%). They suggested that these changes represented a compensatory spinal reflex mechanism triggered by increased bladder wall tension and work necessary to empty the bladder in the presence of outlet obstruction.

Levin et al. 1984 reported a greater than 50% decrease in the response of the obstructed rat bladder both to bethanecol and nerve-mediated stimulation, which is supported by Andersson et al.'s observations (1988) and is at variance with the pig model (Sibley, 1987). This apparent discrepancy may be explained by the suggestion that there is a reduction in the total force exerted by obstructed versus control bladder if allowance is made for the increased bulk of the bladder musculature (Speakman et al. 1988). Alternatively, it may be related to inter-species differences.

Although these animal studies allow the formulation of plausible hypotheses upon which to base a further investigation of the pathophysiology of secondary detrusor instability, they can only be adequately tested on the human detrusor. Such work is extremely difficult to conduct as evidenced by the paucity of literature available on this subject.

Human Studies

Millar (1958) noted smooth muscle hypertrophy as a complication of bladder outlet obstruction. Susset et al. (1978) used biochemical techniques to measure the collagen content of the obstructed bladder and provided evidence of a relative fall in the connective tissue component. Gosling and Dixon (1980), using subjective evaluation of histological sections from both control and obstructed bladders, observed connective tissue infiltration of smooth muscle bundles but no apparent change in muscle cell size or number. The combined use of morphological and morphometric techniques was subsequently applied to the study of the obstructed detrusor by the same group (Gilpin et al. 1985), and demonstrated the importance of an objective technique to the identification of significant changes in muscle cell size. In this study 12 of the 14 patients studied had connective tissue infiltration as previously reported (Gosling and Dixon, 1980) and furthermore, there was significant detrusor smooth muscle hypertrophy; hyperplasia could not be excluded since specimens incorporating a full thickness of the bladder wall were not available. Similar techniques have subsequently been applied to the objective quantification of AChE-positive neurons using the light microscope in patients with no urological or urodynamic abnormality; and have been further validated by the assessment of total neuronal profile using electron microscopy. These studies have demonstrated a significant reduction in neuronal count in the human detrusor with advancing age (Gilpin et al. 1986). Similar quantitative work in the obstructed detrusor using light and electron microscopy with corrections applied for the increased mean profile area of smooth muscle cells (hypertrophy) and increased amounts of connective tissue (collagen infiltration) has demonstrated a highly significant reduction in nerve profiles per square mm in obstructed bladder versus control ($p < 0.01$); with a 56% reduction in AChE-stained nerves (Gosling et al. 1986). It must however be remembered that this study looked at a mixed group of male and female patients who had not undergone detailed urodynamic investigation. Nevertheless, these findings parallel those reported from workers on the pig model (Sibley, 1987; Speakman et al. 1987) and support the suggestion that post-junctional denervation supersensitivity may be contributing to detrusor instability complicating bladder outlet obstruction.

Whilst this hypothesis provides a plausible explanation for the reported findings, a more detailed correlation with the duration and degree of the changes in detrusor function associated with prostatic obstruction and morphological responses of the detrusor to relief of obstruction needs to be carried out. Although a review of the data so far available from the pig model supports the hypothesis of a post-junctional hypersensitivity it does not satisfactorily explain the predilection of some animals to unstable as contrasted to stable detrusor behaviour in the presence of obstruction. This may be related to the small numbers of animals studied, but additional explanations need to be considered. Few previous studies of the responses of the obstructed as contrasted to control human bladder have been reported. Sibley (1985) documented a shift to the left of the dose response curve to acetylcholine at a dose range of 5×10^{-5} M up to 5×10^{-4} M and bladders from obstructed patients exhibited a significant decrease in the response to intramural nerve stimulation. Harrison et al. (1987) only demonstrated significant differences at stimulation frequencies of 30 to 50 Hz and at acetylcholine concentrations in the dose range 10^{-5} M–10^{-4} M. In contrast, Eaton and Bates (1982) reported no differences in the responses of normal and unstable detrusor, but found an exaggerated response to electrical stimulation of muscle in the unstable group. This study equated normal with stable detrusor function and both groups included both male and female patients, the majority having obstructed bladders (42/61).

Other hypotheses advanced to explain a link between detrusor instability and obstruction remain largely speculative. Chalfin and Bradley (1982) suggested that abnormal sensory stimuli from an altered prostatic urethra could provide sufficient afferent input into a local spinal reflex arc to induce detrusor instability. They injected 6 ml of 1% lignocaine into each lobe of the prostate in 15 patients with bladder outlet obstruction (11 unstable, 4 stable) and documented the effects of this procedure on the cystometrogram. Local anaesthetic prostate block eliminated instability in 10 out of 11 patients and had no effect on the 4 patients with a normal CMG. On the basis of these findings they concluded that surgical resection of the prostate may correct detrusor instability via a primary action to reduce afferent neural impulses from the prostate.

Other workers have supported the view that abnormal afferent input from the obstructed bladder may be of importance to the genesis of detrusor instability. For instance, it has been suggested that stretch receptors in the bladder wall may have a lower threshold in patients who subsequently develop detrusor instability (Higson et al. 1979). However, this study failed to produce consistent effects to the application of lignocaine. Reuther et al. (1983) reported that the instillation of lignocaine altered bladder sensation and increased the volume at which uninhibited bladder contractions occurred. This has subsequently been investigated by Sethia and Smith (1987) who reported that the instillation of an alkaline solution into the obstructed unstable bladder resulted in increased capacity and reduced instability. In contrast, lignocaine produced a variable effect on bladder capacity, increasing it in those with a flow rate greater than 10 ml per second and decreasing it in those with a flow rate less than 10 ml per second. In addition, it had little effect on instability and in 3 out of 29 unstable obstructed bladders actually worsened the instability, a finding for which no clear explanation is currently available. Further work is required to clarify these observations before final conclusions can be drawn.

In 1978 Rohner and co-workers reported the results of experiments on the effects of chronic bladder outlet obstruction in dogs. In 7 out of 12 obstructed dogs (58%), they documented a change in response to adrenergic stimulation of detrusor muscle in the bladder body and dome from a relaxant β-adrenoceptor to a contractile α-adrenoceptor response. Rohner et al. observed that the severity of the urethral obstruction was directly related to the muscle strip response, with the greatest contractile effects in dogs with the most severe narrowing of the urethra. They postulated that these pharmacological changes may contribute to the decreased bladder capacity and associated increase in detrusor instability seen in the obstructed bladder. In contrast, Sibley (1987) could not elicit any such alteration in the response of the detrusor muscle to adrenergic stimulation in the obstructed pig model.

A subsequent study of human detrusor muscle obtained from the bladder dome in 47 subjects was reported by Perlberg and Caine (1982). They carried out detailed urodynamic assessment using cystometry in 27 of the patients studied (11 unstable, 16 stable). Of the 11 patients with unstable detrusor behaviour 6 (55%) showed an α-adrenoceptor response, 3 (27%) a β response and in 2 (18%) no response; in contrast, in the stable detrusors 15 (94%) exhibited a β response and 1 (6%) an α response. They reported a correlation between the irritative symptoms reported by the patients and a tendency to a contractile α-adrenergic response. Reuther and Aagaard (1984) reported a small series of 4 patients; in 3 detrusor instability disappeared on treatment with the α-adrenoceptor antagonist phenoxybenzamine and reappeared when treatment was discontinued. They documented the same findings following surgical relief of obstruction in these patients.

Atropine-resistant non-adrenergic, non-cholinergic neurotransmission may be important in the genesis of detrusor instability. Evidence for this suggestion can be found in studies of detrusor muscle strip preparations from patients with prostatic obstruction reported by Sjogren et al. (1982) and Nergardh and Kinn (1983). Subsequent studies have refuted this suggestion. Sibley (1984b) in a study of 5 obstructed patients reported that an atropine-resistant response of 10%–20% persisted at 50 Hz, but appeared to be TTX-resistant, suggesting an increased sensitivity of obstructed bladder muscle to direct stimulation. Similarly Kinder and Mundy (1985b) reported almost total inhibition of the response to nerve-mediated stimulation by atropine in normal bladder and subsequently in idiopathic unstable and hyperreflexic detrusor.

The observation that detrusor muscle might be more excitable (Malmgren et al. 1988; Malmgren, 1989) could be explained by a non-specific increase in muscle excitability in these patients; alternatively there may be a disorder of intrinsic inhibition or neural modulation, which may under normal circumstances be mediated by putative neuropeptide transmitters such as VIP (Gu et al. 1983b; Kinder and Mundy, 1985a; Kinder et al. 1985).

Idiopathic instability cannot be distinguished on the basis of filling cystometry from instability occurring in association with bladder outlet obstruction, although it is not possible to determine to what extent the detrusor instability associated with obstruction is related to idiopathic detrusor instability. Nevertheless, it is informative to document some of the altered physiological responses reported in the context of idiopathic detrusor instability as they provide an additional perspective.

In complete contrast to the findings reported with the obstructed bladder, Eaton and Bates (1982) reported an increased contractile response by detrusor strips from patients with idiopathic and post-obstructive instability to nerve-mediated stimulation but with no change in sensitivity to acetylcholine. Kinder and Mundy (1987) documented an increased sensitivity of detrusor muscle in patients with idiopathic instability and hyperreflexia at lower frequencies of stimulation but with no increase in the maximum contractile response produced. The abnormal muscle exhibited an exaggerated response to stimulation with the agonist acetylcholine at threshold concentrations ($< 3 \times 10^{-8}$ M), and in addition showed a greater tendency to develop spontaneous contractile activity, higher basal tensions and contractions of greater frequency and amplitude, as compared to normal muscle. These findings suggest a primary myogenic abnormality in unstable muscle. Maximal responses could be largely abolished (92.7%–97.4%) following pre-treatment with atropine, suggesting the principal functional neural component to be parasympathetic, with a limited role for non-adrenergic and non-cholinergic mechanisms.

As has been emphasised in this review, no comprehensive synchronous studies of the histological and physiological changes occurring in the obstructed human bladder have previously been reported. The results of such a study with the intention of shedding some light on this complex and controversial subject are presented in the next section.

A Clinical Study of the Pathogenesis of Detrusor Instability in the Obstructed Bladder

We carried out a study with two main aims:

1. Via a combined histochemical and pharmacological investigation to investigate the changes in cholinergic and adrenergic detrusor innervation and in vitro pharmacological responses occurring in the human bladder following prostatic bladder outlet obstruction. These results were correlated with bladder function assessed both clinically and using comprehensive urodynamic investigation.

2. To investigate the normal histological distribution of the putative neurotransmitter peptides NPY, VIP, SP, calcitonin gene-related peptide (CGRP) and somatostatin (Som), which are thought to play an important role in sensorimotor nerves and to document the changes that occur in association with bladder outflow tract obstruction.

There is no doubt that major pathophysiological changes accompany the disruption of normal tissue architecture, as characterised by the collagen infiltration and muscle cell hyperplasia (Gilpin et al. 1985), which occur in the obstructed human bladder. The consequences of bladder outflow obstruction have been extensively studied in animal models, including the rat (Mattiasson and Uvelius, 1982), pig (Sibley, 1985), dog (Rohner et al. 1978) and rabbit (Mayo and Hinman, 1976; Levin et al. 1984, 1986; Kato et al. 1988). The results obtained are invaluable in allowing interpretation of the human condition but must be used with caution in extrapolating to man because of inter-species variation.

It must be remembered that although detrusor instability occurs in a majority of patients with bladder outflow obstruction, there is no quantifiable correlation between the severity of obstruction and the magnitude of instability (Turner-Warwick, 1984). Furthermore, resolution of detrusor instability in the obstructed pig model often occurs without a corresponding change in in vitro parameters (Sibley, 1985; Speakman et al. 1987). Previous studies have considered the autonomic innervation of the bladder to be solely comprised of cholinergic or adrenergic nerves. It is now well recognised that a number of additional transmitters are involved (Burnstock, 1986a, b): neuropeptide Y and adenosine triphosphate (ATP) as well as noradrenaline in sympathetic nerves, vasoactive intestinal polypeptide in addition to acetylcholine in parasympathetic nerves. Furthermore, sensory nerves containing substance P, calcitonin gene-related peptide and ATP may have an important influence on motor function.

A striking feature in this study was the pronounced reduction in AChE-positive nerves in all categories of obstructed bladder, most marked in the chronic retention bladder (89%) (Fig. 4.1). This confirmed the results of a previous study (Gosling et al. 1986) of male and female bladders, which documented a similar reduction in AChE-positive staining. It is of particular interest that the reduction in AChE-positive staining was similar in detrusor muscle from both stable and unstable bladders, a finding corroborated by work from a pig model (Speakman et al. 1987). In view of the absence of significant differences between stable, unstable and acute retention obstructed bladder it has to be concluded that these changes in the density of AChE-positive staining of nerves do not by themselves provide a satisfactory explanation for the altered detrusor function, seen in the obstructed bladder. Although

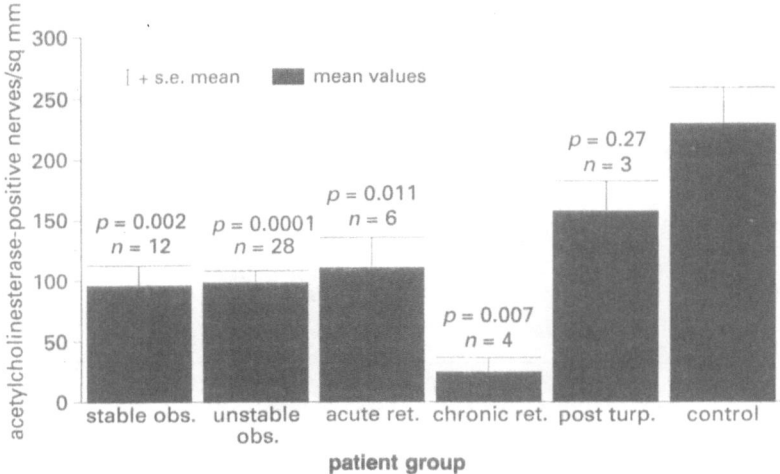

Fig.4.1. Quantification of the density of acetylcholinesterase–positive nerves within human bladder contrasting the findings in the various obstructed groups and following a transurethral resection of the prostate as contrasted to control.

it is tempting to speculate that the regression of the nerve count towards control values seen in the unobstructed post-prostatectomy group represents a reversal of previous damage, this was a small group and their bladders were unlikely to be normal since all of these patients were troubled by urinary frequency and two patients had detrusor instability. The markedly reduced innervation of the chronic retention bladder conforms with the clinical experience of detrusor failure in these patients. In interpreting these results it must be remembered that loss of AChE-stained fibres does not necessarily reflect a loss of cholinergic excitatory nerves alone, since this represents such a non-specific marker; but could also indicate a significant loss of sensorimotor (peptidergic) nerves.

Previous study of the normal human bladder has demonstrated a linear reduction with age in the density of AChE-positive nerves present within the bladder wall (Gilpin et al. 1986). No similar correlation between the neural count and age was evident in the present study (Fig. 4.2), possibly related to the small number of control patients. Alternatively, it might be suggested that a factor other than age was influencing the results. Nevertheless, all patients within the study group were accurately age matched to a carefully selected control population. This is an important consideration since it seems likely that the prevalence of detrusor instability in the human male increases with age (Abrams, 1985). Certainly, study of the rat highlights the important changes in bladder function which occur with increasing age (Chun et al. 1988); an observation supported by evidence of increased sensitivity of detrusor strips to acetylcholine and increased cholinoceptor density in older rats (Kolta et al. 1984).

The phenomenon of increased smooth muscle sensitivity to agonists is known as "supersensitivity" (Trendelenburg, 1963). It is now well recognised that smooth muscle supersensitivity follows experimental damage to

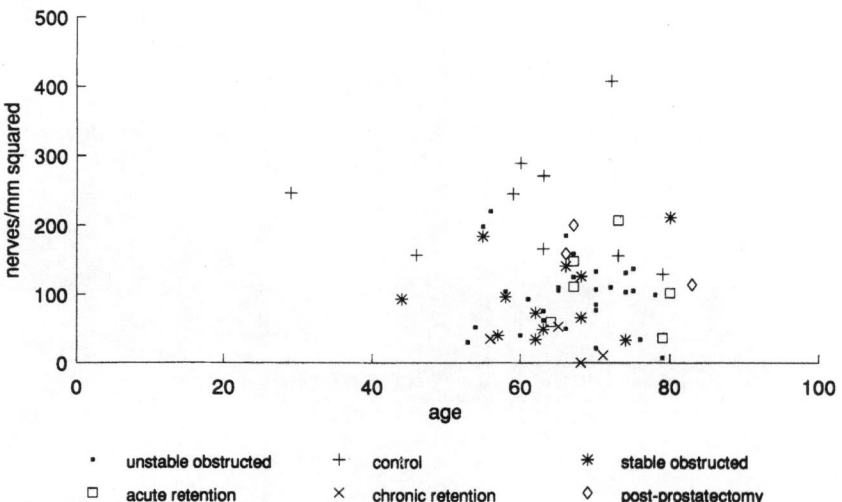

Fig.4.2. Results of quantification of acetylcholinesterase-positive nerves for each of the obstructed groups and post-prostatectomy plotted against patients' age.

its motor innervation (Westfall, 1981). Indeed such observations are not new, and formed the basis of Cannon's law which states that when an organ is deprived of its normal nerve supply it will develop hypersensitivity, in particular to its own neurotransmitter substance (Cannon and Rosenblueth 1949). Two qualitatively distinct manifestations of supersensitivity are recognised, termed pre-junctional and postjunctional (Fleming et al. 1973). Pre-junctional supersensitivity only occurs if presynaptic mechanisms for the control of local agonist concentration are impaired, resulting in more acetylcholine being available at the smooth muscle cells. Post-junctional supersensitivity encompasses a situation where there is reduced contact between agonist and effector cell receptors, and includes situations such as an inhibition of transmitter release, receptor blockade and denervation.

It has been reported that the obstructed pig bladder (Sibley, 1987) contracts more vigorously in response to cholinergic stimulation than normal tissue, with a corresponding reduction in response to nerve-mediated stimulation, findings which were attributed to a post-junctional cholinergic supersensitivity phenomenon. These results remain controversial, since further work using this model has reported that if the increased detrusor response to acetylcholine is related to the tissue mass then there is an overall reduction in the maximum force/gram tissue produced (Speakman et al. 1987), confirming the observations of other workers (Levin et al. 1984). In support of these observations, in our study of a limited number of patients, the maximum tissue contractile responses noted upon stimulation of the obstructed bladder with potassium (Table 4.1) were considerably reduced ($p < 0.05$) as compared to control.

The in vitro pharmacological results obtained in this study confirm that a disruption of normal detrusor muscle responsiveness to both pharmacological and nerve-mediated stimulation occurs in the presence of bladder outflow obstruction. Although an inverse relationship was evident between the responses to acetylcholine and electrical field stimulation in the unstable and stable obstructed (Figs. 4.3, 4.4) groups, compatible with a post-denervation state, the differences were not statistically significant. Nevertheless the trends seen in combination with the morphological studies do provide additional support for the hypothesis that post-junctional cholinoceptor supersensitivity resulting from denervation is important in the development

Table 4.1. Contractile responses of bladder from each of the groups (control, acute retention, stable obstruction, unstable obstruction) demonstrating maximal responses to potassium

Study group	Patients	Mean	±Std error
Control	3	1.758	0.369
Acute retention	4	0.632[a]	0.104
Stable obstruction	3	1.029	0.360
Unstable obstruction	6	0.720	0.253

Maximum response to K^+ (mean ± S.E.M.).
[a] $p \leqslant 0.05$ Mann-Whitney test.

of detrusor instability in the obstructed bladder. It is, however, unlikely to be the sole explanation. Certainly, the suggestion that denervation results in cholinoceptor supersensitivity has been challenged by Nilvebrant (1986). Using observations based on radioligand receptor-binding studies and on measurements of affinity and receptor density, she concluded that muscarinic receptors in the rat urinary bladder are not involved in the development of supersensitivity.

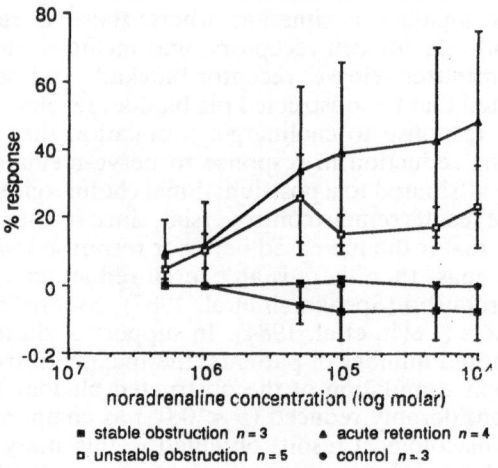

Fig.4.3. Dose response curves of human detrusor for the groups: stable obstruction, unstable obstruction, acute retention and control demonstrating the response to acetylcholine. (Results expressed as a percentage of the maximal response to K+.)

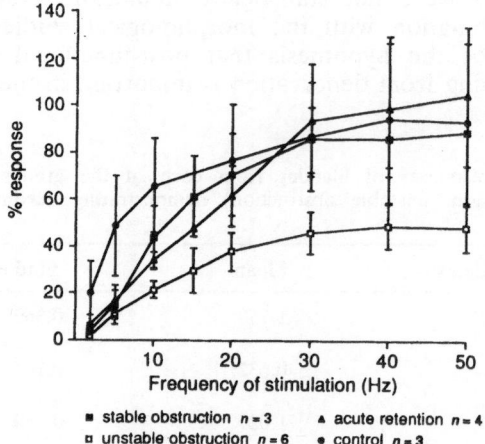

Fig.4.4. Frequency response curves for each of the groups: stable obstruction, unstable obstruction, acute retention and control contrasting the response of the detrusor in each group to neural stimulation in vitro. (Results expressed as a percentage of the maximal response to K+.)

The finding of a reduced response in acute retention bladder to cholinergic stimulation with little corresponding change in nerve-mediated stimulation cannot be explained by a denervation hypothesis (Figs. 4.3, 4.4). Alternative pathophysiological mechanisms therefore need to be considered. Administration of noradrenaline produced an α_1-mediated contractile response in the acute retention bladder, with a smaller but similar response in some preparations from unstable obstructed bladder (Fig. 4.5). However, quantification of dopamine βhydroxylase (DBH)-like immunoreactivity (albeit a relatively non-specific staining method for sympathetic nerves) failed to demonstrate any significant change in adrenergic innervation in the obstructed detrusor (Fig. 4.6). In addition there was no evidence to suggest an increase in adrenergic nerve density similar to that reported in the decentralised human bladder (Sundin et al. 1977). Isometric muscle strip studies demonstrated that prazosin did not antagonise nerve-mediated contraction of detrusor muscle, thereby suggesting that the altered adrenergic response seen in the obstructed bladder resulted from changes in receptor function rather than nerve density. The significant increase in noradrenaline content seen in the unstable obstructed bladder body (Fig. 4.7) is difficult to explain satisfactorily on the basis of current evidence. Unfortunately due to the limited tissue available, further biochemical assays were not possible in the other obstructed subgroups.

Previous experimental studies of adrenoceptor stimulation in the obstructed bladder have produced conflicting results, with documented relaxation in pig bladder (Sibley, 1987) and contractile responses in both dogs (Rohner et al. 1978) and humans (Perlberg and Caine, 1982). The work reported here confirms the observations of Perlberg and Caine demonstrating a correlation between α_1-adrenoceptor-mediated contractile responses and detrusor instability. The observation of a prominent α_1-adrenoceptor-mediated contractile response in the acute retention bladder presented here has not

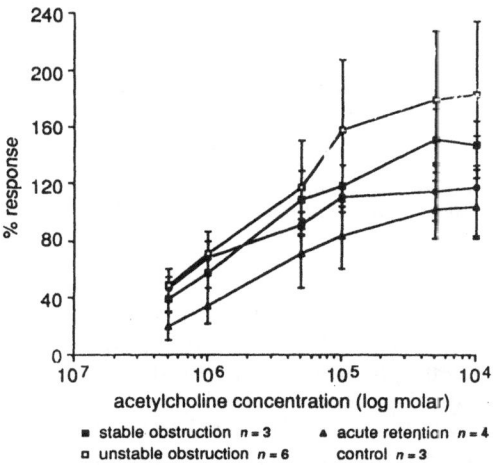

Fig.4.5. Dose response curves for each of the groups: stable obstruction, unstable obstruction, acute retention and control in response to the application of noradrenaline to human detrusor in vitro. (Results expressed as a percentage of the maximal response to K^+.)

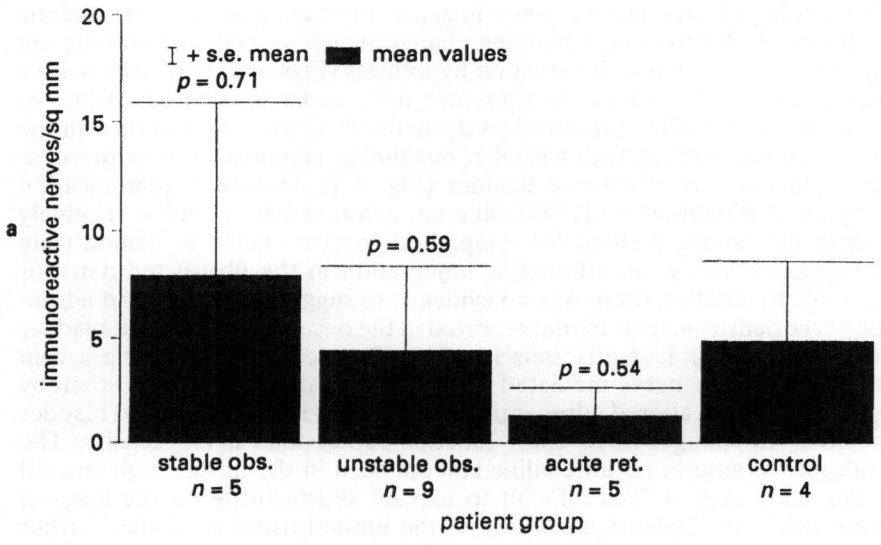

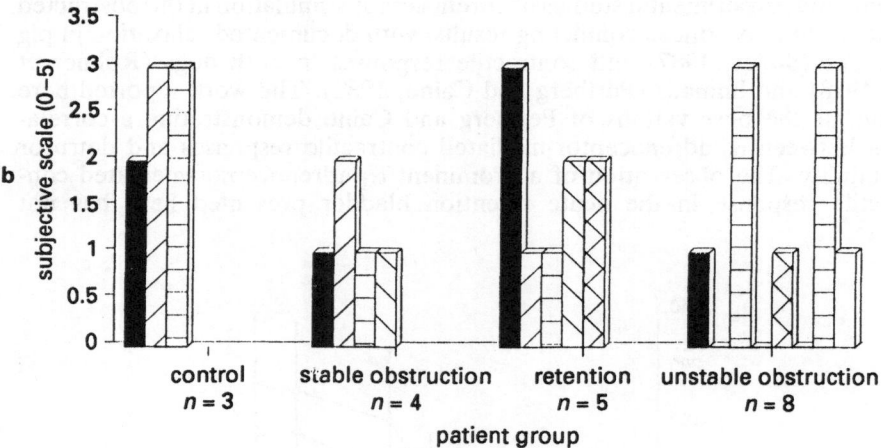

Fig.4.6. Results of **a** objective and **b** subjective quantification of dopamine β-hydroxylase immunoreactive nerves in the groups: control, stable obstruction, unstable obstruction and acute retention.

previously been reported. While this observation is only based on the study of a small number of specimens, an attractive hypothesis is that the altered tissue sensitivity to adrenergic stimulation could explain the unpredictable tendency for a subgroup of patients to develop acute retention in situations of increased sympathetic stimulation. The resultant episode of retention could then be equated to the detrusor–sphincter dyssynergia seen in patients with primary neuropathic disorders.

The potential mechanism of altered adrenoceptor function remains obscure. Certainly changes in receptor function are well recognised elsewhere in the

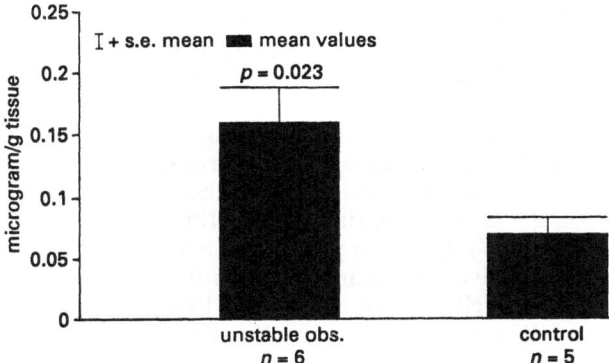

Fig.4.7. Results of biochemical assay of human bladder comparing the groups: unstable obstruction to control for noradrenaline (expressed in micrograms per gram tissue).

body in response to alterations in parameters such as the degree of stretch of muscle fibres (Benson et al. 1975) and hormonal milieu (Levin and Wein, 1981; Anderson and Navarro, 1988). The inconsistent and relatively limited contractions seen in response to the application of noradrenaline in detrusor muscle from unstable obstructed patients suggests that although it may be a contributory factor it is by itself insufficient to explain the pathogenesis of secondary detrusor instability.

An area which remains little explained is the role of the afferent innervation of the bladder and in particular, the effect of obstruction on putative non-adrenergic, non-cholinergic (NANC) sensorimotor neurotransmission. Whilst it is widely recognised that NANC sensorimotor nerves have a limited role, if any, in the function of the normal human detrusor, there is some evidence that its relative importance may be increased in the functionally disturbed bladder.

Despite the potential importance of neuropeptide neurotransmitter mechanisms in the function of the obstructed bladder, there has been little work on the localisation of neuropeptides within the normal human bladder (Gu et al. 1983b, 1984; Chapple et al. 1990). The highest density of neural immunoreactivity in the bladder is to NPY. Although nerve staining for this compound is occasionally seen in the submucosal tissue and around blood vessels, its predominant localisation is in the detrusor muscle layer. VIP is present with a similar distribution. In addition a number of VIP-like immunoreactive nerves are present within the lamina propria and to a lesser extent the submucosa. Both VIP- and NPY-like immunoreactivity are also equally evident in association with blood vessels. No immunoreactive neural ganglia were identified. CGRP-like immunoreactivity is found predominantly in relation to vessels with only isolated nerve fibres being identified in detrusor muscle and submucosal tissues. SP-like immunoreactive nerves, although present in a similar density to CGRP, are principally localised to the mucosa and submucosal layers. In contrast, there are very few Som-like immunoreactive nerves and when present these are localised within the submucosal tissues.

Both NPY- and VIP- immunoreactivity are present with the highest density in the human bladder and although primarily associated with the detrusor muscle, are also located around blood vessels. These findings suggest them to have a primary role in the motor innervation of detrusor muscle, but also suggest that these two peptides may participate in the regulation of blood flow.

At present, the distribution and role of peptides contained in the sensory nerves of the human bladder remains obscure. Previous studies have suggested the sensory innervation to be associated with the prominent AChE-positive nerves seen within the lamina propria of the urethra and bladder (George and Dixon, 1986; Kirby, 1987). In recent years it has been suggested that a number of the peptides are putative neurotransmitters within primary afferent neurons (Gibbins et al. 1987), including SP (Lembeck, 1953; Nicoll et al. 1980), and CGRP, Som and VIP (Jancso et al. 1977; Sundler et al. 1985).

Semi-quantitative assessment on further tissue from the same patient groups studied above suggested there was a significant reduction in immunoreactivity to neuropeptides in the obstructed bladder, with a particularly marked reduction in the density of immunoreactivity of nerves to VIP, CGRP and SP. An age-related reduction in the enkephalinergic nerves of human prostate has been reported (Jungblat et al. 1989), similar to that of the age-related reduction in AChE-positive nerves (Gosling et al. 1986), and sympathetic nerves (Benson et al. 1979). It is most unlikely that age by itself would explain the reduced density of innervation reported here, particularly as the age range of the different groups of patients studied showed considerable overlap and parallel studies of AChE staining on the same tissue did not demonstrate an age-related reduction.

These findings provide the first substantive histological evidence for a disturbance of the afferent and sensorimotor innervation of the obstructed human detrusor. Recently it has been suggested that the afferent limb of the micturition reflex may be more important in influencing bladder function than has been recognised previously. Recent study of a rat model suggests that there is an increase in local afferent spinal reflex activity in the presence of obstruction (Steers and De Groat, 1988). Further studies have suggested that there is hypertrophy of nerves innervating the bladder (Steers et al. 1989). A tempting explanation for this latter observation is that this hypertrophy represents a secondary phenomenon in response to the local detrusor denervation.

It is clear from this discussion that a number of putative neuropeptide transmitters occur in the human detrusor and that their concentration is reduced in the presence of obstruction. Although a fuller interpretation of these findings remains highly speculative and awaits further functional and ultrastructural study, the aetiology of obstructive detrusor instability is clearly related to a more widespread disruption of the normal structure and function of the human detrusor than has been previously recognised. Further study of the localisation of neuropeptides and their pharmacological action within the normal and obstructed human detrusor could possibly provide new therapeutic options for the control of functional disorders of the bladder.

Whilst there is good evidence for a disruption of neural mechanisms, the mechanism of injury to the nerves remains speculative. Raised intravesical pressure could lead to a reduction in blood flow to detrusor muscle, which indeed has been shown to occur in experimental models at surprisingly low intraluminal pressures (Dunn, 1974). Subsequent ischaemia would alter the structural characteristics of both smooth muscle cells and nerve fibres. Such an injury could compromise the function of the membrane bound Na^+ pumps, which require a constant supply of high energy phosphate and which would be particularly susceptible to such damage (Sehn, 1979).

Since none of the neuropathic hypotheses has fully explained the aetiology of detrusor instability, it is likely that there may be an additional functional abnormality of the obstructed detrusor smooth muscle (Malmgren et al. 1987). Certainly, marked structural changes within the human detrusor muscle follow obstruction (Uvelius et al. 1989) and this study demonstrated a reduced maximal contractile response of obstructed human detrusor to high-dose potassium, confirming previous animal studies (Levin et al. 1984; Uvelius et al. 1988).

Experimental study of denervated smooth muscle has revealed important neurophysiological changes rendering the cell more susceptible to stimuli (Fleming and Westfall, 1975). Westfall (1981) demonstrated partial depolarisation of the muscle cell membrane following chronic denervation of the guinea pig vas deferens. If similar changes occur in the obstructed human detrusor this would tend to increase the sensitivity of the smooth muscle cell to any agonist which induces contraction by depolarising the cell membrane, thereby non-specifically increasing responsiveness to stimuli unrelated to the naturally occurring neurotransmitter. Post-junctional supersensitivity arising from a disruption of cholinergic innervation, altered adrenergic neural control, an abnormality of normal inhibitory mechanisms (Kinder and Mundy, 1985a, b) and altered local spinal reflex activity (Chalfin and Bradley, 1982; Steers and De Groat, 1988) could all lead to changes in the physiological responses of smooth muscle cells.

Potentially, such detrusor muscle supersensitivity could facilitate the spread of waves of contraction throughout the detrusor muscle. Support for this suggestion is provided by the in vitro demonstration of exaggerated responsiveness of obstructed as compared to control bladder upon direct electrical stimulation of the pig (Sibley, 1985) and rat (Malmgren et al. 1988) detrusor muscle. Indeed, detrusor electromyography has demonstrated an abnormally hyperactive pattern of voltage fluctuation in the detrusor muscle of patients with primary detrusor instability (Doyle and Hill, 1976).

Summary

The current literature supports a number of hypotheses, advanced to explain the development of detrusor instability in association with bladder outlet obstruction. These can best be considered in two categories, myopathic and neuropathic.

Support for a primary myopathic abnormality is provided by the well-documented histological changes which occur in the obstructed bladder; the interpretation of the pharmacological studies remains controversial. In vitro animal studies have demonstrated both detrusor underactivity and hyperexcitability. Recent animal models using the rat, lend particular support to the suggestion that increased muscle excitability results from outlet obstruction. This observation is supported by in vitro muscle strip studies in the human.

Neuropathic hypotheses encompass both changes in local spinal reflex pathways and the local bladder innervation, to explain the altered detrusor function associated with detrusor instability. Recent evidence from a rat model suggests that local spinal reflexes are augmented in the presence of bladder obstruction, with exaggerated local spinal reflexes to electrical stimulation of afferent nerves. Histological study suggests that the obstructed bladder undergoes a cholinergic denervation. In vitro pharmacological isometric muscle strip studies have demonstrated post-junctional cholinergic denervation supersensitivity, an increase in NANC-mediated detrusor contractile activity, reduced contractile responses to substance P and reversed responsiveness of obstructed detrusor to adrenergic stimulation.

Bladder outflow obstruction leads to marked changes in the function of the human bladder with concomitant abnormalities seen in both ultrastructural and in vitro neuropharmacological studies. The results discussed here suggest the interplay and summation of a number of different pathophysiological mechanisms and support the view that a global disruption of neural function accompanies the marked ultrastructural changes seen in the obstructed detrusor muscle. These observations lend credence to the suggestion that both drugs which stabilise muscle cell membranes (Malmgren 1989) and α_1 antagonists (Chapple et al. 1989) may have a potential therapeutic role in the treatment of obstructive detrusor instability. Further studies of obstructed human bladder are necessary to investigate the role of changes in receptor density, affinity and distribution, agonist release and degradation and the ultrastructural and physiological alterations following the relief of obstruction.

References

Abrams, P.H. 1985. Detrusor instability in bladder outlet obstruction. Neurourol. Urodynamics 4:317–328

Anderson, G.F., Navarro, S.P. 1988. The response of autonomic receptors to castration and testosterone in the urinary bladder of the rabbit. J. Urol. 140:885–889

Andersson, P.O., Andersson, K.E., Fahrenkrug, J., Mattiasson, A., Sjogren, C., Uvelius, B. 1988. Contents and effects of substance P and vasoactive intestinal polypeptide in the bladder of rats with and without infravesical outflow obstruction. J. Urol. 140:168–172

Benson, G.S., Raezer, D.M., Wein, A.J., Carriere, J.N. 1975. Effect of muscle length on adrenergic stimulation of canine detrusor. Urology 5:769–772

Benson, G.S., McConnell, J.A., Wood, J.G. 1979. Adrenergic innervation of the human bladder body. J. Urol. 122:189–191

Brent, L., Stephens, F.D. 1975. The response of smooth muscle cells in the rabbit urinary bladder to outflow obstruction. Invest. Urol. 12:494–502

Burnstock, G. 1986a. The changing face of autonomic neurotransmission. Acta Physiol. Scand. 126:67–91

Burnstock, G. 1986b. Autonomic neuromuscular junctions: current developments and future directions. J. Anat. 146:1–30

Cannon, W.B., Rosenblueth, A., 1949. The supersensitivity of denervated structures: a law of denervation. New York, Macmillan, p 245

Carpenter, F.G., Rubin, R.M., 1967. The motor innervation of the rat urinary bladder. J. Physiol. 192:609–617

Chalfin, S.A., Bradley, W.E. 1982. The aetiology of detrusor hyperreflexia in patients with infravesical obstruction. J. Urol. 127:938–942

Chapple, C.R., Aubry, M., Greengrass, P. et al. 1989. Characterisation of human prostatic adrenoceptors using pharmacological receptor binding and localisation. Br. J. Urol. 63:487–496

Chapple, C.R., Gilphin, S.A., Moss, H. et al. 1990. The role of neural factors in the aetiology of detrusor instability associated with prostatic obstruction. Eur. Urol. 18 (Suppl.l):20, 35A

Chapple, C.R., Milner, P., Moss, H., Burnstock, G. 1992. Loss of sensory nerves in the obstructed bladder. Br. J. Urol. 70:373–381.

Chun, A.L., Wallace, L.J., Gerald, M.C., Levin, R.M., Wein, A.J. 1988. Effect of age on in vitro urinary bladder function in the rat. J. Urol. 139:625–627

Creevy, C.D. 1934. Distension of the urinary bladder. I. Haematuria and sudden emptying; an experimental and clinical study. Arch. Surg. 28:948–973

Doyle, P.T., Hill, D.W. 1976. Detrusor electomyography. In: Scientific foundations of urology. Williams, D.J., Chisholm, G.D., eds. London, Heinemann

Duncan, G.W., Goodwin, W.E. 1949. Experimental urinary tract obstruction produced by cellophane sclerosis. Surgery 25:113–116

Dunn, M. 1974. A study of the bladder blood flow during distension in rabbits. Br. J. Urol. 46:67–72

Eaton, A.C., Bates, C.P. 1982. An in vitro physiological study of normal and unstable human detrusor muscle. Br. J. Urol. 54:653–657

Ekstrom, J., Malmberg, L., Wallin, A. 1986. Transient supersensitivity in the hypertrophied rat urinary bladder. Acta Physiol. Scand. 126:365–370

Elmer, M. 1974. Action of drugs on the innervated and denervated urinary bladder of the cat. Acta Physiol. Scand. 91:289–297

Fleming, W.W., McPhillips, J.J., Westfall, D.P. 1973. Postjunctional supersensitivity and subsensitivity of excitable tissues to drugs. Rev. Physiol. 68:55–119

Fleming, W.W., Westfall, D.P. 1975. Altered resting membrane potential in the supersensitive vas deferens of the guinea pig. J. Pharmacol. Exp. Ther. 192:381–389

George, M.J.R., Dixon, J.S. 1986. In: Sensory disorders of the bladder and urethra. George, N.J.R., Gosling, J.A., eds. Berlin, Heidelberg, New York, Springer

Ghoneim, G.M., Regnier, C.H., Biancani, P., Johnson, L., Susset, J.G. 1986. Effect of vesical outlet obstruction on detrusor contractility and passive properties in rabbits. J. Urol. 135:1284–1289

Gibbins, I.L., Furness, J.B., Costa, M. 1987. Pathway-specific patterns of the co-existence of substance P, calcitonin gene-related peptide, cholecystokinin and dynorphin in neurones of the dorsal root ganglia of the guinea pig. Cell Tissue Res. 248:417–437

Gilpin, S.A., Gosling, J.A., Barnard, R.J. 1985. Morphological and morphometric studies of the human obstructed trabeculated urinary bladder. J. Urol. 57:525–529

Gilpin, S.A., Gilpin, C.J., Dixon, J.S., Gosling, J.A., Kirby, R.S. 1986. The effect of age on the autonomic innervation of the urinary bladder. Br. J. Urol. 58:378–381

Gosling, J.A., Dixon, J.S., Dunn, M. 1977. The structure of the rabbit urinary bladder after experimental distension. Invest. Urol. 14:386–389

Gosling, J.A., Dixon, J.S. 1980. Structure of trabeculated detrusor smooth muscle in cases of prostatic hypertrophy. Urol. Int. 35:351–355

Gosling, J.A., Gilpin, S.A., Dixon, J.S., Gilpin, C.J. 1986. Decrease in the autonomic innervation of human detrusor muscle in outflow obstruction. J. Urol. 136:501–503

Gu, J., Restorick, J.M., Blank, M.A., et al. 1983a. Vasoactive intestinal polypeptide in the normal and unstable bladder. Br. J. Urol. 55:645–647

Gu, J., Polak, J.M., Polak, P.L. 1983b. Peptidergic innvervation of the human genital tract. J. Urol. 130:386–391

Gu, J., Blank, M.A., Huang, W.M., et al. 1984. Peptide containing nerves in human urinary bladder. Urology 24:353–357

Guyon, F., Albarron, J. 1890. Anatomie et physiologie pathologiques de la retention d'urine. Arch. de Med. Exper. Anat. Pathol. 2:181–221

Harrison, S.C.W., Hunnam, G.R., Farman, P., Ferguson, D.R., Doyle, P.T. 1987. Bladder instability and denervation in patients with bladder outflow obstruction. Br. J. Urol. 60:519–522

Higson, R.H., Smith, J.C., Hills, W. 1979. Intravesical lignocaine and detrusor instability. Br. J. Urol. 51:500–503

Jancso, G., Kiraly, E., Jancso-Gabor, A. 1977. Pharmacologically induced selective degeneration of chemo-sensitive primary sensory neurons. Nature 270:741–742

Jorgensen, T.M., Djorhuus, J.C., Jorgensen, H.S., Sorensen, S.S. 1983. Experimental bladder hyperreflexia in pigs. Urol. Res. 11:239–240

Jungblat, T., Melchior, H., Aumueller, G., Malek, B. 1989. Age-dependency and regional distribution of enkephalinergic nerves in human prostate. J. Urol. 141:307A

Kato, K., Wein, A.J., Kitada, S., Haugaard, N., Levin, R.M. 1988. The functional effect of mild outlet obstruction in the rabbit urinary bladder. J. Urol. 140:880–884

Kinder, R.B., Mundy, A.R. 1985a. Inhibition of spontaneous contractile activity in isolated human detrusor muscle strips by vasoactive intestinal polypeptide. Br. J. Urol. 57:20–23

Kinder, R.B., Mundy, A.R. 1985b. Atropine blockade of nerve-mediated stimulation of the human detrusor. Br. J. Urol. 57:418–421

Kinder, R.B., Restorick, J.M., Mundy, A.R. 1985. Vasoactive intestinal polypeptide in the hyperreflexic neuropathic bladder. Br. J. Urol. 57:289–291

Kinder, R.B., Mundy, A.R. 1987. Pathophysiology of idiopathic detrusor instability and detrusor hyperreflexiain an in vitro study of human detrusor muscle. Br. J. Urol. 60:509–515

Kirby, R.S. 1987. MD Thesis, University of Cambridge

Kolta, M.G., Wallace, L.J., Gerald, M.C. 1984. Age-related changes in sensitivity of rabbit urinary bladder to autonomic agents. Mechanisms of ageing and development. 27:183–188

Lembeck, F. 1953. Zur Frage der zentralen Übertragung afferenter Impulse. III. Das Vorkommen und die Bedeutung der Substanz p in den dorsalen Wurzeln des Ruckenmarks. Naunyn Schmiedebergs Arch. Pharmakol. 219:197–213

Levin, R.M., Wein, A.J. 1981. Effect of vasoactive intestinal polypeptide on the contractility of the rabbit urinary bladder. Urol. Res. 9:217–218

Levin, R.M., High, J., Wein, A.J. 1984. The effect of short-term obstruction on urinary bladder function in the rabbit. J. Urol. 132:789–791

Levin, R.M., Malkowicz, S.B., Wein, A.J., Atta, M.A., Elbadawi, A. 1985. Recovery from short-term obstruction of the rat urinary bladder. J. Urol. 134:388–390

Levin, R.M., Memberg, W., Ruggieri, M.R., Wein, A.J. 1986. Functional effects of in vitro obstruction on the rabbit urinary bladder. J. Urol. 135:847–851

Malmgren, A., Sjogren, C., Uvelius, B., Mattiasson, A., Andersson, K.E., Andersson, P.O. 1987. Cystometrical evaluation of bladder instability in rats with infravesical outflow obstruction. J. Urol. 137:1291–1294

Malmgren, A., Uvelius, B., Andersson, K.E., Andersson, P.O. 1988. Disappearance of detrusor instability in rats after removal of infravesical outflow obstruction. Neurourol. Urodynamics 7:252–253

Malmgren, A. 1989. On the nature of bladder instability associated with outflow obstruction – an experimental study in the rat. Doctoral Dissertation, Lund University, pp 1–61

Mattiasson, A., Uvelius, B. 1982. Changes in contractile properties in hypertrophic rat urinary bladder. J. Urol. 128:1340–1342

Mattiasson, A., Andersson, K.E., Sjogren, C., Sundin, T., Uvelius, B. 1983. Supersensitivity to carbachol in the parasympathetically decentralised feline urinary bladder. Proc. 2nd. Int. Continence Soc., pp 77–79

Mayo, M.E., Hinman, F. 1976. Structure and function of the rabbit bladder altered by chronic obstruction or cystitis. Invest. Urol. 14:6–9

Melick, W.F., Naryka, J.J., Schmidt, J.H. 1978. Experimental studies of urethral peristaltic patterns of the pig. I. Similarity of pig and human ureter and bladder physiology. J. Urol. 85:145–148

Millar, J. 1958. The aetiology and treatment of diverticulum of the bladder. Br. J. Urol. 30:43–56

Nergardh, A., Kinn, A.C. 1983. Neurotransmission in activation of the contractile response in the human urinary bladder. Scand. J. Urol. Nephrol. 17:135–137

Nicoll, R.A., Schenker, C., Leeman, S.E. 1980. Substance P as a transmitter candidate. Am. Rev. Neuro. Sci. 3:227–268

Nilvebrant, L. 1986. On the muscarinic receptors in the urinary bladder and the putative subclassification of muscarinic receptors. Acta Pharmacol. Toxicol. 59 (suppl 1):1–45

Perlberg, S., Caine, M. 1982. Adrenergic response of bladder muscle in prostatic obstruction. Urology 20:524–527

Reuther, K., Aagaard, J., Sander Jensen, K. 1983. Lignocaine test and detrusor instability. Br. J. Urol. 55:493–494

Reuther, K., Aagaard, J. 1984. Alpha-adrenergic blockade in the diagnosis of detrusor instability secondary to intravesical obstruction. Urol. Int. 39:312–313

Rohner, T.J., Hannigan, J.D., Sanford, E.J. 1978. Altered in vitro adrenergic responses of dog detrusor muscle after chronic bladder outlet obstruction. Urology 11:357–361

Sehn, J.T. 1978. Anatomic effect of distension therapy in unstable bladder: new approach. Urology 11:581–587

Sehn, J.T. 1979. The ultrastructural effect of distension on the neuromuscular apparatus of the urinary bladder. Invest. Urol. 16:369–375

Sethia, K.K., Smith, J.C. 1987. The effect of pH and lignocaine on detrusor instability. Br. J. Urol. 60:516–518

Shigematsu, H. 1928. Etude experimentale de la retention d'urine. J. Urol. (Paris) 25:16–21

Sibley, G.N.A. 1984a. A comparison of spontaneous and nerve-mediated activity in bladder muscle from man, pig and rabbit. J. Physiol. (Lond) 354:431–443

Sibley, G.N.A. 1984b. The response of the bladder to lower urinary tract obstruction. DM Thesis, University of Oxford

Sibley, G.N.A. 1985. An experimental model of detrusor instability in the obstructed pig. Br. J. Urol. 57:292–298

Sibley, G.N.A. 1987. The physiological response of the detrusor muscle to experimental bladder outflow obstruction in the pig. Br. J. Urol. 60:332–336

Sjogren, C., Andersson, K.E., Husted, S., Mattiasson, A., Moller-Madsen, B. 1982. Atropine resistance of transmurally stimulated isolated human bladder muscle. J. Urol. 128:1368–1371

Speakman, M.J., Brading, A.F., Gilpin, C.J., Dixon, J.S., Gilpin, S.A., Gosling, J.A. 1987. Bladder outflow obstruction – a cause of denervation supersensitivity. J. Urol. 138:1461–1466

Speakman, M.J., Walmsley, D., Brading, A.F. 1988. An in vitro pharmacological study of the human trigone: a site of non-adrenergic, non-cholinergic neurotransmission. Br. J. Urol. 61:304–309

Steers, W.D., De Groat, W.C. 1988. Effect of bladder outlet obstruction on micturition reflex pathways in the rat. J. Urol. 140:864–871

Steers, W.D., Ciambotti, J.A., Etzel, B., Erdman, B., Erdman, S., De Groat, W.C. 1989. Morphological changes in afferent and efferent pathways to the urinary bladder following urethral obstruction in the rat. J. Urol. 141:323A

Sundin, T., Dahlstrom, A., Norlen, L., Svedmyr, N. 1977. The sympathetic innervation and adrenoceptor function of the human lower urinary tract in the normal state and after parasympathetic denervation. Invest. Urol. 14:328–332

Sundler, F., Brodin, E., Ekblad, E., Hakansson, R., Uddman, R. 1985. Sensory nerve fibres distribution of substance P, neurokinin A and calcitonin gene-related peptide. In: Tachykinin antagonists. Hakansson, R., Sundler, F., eds. Amsterdam, Elsevier, pp 3–14

Susset, J.G., Serlot-Viguier, D., Lamy, F., Madernas, P., Black, R. 1978. Collagen in 155 human bladders. Invest. Urol. 16:204–206

Trendelenburg, U. 1963. Supersensitivity and subsensitivity to sympathomimetic amines. Pharmacol. Rev. 18:629–640

Turner-Warwick, R.T. 1984. Bladder outflow obstruction in the male. In: Urodynamics: principles, practice and application. Mundy, A.R., Stephenson, T.P., Wein, A.J., eds. Churchill Livingstone, London, pp 183–204

Uvelius, B., Persson, L., Mattiasson, A. 1984. Smooth muscle cell hypertrophy and hyperplasia in the rat detrusor after short-term infravesical outflow obstruction. J. Urol. 131:173–176

Uvelius, B., Arner, A., Malmquist, U. 1988. Influence of hypoxia on metabolic rates and contraction in urinary bladder from rats with infravesical outflow obstruction. Neurourol. Urodynamics 7:245–246

Uvelius, B., Arner, A., Malmquist, U. 1989. Contractile and cytoskeletal proteins in detrusor muscle from obstructed rat and human bladder. Neurourol. Urodynamics 8:396–398

Westfall, D.P. 1981. In: Supersensitivity of smooth muscle: an assessment of current knowledge. Bulbring, E., Brading, A.F., Jones, A.W., Tomitat, T., eds. London, Edward Arnold

Chapter 5

Anatomy and Innervation of the Prostate Gland

C.R. Chapple

Introduction

Although its true function is unknown, it is likely that the human prostate gland plays a vital role in reproductive physiology. Persistent debate in the literature over both structure and terminology have limited our understanding of prostatic anatomy until recent years. Morgagni (1769) was amongst the first to recognise the predilection of prostatic disease for older men and both benign and malignant prostatic enlargement are important clinical problems from the sixth decade of life onwards.

Anatomy

The prostate gland has been forgotten and rediscovered a number of times during recorded medical history. The term prostate is attributed to Herophilus *c.* 300 BC (Galen) and was applied by him to the structures now called seminal vesicles. Accurate anatomical studies by Nicolo Massa of Padua (*c.* 1550) and Vesalius depicting the prostate gland first appeared in the sixteenth century (Shelley, 1969), but it was noticeably absent from the anatomical drawings of Leonardo da Vinci (O'Malley et al. 1952).

Lowsley (1912) was the first to publish a detailed description of the anatomy of the prostate; he described five prostatic lobes and this system of anatomical subdivision still remains in common use today. This work is based on a study of foetal prostates and it is therefore difficult to justify the extrapolation of such results to the interpretation of adult anatomy; for example, the anterior lobe described by Lowsley atrophies before birth. Franks (1954) modified Lowsley's formulation, introducing the concept of central and peripheral prostate with benign hyperplasia arising in the central zone and carcinomatous disease in the peripheral zone.

McNeal (1972) has carried out the most detailed study of prostatic anatomy to date. He documented anatomical heterogeneity within the prostate and expanded the concept of central and peripheral zones, to include a subdivision of the central zone encompassing periurethral glands, the transitional zone; which he suggested as the site of origin of benign prostatic hyperplasia (McNeal, 1978; see Fig. 5.1). He described a cylindrical sphincter of smooth muscle surrounding the urethra from the upper end of the verumontanum to the bladder neck, the pre-prostatic sphincter. Gosling et al. (1983) confirmed the presence of a circularly disposed smooth muscle collar around the pre-prostatic urethra which was continuous proximally with the bladder neck and merged distally with the capsule of the prostate gland and contributed a fibromuscular covering around the prostate gland.

Tisell and Salander (1975), in a study based on the dissection of gross specimens, reported cleavage planes which separated three regions with microscopically different appearances, which they named middle, lateral and posterior lobes. These lobes are different to those reported by Lowsley but can be equated with the work of McNeal, the middle lobe corresponding to the central zone and the posterior or lateral lobes to the peripheral zone (McNeal, 1980).

The prostatic urethra is continuous above with the pre-prostatic urethra and emerges from the prostate slightly anterior to the apex of the gland. Throughout most of its length there is a midline posterior ridge, the urethral crest, which is most prominent at its midpoint, the verumontanum which is situated at the proximal end of the distal urethral sphincter mechanism (Gosling et al. 1983). The prostatic urethra takes its name from the surrounding prostate gland which contains a prominent muscular component which is particularly marked in benign prostatic hyperplasia (Bartsch 1979). Slender, smooth muscle bundles occur in the proximal part of the urethral crest continuous above with the superficial trigone and below with the prostatic urethra where they merge with the muscle coat of ejaculatory ducts. Distally the prostatic urethra possesses a thin, smooth muscle coat comprising circular and longitudinal muscle and merging with the prostatic musculature, enhanced by an outer circular coat of striated muscle continuous with the distal sphincter mechanism (Gosling and Dixon, 1975; Benoit et al. 1988).

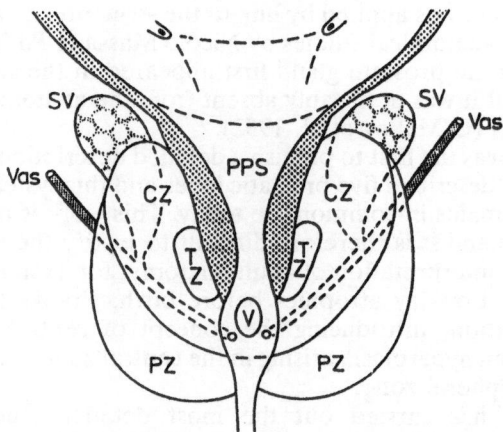

Fig. 5.1. Schematic diagram of adult prostate showing peripheral zone (PZ), central zone (CZ) and transitional zone (TZ) at apex of pre-prostatic sphincter (PPS). Seminal vesicles (SV) and vasa deferentia fuse to form ejaculatory ducts to open alongside verumontanum (V).

Obstruction arising in association with benign prostatic hyperplasia is an important clinical problem, which has been traditionally attributed solely to the mechanical effect of prostatic enlargement. Recent work has suggested that nearly 50% of prostatic outflow obstruction is mediated via neural pathways acting on the smooth muscle of bladder neck, pre-prostatic and prostatic smooth muscle (Furuya et al. 1982). This has renewed interest in a therapeutic role for α-adrenoceptor blockade in the treatment of benign prostatic hyperplasia, a subject which is considered in some detail in Chapter 12.

Innervation

Early investigations dealt almost exclusively with the extrinsic innervation of the gland (Langley and Anderson, 1894, 1895a–c, 1896). Later studies turned to the intrinsic innervation of the prostate and numerous authors sought to describe the various nerve types within the prostate (Casas, 1958), but were limited by lack of suitable staining techniques. It was widely held that some of these nerves were sensory (Seto, 1954), whilst others were motor to blood vessels and stroma (Mori, 1955). The advent of histochemical techniques for the demonstration of catecholamines (Corrodi and Jonsson, 1967) and acetylcholinesterases (Koelle, 1951; Gomori, 1952), made possible the localisation of these nerve types and subsequent work in the last two decades has introduced a separate group of non-adrenergic, non-cholinergic sensorimotor nerves. It is now recognised that the human prostate gland is innervated by short adrenergic sympathetic nerves whose cell bodies lie in the pelvic plexuses (Baumgarten et al. 1968), cholinergic parasympathetic nerves (Duzendorfer et al. 1976) and peptidergic sensorimotor nerves (Larsson et al. 1977; Alm et al. 1977; Gu et al. 1983).

Despite the clinical importance of the prostate gland, few comprehensive studies of the innervation and ultrastructure of the human prostate and associated prostatic urethra have been reported. It is of interest that the human prostate gland receives a considerably less dense innervation than most laboratory animals (Baumgarten et al. 1968; Shirai et al. 1973). This highlights the importance of exercising caution in extrapolating results from animal studies to man.

It has been suggested that although microscopically there is dual innervation to all parts of the prostate: the glandular acini are principally supplied with secretomotor cholinergic parasympathetic nerves and the predominant motor control of prostatic muscle is via sympathetic adrenergic neurons (Gosling, 1983). This suggestion has however been challenged by Vaalasti and Hervonen (1980a), who dispute that there is a significant sympathetic or parasympathetic nerve supply to acinar epithelium. As mentioned above there is a third group of nerves containing putative peptide neurotransmitters. These have been reported to innervate the prostate both in man (Gu et al. 1983; Crowe et al. 1991) and the cat (Alm et al. 1980).

In a recent study a detailed characterisation of the neural innervation of the human prostate has been carried out (Crowe et al. 1991). The distribution and density of nerve fibres found in the prostate gland are summarised in Table 5.1. In all regions of the prostate studied, the nerve fibres were found around alveoli and within the stroma in association with the smooth muscle. The greatest density of nerves was AChE-positive followed (in decreasing order) by nerves immunoreactive to NPY; VIP and DBH; l-Enk and 5-HT; CGRP; m-Enk; SP; and somatostatin. NPY-, VIP- and DBH-immunoreactive nerves were also observed on the adventitial/medial border of blood vessels. The overall neural density of AChE-positive nerves was very variable from one patient to another and could vary quite markedly within the tissue from an individual; therefore, a number of representative fields (minimum 10), were examined for each patient (Fig. 5.2). Similar results were obtained using both the quantitative and semi-quantitative techniques to assess AChE staining. AChE-positive nerves were thicker and exhibited a tendency to form nerve bundles within the prostatic stroma, with finer ramifications passing between acini. Although the density of AChE-stained and VIP- and NPY-immunoreactive nerves remained similar in each region studied, that of the other nerve types varied in the different areas of the prostate studied (see Table 5.1).

The complete absence of any physiological or pharmacological data on the action of the neuropeptides and 5-HT within the human prostate means that their precise role is a matter for speculation at present. Nevertheless, the number and widespread distribution of these putative neurotransmitters within prostatic nerves and the presence of numerous intramural ganglia suggests that these substances play an important functional role within the prostate gland. The precise role of these nerves is obscure at present although, based on other observations, it is likely that they have an important role in controlling vascular tone. In addition, they may be important in neuromodulation, since VIP and NPY are known to coexist with classical transmitters within cholinergic and adrenergic nerves respectively.

The motor control of the pre-prostatic and prostatic urethra appears to be similar to that of the adjacent prostate and is mediated predominantly via the sympathetic nervous system (Andersson et al. 1983). It is, however, difficult to equate this observation with ultrastructural studies. These demonstrate that the human urethra receives a sparse supply of adrenergic nerves, a rich

Table 5.1. Distribution of immunoreactive nerves within the human prostate contrasting the anterior capsule, peripheral zone and distal and proximal central zones

Prostatic area	VIP	SP	Som	m-Enk	NPY	CGRP	5-HT	DBH	l-Enk
Anterior capsule	+++	+	+/−	+	+++++	++ NB	−	++++	+++
Peripheral zone	+++	+	−	−	+++++	++ NB	++++	+	−
Distal central zone	+++	+/−	+/−	+	+++++	+	+	+++	++
Proximal central zone	++++	++ NB	−	+++	+++++	+++	+++	+++++	+++

+, sparse; ++, sparse/moderate; +++, moderate; ++++, moderate/dense; +++++, dense; NB, nerve bundle.

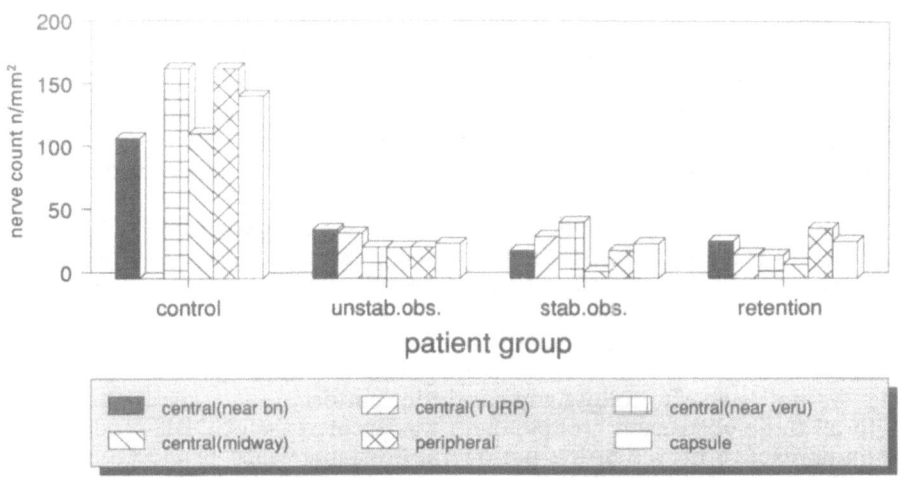

Fig. 5.2. Results of quantitative assessment of acetylcholinesterase staining expressed as nerves/mm² in human prostate from control, unstable obstruction, stable obstruction and acute retention patients.

supply of AChE-positive neurons (Ek et al. 1977) and also contains peptides such as VIP (Alm et al. 1980) and NPY. The adrenergic nerve supply and presumably other nerves enter the prostate alongside the ejaculatory ducts and then ramify superiorly towards the bladder neck and inferiorly to innervate the infra-montanal prostatic urethra (Benoit et al. 1988).

Autonomic ganglia staining for AChE (Gosling, 1983; Kluck, 1980) and noradrenaline (Gosling and Thompson, 1977) have been described in the prostatic capsule, and AChE-positive ganglia have been described within the prostatic stroma (Dunzendorfer et al. 1976). In a detailed study of the ganglia within the human prostate, the nerve fibres and cell bodies contained DBH, AChE and all of the peptides studied except somatostatin and SP. 5-HT immunoreactivity was observed to be associated with the neuroendocrine cells of the prostatic glandular epithelial layer. These cells are characterised by dendritic processes that extend between the epithelial cells (Di Sant' Agnese and De Mesy Jensen, 1984; Di Sant' Agnese et al. 1985) (Fig. 5.2).

Two studies have reported that there is a reduced cholinergic and adrenergic innervation of adenomatous as contrasted to normal prostate (Dunzendorfer et al. 1976; Vaalasti and Hervonen 1980a). This could result from either a dilution of neural structures by the marked increase in muscular and to a lesser extent glandular components within the hyperplastic gland (Bartsch et al. 1979), or could represent a true reduction in innervation. Further support for this suggestion is provided by in vitro isometric studies which have demonstrated an exaggerated response to adrenergic agonists of hyperplastic as compared to normal prostatic tissue, suggestive of a post-junctional supersensitivity (Kitada and Kumazawa 1987). This supersensitivity may contribute to the clinical picture of prostate obstruction.

We have recently investigated the distribution and density of classical and putative neurotransmitters within the human prostate gland and correlated this with regional prostatic heterogeneity and the clinical and urodynamic features of prostatic obstruction. The overall distribution of nerve fibres and nerve cell bodies containing AChE, DBH, 5-HT and the peptides VIP, m-Enk, l-Enk, NPY, SP and CGRP in the prostatic regions from patients with bladder outlet obstruction were similar to those in control patients. There was, however, a reduction in the density of these nerves in the obstructed bladder (Figs 5.2–5.7).

The quantitative assessment demonstrated this very clearly for AChE-positive nerves (Fig. 5.2). Statistical analysis suggested that these data were not normally distributed, therefore non-parametric analysis was carried out using a two-tailed Mann-Whitney U test. All of the obstructed groups showed a significant reduction in the density of nerves within the prostate as compared with controls ($p < 0.0001$). There was significant intraprostatic variation, but this did not appear to follow any consistent pattern.

In all three obstructed groups, there was an increase of DBH- and l-Enk-immunoreactive nerves in the peripheral prostate, whilst in the group with acute urinary retention there was also an increase of VIP- and CGRP-immunoreactive nerves in this region. Most other prostatic regions from patients in all three obstructed groups showed a decrease in nerve density when compared with control patients. There were, however, the following exceptions:

1. In the stable obstructed patients, the densities of VIP-immunoreactive nerves in the anterior capsule and peripheral prostate, SP-immunoreactive nerves in the peripheral prostate and proximal central prostate and CGRP-immunoreactive nerves in the anterior capsule were the same as in the control group.

2. In the unstable obstructed group, the densities of VIP- and NPY-immunoreactive nerves in the anterior capsule, and CGRP-immunoreactive nerves in the proximal central prostate were the same as in the controls.

3. In the acute retention group, the densities of SP- and NPY-immunoreactive nerves in the peripheral prostate and NPY-immunoreactive nerves in the distal central prostate remained the same as in the controls.

The mechanism underlying this increase in density may be either an increase in the synthesis of DBH and neuropeptides or a reduction in axonal transport and release. "Blind" quantitative assessment of prostatic tissue using a point-counting technique revealed similar mean proportions of muscular and glandular tissue in both control prostate and that obtained from patients undergoing surgery for benign prostatic hyperplasia. Although tissue hyperplasia would tend to favour a reduction in nerve density and would explain the patchy variation in the neural distribution, the quantitative technique used minimised errors by a process of averaging. It therefore seems likely that the reduction in neural density was not solely a consequence of prostatic hyperplasia. We found no evidence of the abnormal, thin, coiled AChE-positive nerves described previously in the hyperplastic gland (Baumgarten et al. 1968).

Similar controversy surrounds the subject of urethral innervation, with little available information as to the functional importance of cholinergic and neuropeptide-containing neurons. Investigations both in vivo and in

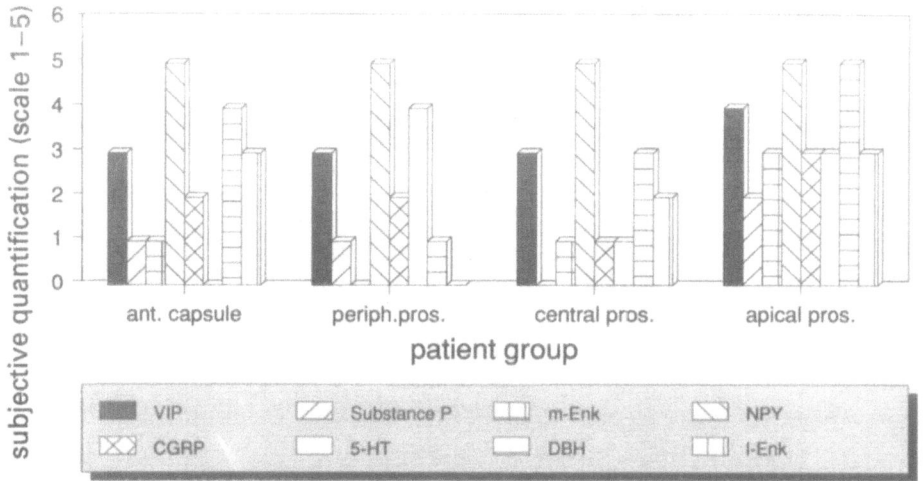

Fig. 5.3. Results of subjective quantification assessed on an arbitrary scale of 1–5 for nerves immunoreactive to DBH, 5-HT and the putative neuropeptides VIP, SP, m-Enk, l-Enk, NPY and CGRP, in "normal" control prostate. A number of areas of the prostate were studied, namely, anterior capsule (ant. capsule), peripheral zone (periph.pros.), central (midway between bladder neck and apex of prostate (central pros.)) and distal (apical prostate) central zone.

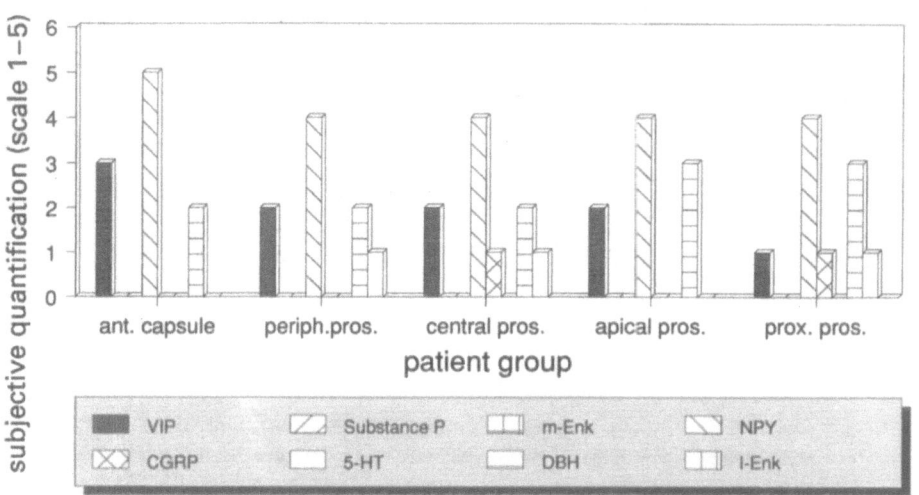

Fig. 5.4. Results of subjective quantification assessed on an arbitrary scale of 1–5 for nerves immunoreactive to DBH, 5-HT and the putative neuropeptides VIP, SP, m-Enk, l-Enk, NPY and CGRP, in prostate from patients presenting with acute retention. A number of areas of the prostate were studied: anterior capsule (ant. capsule), peripheral zone (periph.pros.), central zone (proximal pros.), distal (apical pros.) and sampled from a point midway between these two sites (central pros.).

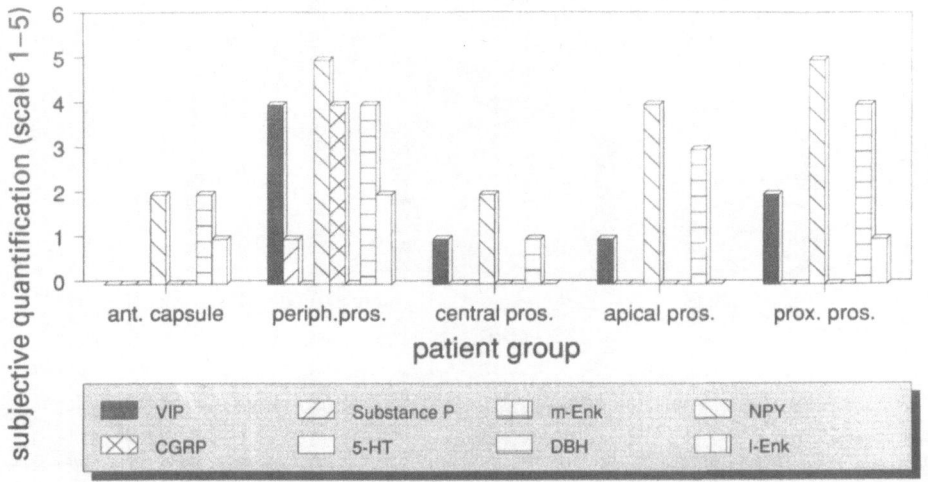

Fig. 5.5. Results of subjective quantification assessed on an arbitrary scale of 1–5 for nerves immunoreactive to DBH, 5-HT and the putative neuropeptides VIP, SP, m-Enk, l-Enk, NPY and CGRP, in prostate from patients presenting with unstable prostatic obstruction. A number of areas of the prostate were studied: anterior capsule (ant. capsule), peripheral zone (periph. pros.) and central zone – proximal (prox. pros.), distal (apical pros.) and sampled from a point midway between these two sites (central pros.).

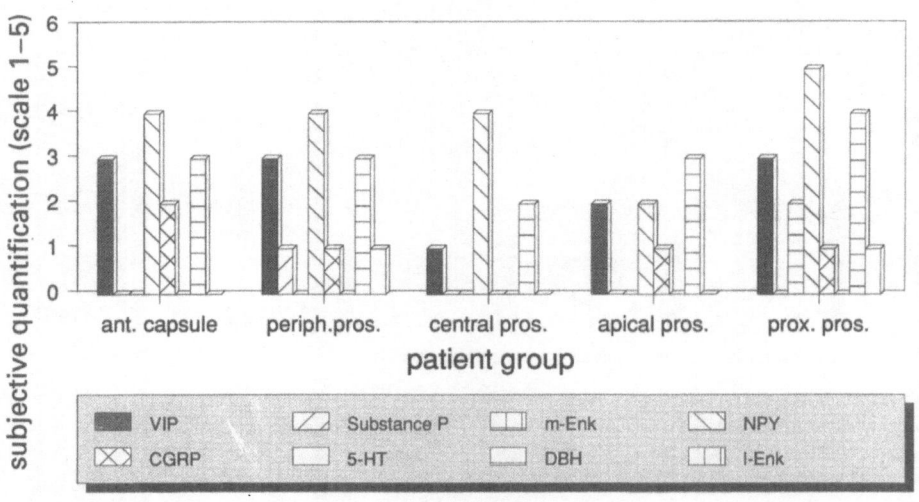

Fig. 5.6. Results of subjective quantification assessed on an arbitrary scale of 1–5 for nerves immunoreactive to DBH, 5-HT and the putative neuropeptides VIP, SP, m-Enk, l-Enk, NPY and CGRP, in prostate from patients presenting with stable prostatic obstruction. A number of areas of the prostate were studied: anterior capsule (ant. capsule), peripheral zone (periph.pros.), and central zone – proximal (prox. pros.), distal (apical pros.) and sampled from a point midway between these two sites (central pros.).

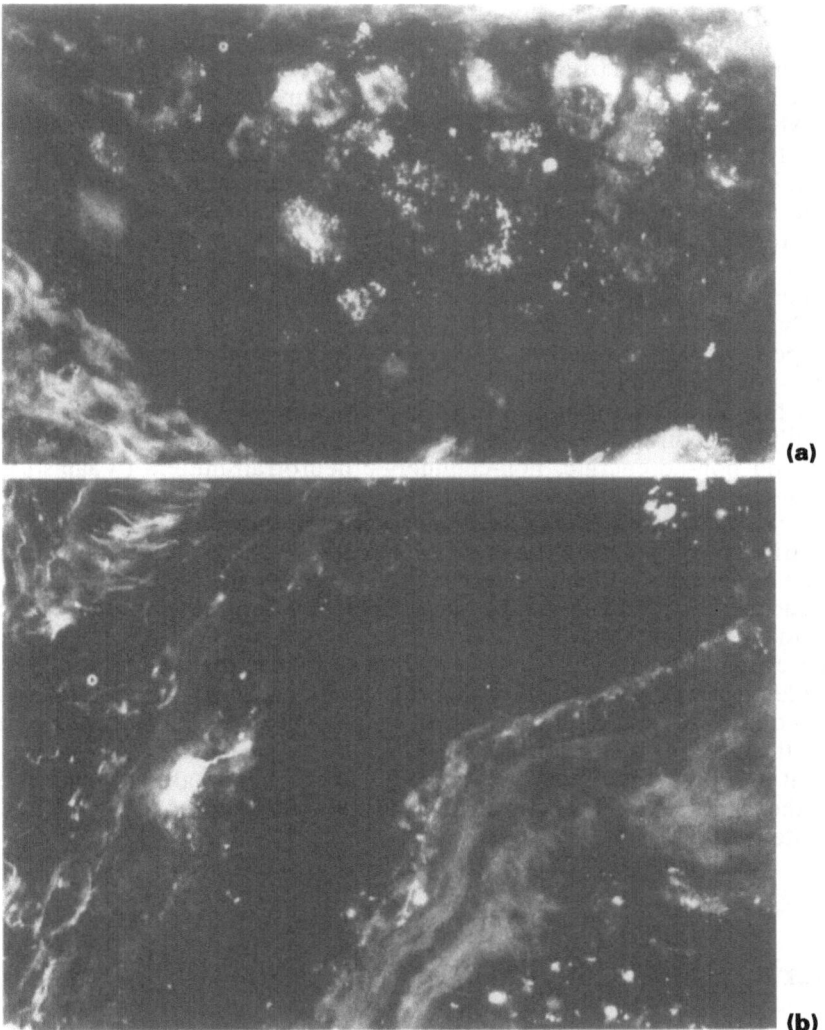

Fig. 5.7. 5-HT-immunoreactivity in sections of human prostate gland. **a** A ganglion containing 5-HT-immunoreactive nerve cell bodies is seen in the distal central prostate. **b** A 5-HT-immunoreactive prostatic paracrine-endocrine cell, located in tissue adjacent to a glandular acinus; note the dendritic process passing towards the acinar epithelium.

vitro have suggested that the smooth muscle of the human urethra contains both adrenoceptors and muscarinic receptors (Andersson and Sjogren, 1982). Whilst adrenergic stimulation has been demonstrated to produce a contractile response, neither muscarinic receptor agonists nor antagonists have any significant effect on intra-urethral pressure (Ek et al. 1978).

Some evidence has accumulated to support NANC neurotransmission in the control of urethral function. Andersson et al. (1983) reported that electrically induced TTX-sensitive relaxant responses both in human inframontanal urethra precontracted with noradrenaline and in corresponding rabbit experiments supported a NANC sensorimotor mechanism of action. Further experiments reported by Mattiasson et al. (1985) demonstrated an electrically induced contraction in both rabbit and human urethra which was suggestive of NANC neurotransmission, but which could not be blocked in all cases with TTX. Non-adrenergic, non-cholinergic neurotransmitters may be contained within interneurons between the cholinergic and adrenergic systems, playing a role as neuromodulators, functioning as co-transmitters, or producing a local trophic effect.

It is likely that there is a functional interaction between cholinergic and adrenergic nerves in the prostate, urethra and bladder neck (Nergardh, 1975; Mutoh et al. 1987; Ek et al. 1977) and the other populations of neural subtypes. Previous workers have identified adrenergic terminals related to AChE-positive ganglia within the prostatic capsule (Kluck, 1980) and have noted the close juxtaposition of nerve fibres which on electron microscopy have ultrastructural appearances suggestive of the presence of noradrenaline, ACh and non-adrenergic, non-cholinergic neurotransmitters (Vaalasti and Hervonen, 1980a,b; Vaalasti et al. 1980, 1986). Mattiasson et al. (1984) in a study conducted on the isolated human urethra showed that stimulation of muscarinic receptors caused a significant decrease of the electrically induced release of ^3H noradrenaline, suggesting that activity in cholinergic parasympathetic nerves could influence sympathetically controlled noradrenaline-dependent urethral tone.

It is evident from this brief review that there are a number of questions as to the role of the adrenergic and cholinergic and in particular the NANC innervation of the prostate/urethral complex which at present remain unanswered. Until the role of the various neural components in the innervation of the normal prostate is clarified, it is unlikely that we will be able to understand fully the significance of this reduction in the innervation of the hyperplastic prostate gland.

References

Alm, P., Alumets, J., Hakanson, R., Sundler, F. 1977. Peptidergic (vasoactive intestinal polypeptide) nerves in the genitourinary tract. Neuroscience 2:751–754

Alm, P., Alumets, J., Hakanson, R., et al. 1980. Origin and distribution of vasoactive intestinal polypeptide (VIP) nerves in the genito-urinary tract. Cell Tissue Res. 205:337–347

Andersson, K.E., Sjogren, C. 1982. Aspects on the physiology and pharmacology of the bladder and urethra. Progr. Neurobiol. 19:71–89

Andersson, K.E., Mattiasson, A., Sjogren, C. 1983. Electrically induced relaxation of the noradrenaline contracted isolated urethra from rabbit and man. J. Urol. 129:210–213

Bartsch, G., Muller, H.R., Oberholzer, M., Rohr, H.P. 1979. Light microscopic stereological analysis of the normal human prostate and of benign prostatic hyperplasia. J. Urol. 122:487–491

Baumgarten, H.G., Falck, B., Holstein, A.F., Owman, C.H., Owman, T. 1968. Adrenergic innervation of the human testis epididymis ductus deferens and prostate. A fluorescence microscopic and fluorimetric study. Z. Zellforsch. 90:81–95

Benoit, G., Quillard, J., Jardin, A. 1988. Anatomical study of the inframontanal urethra in man. J. Urol. 139:866–868

Casas, A.P. 1958. Die Innervation der menschlichen Vorsteherdruse. Z. Mikrosk. Anat. Forsch. 64:608–633

Corrodi, H., Jonsson, G. 1967. The formaldehyde fluorescence method for the histochemical demonstration of biogenic amines. A review on the methodology. J. Histochem. Cytochem. 15:65–78

Crowe, R., Chapple, C.R., Burnstock, G. 1991. The human prostate gland: a histochemical and immunohistochemical study of neuropeptides, serotonin, dopamine β-hydroxylase and acetylcholinesterase in autonomic nerves and ganglia. Br. J. Urol. 68:53–61

Di Sant'Agnese, P.A., De Mesy Jensen, K.L. 1984. Endocrine-paracrine cells of the prostate and prostatic urethra. Hum. Pathol. 15:1034–1041

Di Sant'Agnese, P.A., De Mesy Jensen, K.L., Churukian, C.J., Agarwal, M.M. 1985. Human prostatic endocrine-paracrine (APUD) cells. Arch. Pathol. 109:607–612

Dunzendorfer, U., Jonas, D., Weber, W. 1976. The autonomic innervation of the human prostate. Histochemistry of acetylcholinesterase in the normal and pathologic states. Urol. Res. 4:29–31

Ek, A., Alm, P., Andersson, K.E., Persson, C.G.A. 1977. Adrenergic and cholinergic nerves of the human urethra and urinary bladder. A histochemical study. Acta Physiol. Scand. 99:345–352

Ek, A., Andersson, K.E., Ulmsten, U. 1978. The effects of norephedrine and bethanecol on the human urethral closure pressure profile. Scand. J. Urol. Nephrol. 12:97–104

Franks, L.M. 1954. Benign nodular hyperplasia of the prostate: a review. Ann. R. Coll. Surg. Engl. 14:92–106

Furuya, S., Kumamoto, Y., Yokoyama, E. et al. Alpha-adrenergic activity and urethral pressure profilometry in prostatic zone in benign prostatic hypertrophy. J. Urol. 128:835–839

Gomori, G. 1952. Microscopy histochemistry: principles and practice. Chicago, University of Chicago Press, pp 208–214

Gosling, J.A., Dixon, J.S. 1975. Structure and innervation of smooth muscle in the wall of the bladder neck and proximal urethra. J. Urol. 47:549–558

Gosling, J.A., Thompson, S.A. 1977. A neurohistochemical and histological of peripheral autonomic neurones of the human bladder neck and prostate. Urol. Int. 32:269–276

Gosling, J.A. 1983. Autonomic innervation of the prostate. In: Benign prostatic hypertrophy. Hinman, F.,Jr., ed. Berlin, Heidelberg, New York, Springer, pp 349–360

Gosling, J.A., Dixon, J.S., Humpherson, J.R. 1983. Functional anatomy of the urinary tract. Edinburgh, Churchill Livingstone.

Gu, J., Polak, J.M., Polak, P.L. 1983. Peptidergic innvervation of the human genital tract. J. Urol. 130:386–391

Kitada, S., Kumazawa, J. 1987. Pharmacological characteristics of smooth muscle in benign prostatic hyperplasia and normal prostatic tissue. J. Urol. 138:158–160

Kluck, P. 1980. The autonomic innervation of the human urinary bladder, bladder neck and urethra: a histochemical study. Anat. Rec. 198:439–447

Koelle, G.B. 1951. The elimination of enzymatic diffusion artefacts in the histochemical localisation of cholinesterases and a survey of cellular distributions. J. Pharmacol. Exp. Ther. 103:153–171

Langley, J.N., Anderson, H.K. 1894. The constituents of the hypogastric nerves. J. Physiol. (Lond) 17:177–191

Langley, J.N., Anderson, H.K. 1895a. The innervation of the pelvic and adjoining viscera. Part 2. The bladder. J. Physiol. (Lond) 19:85–139

Langley, J.N., Anderson, H.K. 1895b. The innervation of the pelvic and adjoining viscera. Part 1. J. Physiol. (Lond) 19:71–84

Langley, J.N., Anderson, H.K. 1895c. The innervation of the pelvic and adjoining viscera. Part 4. The internal generative organs. Part 5. Position of the nerve cells on the course of the efferent nerve fibres. J. Physiol. (Lond) 18:122–139

Langley, J.N., Anderson, H.K. 1896. The innervation of the pelvic and adjoining viscera. Part 6. Anatomical observations. J. Physiol. (Lond) 20:372–406

Larsson, L.I., Fahrenkrug, J., Schaffalitzkyde de Muckadell, O.B. 1977. Occurrence of nerves containing VIP-immunoreactivity in the male genital tract. Life Sci. 21:503–508

Lowsley, O.S. 1912. The development of the human prostate gland with reference to the development of other structures at the neck of the urinary bladder. Am. J. Anat. 13:299–349

Mattiasson, A., Andersson, K.E., Sjogren, C. 1984. Adrenoceptors and cholinoceptors controlling noradrenaline release from adrenergic nerves in the urethra of rabbit and man. J. Urol. 131:1190–1195

Mattiasson, A., Andersson, K.E., Sjogren, C. 1985. Adrenergic and non-adrenergic contraction of isolated urethral muscle from rabbit and man. J. Urol. 133:298–303
McNeal, J.E. 1972. The prostate and prostatic urethra: a morphological synthesis. J. Urol. 107:1008–1016
McNeal, J.E. 1978. Origin and evolution of benign prostatic enlargement. Invest. Urol. 15:340–345
McNeal, J.E. 1980. Anatomy of the prostate; an historical survey of divergent views. Prostate 1:3–13
Morgagni, G. 1769. The seats and causes of disease. In: Investigated by Anatomy. Book 3. Miller, A., Cadell, T., eds. London, Johnson & Payne, pp 46–462
Mori, J. 1955. Histology and innervation of prostate and pars pelocina urethrae in cat. Arch. Hist. Jpn. 8:227–241
Mutoh, S., Ueda, S., Fukumoto, Y., Machida, J., Ikegami, K. 1987. Effect of adrenergic and cholinergic drugs on the noradrenergic transmission in bladder neck smooth muscle. J. Urol. 138:212–215
Nergardh, A. 1975. Autonomic receptor functions in the lower urinary tract: a survey of recent experimental results. J. Urol. 113:180–185
O'Malley, C.D., Saunders, J.B., De, C.M. 1952. Leonardo da Vinci on the human body (genitourinary system).
Seto, H. 1954. Histological studies on the sensory terminations distributed in the circulatory system and the urogenital organs. Arch. Hist. Jpn. 6:665–678
Shelley, H.S. 1969. The enlarged prostate, a brief history of its treatment. J. Hist. Med. 20:452–473
Shirai, M., Sasaki, K., Rikimaru, A. 1973. A histochemical investigation of the distribution of adrenergic and cholinergic nerves in the human male genital organs. Tohoku J. Exp. Med. 111:281–291
Tisell, L.E., Salander, H. 1975. The lobes of the human prostate. Scand. J. Urol. Nephrol. 9:185–191
Vaalasti, A., Hervonen, A. 1980a. Autonomic innervation of the human prostate. Invest. Urol. 17:293–297
Vaalasti, A., Hervonen, A. 1980b. Nerve endings in the human prostate. Am. J. Anat. 157:41–47
Vaalasti, A., Linnoila, I., Hervonen, A. 1980. Immunohistochemical demonstration of VIP and enkephalin immunoreactive nerve fibres in the human prostate and seminal vesicles. Histochemistry 66:89–98
Vaalasti, A., Tainioh, H., Pelto-Huikko, M., Hervonen, A. 1986. Light and electron microscope demonstration of VIP- and enkephalin-immunoreactive nerves in the human male genitourinary tract. Anat. Rec. 215:21–27

Section B
Contemporary Management of Bladder Outflow Obstruction

Chapter 6

Bladder Outflow Obstruction in the Male

R. Turner-Warwick

Introduction

It is important to analyse carefully the symptoms associated with bladder outflow obstruction:

1. The basic effect of partial restriction of the outflow of the bladder, irrespective of its cause, is simply its effect on the voiding flow – a slow start, a poor intermittent stream and terminal dribble – no more.

2. The symptoms of frequency, urgency and nocturia are not directly created by outflow obstruction except in the occasional case of a large residual urine associated with borderline retention; they sometimes result from hypersensitive conditions such as urine infection or vesical calculi but, very much more commonly, they are the result of unstable detrusor contractions which create an erroneous premature sensation of bladder fullness. However, unstable detrusor dysfunction is not unusual in many who void efficiently so these symptoms should not, on their own, be regarded as indicative of outflow obstruction (Turner-Warwick et al. 1973a).

Detrusor Function and Dysfunction

Normal Bladder Function

The bladder detrusor is unique: it is the only autonomically innervated smooth muscle that is under complete voluntary control; we do not yet understand the mechanism of this. A normally functioning detrusor contracts during voluntary voiding and at no other time; this controlled behaviour is conveniently referred to as "stable"; however, by definition, it cannot be designated as stable without objective urodynamic proof.

Instability and Myth of "Prostatism"

About 10%–15% of normal males and females never achieve full inhibitory control over their sacrovesical reflex mechanisms so that their bladders develop involuntary "unstable" contractions between voiding; these contractions increase the intravesical pressure long before the bladder is fully distended and they usually cause a premature sensation of bladder fullness, hence the symptoms of frequency, urgency and nocturia. The natural incidence of idiopathic unstable detrusor behaviour seems to increase with age, in the absence of obstruction, to about 20% in the eighth and ninth decade in both males and females (Turner-Warwick et al. 1973a); the apparent increase in males is higher because of the additional age related increase in outflow obstruction (vide infra).

Detrusor Response to Obstruction

In men, detrusors that were previously stable often develop unstable behaviour in association with bladder outflow obstruction so that, in addition to flow-restriction symptoms of the slow start, poor stream and terminal dribble, 75%–80% of men with prostatic obstruction also have secondary detrusor symptoms of frequency, urgency and nocturia. This secondary symptom complex is widely referred to as prostatism but this is entirely erroneous and often misleading in concept because:

1. the same symptoms commonly arise from unstable detrusor behaviour in the absence of obstruction;
2. the obstruction may be the result of a dyssynergic bladder neck mechanism or a distal stricture not the prostate; and
3. the symptoms are not referred to as prostatism when they occur in females.

These observations emphasise the importance of proving objectively whether a patient with prostatic enlargement and symptoms of frequency, urgency and nocturia resulting from unstable detrusor behaviour does or does not have bladder outflow obstruction before advising a prostatectomy (Turner-Warwick et al. 1973a).

In the male the detrusor muscle reacts to outflow obstruction in a variety of ways – not all detrusors are equal (Turner-Warwick et al. 1973a). Some respond by developing an increased contraction pressure to "compensate" for an increased outflow resistance, and others do not.

In some the voiding detrusor contraction is normally sustained so that the bladder empties completely; in others it fades before the bladder is empty, leaving a residual urine. This prematurely fading contraction should be accurately described as an "unsustained" voiding contraction; it should not be described as a "decompensated bladder" because such a conceptual term is based on the supposition that an unsustained contraction is the result of failure of the bladder to compensate for obstruction and, although sometimes this may be true, it is often inaccurate because an unsustained detrusor contraction is also a characteristic of one of many types of unobstructed neuropathic detrusor dysfunction. This emphasises the importance of describing all urodynamic findings accurately and objectively without prejudgement or conceptualisation.

Occasionally an outflow obstruction evokes little or no detectable detrusor response: the bladder gradually becomes over-distended and progressively fails to empty. This retention is of course an entirely different situation from that of a bladder that has been achieving a reasonable voiding balance by compensating for a significant outlet obstruction but which is precipitated into retention by a single episode of over-distension because overstretched muscle fibres cannot generate their maximum contraction force; however, both may create the important warning symptom of increased difficulty in voiding when the bladder is overfull.

Response of Unstable Detrusor Symptoms to the Relief of Obstruction

About 80% of men with prostatic obstruction have secondary symptoms of frequency, urgency and nocturia resulting from unstable detrusor behaviour. The effective relief of a proven outflow obstruction leads to reversion of unstable muscle behaviour to stable in about three quarters of these; in the remaining quarter, the unstable behaviour persists (Turner-Warwick, 1979). Such an incidence of persistent unstable behaviour approximates to the natural incidence in this age group and it would be unreasonable to expect that it would be less.

It should be explained to every patient presenting with proven outflow obstruction and symptoms of instability that although surgery should certainly resolve the obstruction, the chances that the relief of this obstruction will result in resolution of their detrusor instability symptoms is only about 70%. This is a most important pre-operative communication because otherwise a patient who presented with symptoms of detrusor instability will return saying that he "had the prostate operation but it failed"; he will not be satisfied with the restoration of his competitive voiding stream if he had been allowed to expect that his more troublesome symptoms would be resolved. Fortunately when instability persists after the relief of a proven obstruction the symptoms are usually less severe.

It is also important to appreciate that unstable detrusor behaviour is occasionally asymptomatic. Routine pre-operative urodynamic evaluation shows that a proportion of male patients presenting with proven outflow obstruction and simple flow reduction symptoms of slow flow, poor stream and terminal dribble have asymptomatic involuntary unstable detrusor behaviour (Fig. 6.1) (Turner-Warwick, 1979). After a prostatic resection, sensitivity sometimes seems to increase so that if detrusor instability persists, the patient may subsequently become aware of his involuntary contractions for the first time and develop the appropriate symptoms; if such a patient is investigated by cystometry for the first time post-operatively it should not be assumed that his bladder has become unstable as a result of the operation; in fact this is rare (Turner-Warwick, 1979).

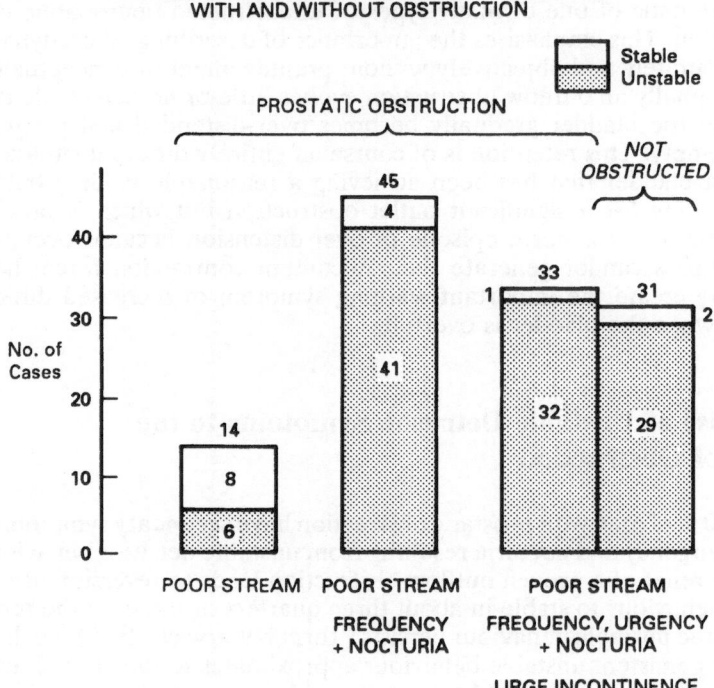

Fig. 6.1. The close relationship between symptoms and unstable detrusor behaviour: the poor relationship between symptoms and the incidence of obstruction (Turner-Warwick et al. 1973a).

The Cause of Unstable Detrusor Behaviour in Male Bladder Outflow Obstruction

Stable detrusor function is fundamentally dependent upon positive, inhibitory control of the sacrovesical reflex mechanism. However, although stability must be neurologically mediated, it is not clinically helpful to conceive unstable detrusor dysfunction as essentially neuropathic; furthermore, neuropathy may result in a variety of detrusor dysfunctions and it is irrational to use the term "neurogenic bladder" to indicate a particular dysfunction such as instability (Thomas, 1979).

For clinical purposes unstable detrusor behaviour is best regarded as idiopathic, neuropathic or obstructive in origin but it is not possible to distinguish between these on the basis of detrusor response measurements. Thus if a patient with proven bladder outflow obstruction has a mild neuropathy one cannot determine pre-operatively whether there is a chance that relief of the obstructive element could result in reversion of an unstable detrusor dysfunction to stability. We do not know exactly why bladder outflow obstruction in the male is associated with such a high incidence of detrusor instability; the common factor in most cases seems to be a high resistance outflow obstruction, but why an obstruction during the voiding phase should cause an abnormality of detrusor function during the storage phase is not clear. However, obstruction instability is unique in that it is the only type of unstable detrusor behaviour that can often be reverted to stability by a local operative procedure; this is clear proof that some local factors are involved and it should further dissuade us from assuming that the only significant aetiological factor is impairment of central control.

It has been suggested that an increase in afferent impulses, possibly due to "tension arising in the prostatic capsule" may play an important role in the development of instability. However, in general, hypersensitive conditions such as cystitis, interstitial cystitis and prostatitis, associated with a massive increase in afferent neuron activity, do not result in a significant increase in the natural incidence of instability.

There is a close correlation between the effective relief of bladder outflow obstruction and reversion to stability, irrespective of the actual operative procedure that is used: thus the removal of a large proportion of the bulk of a prostatic enlargement may not be sufficient if a small remnant of apical tissue causes persistent outlet obstruction. On the other hand, the reversion rate after the simple selective endoscopic incision of a dyssynergic bladder neck obstruction in the absence of any prostatic enlargement is comparable with that resulting from the effective resection of a large obstructive prostate. Furthermore, although the incidence of instability resulting from obstruction due to an anterior urethral stricture is, in fact, somewhat less than that due to a posterior urethral obstruction, it approximates to the natural incidence after the relief of obstruction (Turner-Warwick, 1979).

It might be reasonable to suppose that the likelihood of reversion to stability might diminish in patients who had had bladder outlet obstruction for a long time but Arnold (1980) found no evidence to support this. Similarly he found little correlation between the severity of an obstruction, the incidence of instability and the incidence of its reversion after relief of the obstruction. However, this raises the interesting question: what degree of obstruction has to be present to offer a worthwhile chance of reversion to stability after the relief of marginally obstructive states? This question still remains to be answered.

Should the Natural Age-Related Diminution of the Voiding Flow be Regarded as Normal?

So well recognised is the age-related diminution of the voiding flow and the increase in diurnal and nocturnal frequency that men commonly accept this as their natural burden. The average flow pattern diminishes in each decade after the age of 50 years; however, it is highly questionable whether this should be regarded as normal because, in the majority of males, this natural diminution of flow is the result of a positive increase in the outflow resistance, either as a result of a natural age-related increase in prostatic size or progressive increase in a subclinical dyssynergic bladder neck obstruction, or a combination of both. The accuracy of this observation is self-evident from the fact that effective operative relief of the underlying obstruction restores the youthful stream with the usual incidence of reduction of the associated detrusor frequency/urgency symptoms. While some men prefer to procrastinate and live with their increasing symptoms, others are philosophically inclined towards a definitive procedure to resolve their increasingly symptomatic obstruction and it is unreasonable to dissuade them from this on the basis of the natural incidence of symptoms resulting from age-related obstruction, supposing this to be "normal".

Bladder Neck Obstruction

The term "bladder neck obstruction" is open to misinterpretation:

1. it can be used in a specific sense to indicate that the bladder neck mechanism itself is obstructive;
2. it can be used generally to indicate that the site of obstruction is located in the neck of the bladder, i.e. the internal meatus (this, of course, includes all forms of obstruction at this level such as prostatic enlargement and carcinoma); and
3. it is still sometimes used clinically to denote a bladder outflow obstruction in general without any distinction between proximal and distal location, but this is archaic.

Bladder Outflow Obstruction and "Relative Obstruction"

Efficient voiding is fundamentally dependent on the balance between the detrusor and the abdominal components of the voiding pressures on the one hand (which are easy to quantify and evaluate) and the outlet resistance on the other (the functional components of which are difficult to measure accurately).

Urodynamically, the term "bladder outflow obstruction" should not be conceptually restricted to patients with a positive increase in outflow resistancepartly because even when this is identifiable there may be an additional bladder deficiency component and partly because voiding inefficiency commonly proves to be a relative imbalance in which the element of outflow resistance, is not abnormally increased. An example of this is after a bowel cystoplasty in which the sphincter mechanisms were, and remain, quite normal but an adjustment may be required to resolve the imbalance that results from the substitution of a normal detrusor with the functionally inappropriate characteristics of bowel peristalsis (Turner-Warwick and Handley-Ashken, 1967).

Voiding Inefficiency

There are two important factors in the evaluation of voiding inefficiency:

1. the identification of voiding inefficiency and its quantification; and
2. the actual site of the outflow occlusion and its cause, which is fundamental to appropriate treatment.

Normal Bladder Neck Function

The bladder neck sphincter mechanism is formed by a concentration of detrusor smooth muscle around the internal meatus extending down to the level of the verumontanum. It is easy to show, by synchronous video-pressure studies, that it creates an occlusive cough-competent sphincter mechanism while the detrusor is at rest; however, its competence is dependent upon stable detrusor behaviour because it funnels open in association with a detrusor contraction.

The actual mechanism of normal bladder neck opening is also incompletely understood but certainly it is not explained by Hutch's over-simplistic base-plate concept. Tanagho (1978) has shown that bladder neck opening slightly precedes detrusor contraction and that it is reflex mediated.

Bladder Neck Dyssynergia

Varying degrees of failure of the bladder neck to open normally in association with a voiding detrusor contraction are not uncommon in the male although this is exceedingly rare in the female (Turner-Warwick, 1970, 1979; Turner-Warwick et al. 1973a); they range from inefficient opening associated with a marginally poor flow rate to grossly self-obstructive dyssynergic contraction. The fact that a clinically significant dyssynergic bladder neck obstruction in the male is caused by progressive positive contraction of the bladder neck rather than by a simple failure of its opening is shown by the simple observation of Bates et al. (1973) that although the resting closing pressure of a dyssynergic mechanism on a simple profile study is not abnormally elevated (about 10 cm H_2O) it can be seen on synchronous video-pressure studies to maintain an effective closure that progressively exceeds the intravesical pressures created by a voiding detrusor contraction and we have examples of this greater than 100 cm H_2O.

The mechanism of dyssynergic contraction of the bladder neck muscle is presently as poorly understood as the mechanism of its normal synergic opening; however, a number of relevant facts emerge:

1. Although the smooth muscle fibres of the concentric bladder neck sphincter mechanism of the female and the proximal part of the male

bladder neck are morphological extensions of the cholinergically innervated detrusor fibres, Gosling has shown that the innervation of the male bladder neck mechanism, like the seminal vesicles, is adrenergic whereas that of the female, like the detrusor of both the male and the female, is cholinergic (Gosling et al. 1977). The smooth muscle fibres of the distal part of the bladder neck are morphologically distinct from the detrusor fibres being smaller, aggregated into smaller muscle bundles and separated by a greater proportion of collagen than detrusor bundles. They are derived from the "prostatic capsule" and form a proximal sex-orientated procreative mechanism which prevents reflux seminal emission by orgasmic contraction synchronous with that of the seminal vesicles. It is probable that this differential innervation and function explains why dyssynergic bladder neck dysfunction is common in the male but virtually never occurs in the female; it also explains why the sympathetic blocker phenoxybenzamine relaxes dyssynergic bladder neck obstruction in the male.

2. Although opening of the bladder neck mechanism is almost always associated with a voiding detrusor contraction and vice versa, Tanagho (1978) has shown that it is not only reflex mediated, but that it marginally precedes the detrusor pressure rise; thus it is most unlikely that either a normal synergic opening or an abnormal dyssynergic closure are the simple result of a normal or abnormal morphological arrangement of the component fibre bundles.

3. Although the bladder neck mechanism is reflex mediated, dyssynergic dysfunction of this should not be regarded as neuropathic; indeed it is interesting that dyssynergic contraction of the neck mechanism is a dysfunction which very rarely develops as a result of overt neuropathy (Turner-Warwick, 1979).

4. Although opening and closing of the bladder neck is associated with detrusor contraction, they are not functionally related to the actual contraction pressure; synchronous video-pressure voiding studies often show that the detrusor pressure at the time of its opening is quite different from that at the time of its closing (Turner-Warwick and Whiteside, 1982).

5. The weight of evidence suggests that the characteristic behaviour of a particular bladder neck mechanism rarely changes. Although the obstruction caused by a dyssynergic mechanism may increase somewhat with age, its characteristic dysfunction usually can be traced back to childhood. The unequivocal conversion of an overtly synergic mechanism to dyssynergia is exceedingly rare, except possibly in diabetes, and its behaviour is not significantly affected by a generalised hypertrophy in response to a distal obstruction.

Symptoms and Presentation of Dyssynergic Bladder Neck Obstruction

There are wide variations in the degree of obstruction that dyssynergic bladder neck behaviour causes; the most severe require treatment in childhood and moderate degrees are much the most common cause of obstruction up to the age of 50 years. After this the apparent incidence appears to fall because outflow obstruction is then ᵪmmonly ascribed solely to coincidental prostatic enlargement, however mini .ial, and the significance of a tight circular bladder neck proximal to it, indicating that it is dyssynergic, is still not generally recognised (Turner-Warwick, 1979, 1983).

Because dyssynergic bladder neck obstruction is usually a life-long condition, few patients complain of the classic symptoms of outflow restriction: slow start, poor flow and terminal dribble; even a detailed enquiry can be a misleading substitute for uroflowmetry because many patients regard their pathetically poor flow as normal for them and commonly report it as good. The commonest feature is an admission that their voiding flow has always been non-competitive (they could never play that game at school); but this information has to be sought, as it is never volunteered. Some patients complain of being unable to void in the company of others at a public urinal. This particular symptom sometimes causes considerable distress. It is not unusual for patients to have consulted a psychiatrist (without avail) and some have embarrassing memories such as missing the last act of an opera because they could not urinate in the crowded toilet during the interval. Such symptoms should never be regarded as functional until an organic cause has been excluded urodynamically. A few patients primarily complain of hesitancy bordering upon retention when the bladder is over-distended. The development of unexpected retention of urine after an incidental operative procedure such as a hernia repair in the younger age group is commonly the result of unsuspected long-standing dyssynergic bladder neck obstruction. However, unlike retention due to large prostates, natural voiding is usually restored by a short period of catheter drainage.

Secondary Symptoms

The majority of patients with dyssynergic bladder neck obstruction develop unstable detrusor behaviour sooner or later and most of these then have the characteristic symptoms of frequency, urgency and nocturia with the usual incidence of reversion after effective relief of the obstruction. Urinary infection in the male always suggests outflow obstruction and a dyssynergic bladder neck is much the commonest cause of this before the age of 50 years (Turner-Warwick, 1979).

Prostatitis and the Dyssynergic Bladder Neck

Overlap of somewhat non-specific symptoms sometimes makes it difficult to differentiate clinically between dyssynergic bladder neck obstruction and hypersensitive prostatitis; furthermore, when the two conditions coexist it is virtually impossible to apportion them. Thus, the flow rate of every patient with suspected prostatitis should be recorded to avoid failure to identify a treatable element of obstruction which, in an average series, may be found in about 1 in 10 cases (Turner-Warwick, 1979). However, in the case of infected prostatitis, it is important that the flow rate should be checked between exacerbations of inflammation which may themselves create a mild obstruction.

When an element of dyssynergic bladder neck obstruction is identified in a patient with equivocal prostatitis symptoms, treatment should be discussed on the basis that the relief of the obstruction may improve matters to some extent, and possibly to a considerable extent, but that, by the nature of things, it may not. If the result is satisfactory then patients are only marginally more delighted that they are relieved of the burden than is the urologist.

Synergic Bladder Neck Obstruction: Detrusor Dysfunction

Although for reasons already discussed, bladder neck opening is not a direct effect of detrusor contraction, it is closely associated with it. Thus a detrusor contraction failure is generally associated with failure of opening of a normal occlusive synergic mechanism; urodynamically this can be regarded as a voiding imbalance in which the outlet is occluded at the bladder neck.

A variety of detrusor dysfunctions may result in failure or inadequacy of bladder neck opening:

1. The detrusor may be acontractile.

2. The patient may be unable voluntarily to initiate a contraction of an otherwise functional detrusor and this disability may be occasional or complete.

3. An unsustained voiding detrusor contraction commonly results in premature closure of a synergic bladder neck which initially opened widely, resulting in residual urine due to terminal bladder neck occlusions. This is a common neuropathic dysfunction but it is not unusual in the absence of neuropathy.

4. An indifferent low-pressure detrusor contraction may be associated with an indifferent opening of the bladder neck mechanism. Synchronous video-pressure studies may be required to distinguish this from dyssynergic bladder neck obstruction in the male, because both conditions are characterised by a prolonged poor flow rate and a poorly opening bladder neck mechanism on cystography with a considerable symptom overlap. However, a true dyssynergic bladder neck obstruction usually results in the development of an elevated detrusor pressure before the third decade.

5. The results of treating "relative outflow obstruction" associated with low-pressure detrusor dysfunction by endoscopic bladder neck incision are relatively poor, particularly when this is the result of neuropathy such as progressive autonomic failure (PAF), of which the Shy–Drager syndrome is but one variety. (This condition may present as a urodynamic dysfunction and its accurate diagnosis in the early stages depends upon a high level of suspicion and appropriate investigation (Kirby et al. 1983).)

6. Dyssynergic bladder neck obstruction almost never occurs in females. Not only is outflow obstruction located at the bladder neck itself relatively rare, but when present it is almost invariably associated with a primary detrusor

contraction failure that is rarely the result of overt neuropathy (Brown and Turner-Warwick, 1979).

Diagnosis of Dyssynergic Bladder Neck Obstruction

Whether they recognise it or not, the great majority of patients with dyssynergic bladder neck obstruction have a grossly impaired voiding flow pattern. The fact that many have difficulty in voiding in the company of others or under strange circumstances, emphasises the shortcomings of trying to identify it by the classic exercise of watching them void. This is often most difficult to achieve with those for whom it matters most. The importance of routine uroflowmetry cannot be over-emphasised because without it the condition is inevitably under-diagnosed.

Many patients are referred for a second opinion on troublesome symptoms that prove to be the result of a severe and easily relieved dyssynergic bladder neck obstruction when obstruction supposedly had been excluded by previous routine urological findings of a prostate that is not enlarged, the absence of a residual urine and normal appearances on endoscopy. More than 10 years after the unequivocal demonstration of the importance of objective urodynamic evaluation in the accurate diagnosis and treatment of disorders of lower urinary tract function, this simply should not happen; it is virtually impossible to justify the treatment of voiding disorders in the male without routine pre- and post-operative uroflow records.

Many patients present with a reasonable flow pattern and a peak flow which appears within the equivocal range of 10–20 ml/sec; as previously emphasised, pressure studies are required to identify those that are the result of elevated pressure obstruction. Occasionally, patients present with a peak flow of over 20 ml/sec which is nevertheless the obstructed result of a grossly elevated detrusor contraction pressure of over 100 cm H_2O; the identification of these is easily missed and is dependent upon a particularly high level of suspicion.

It is fundamentally important to appreciate that there are no endoscopic appearances by which a dyssynergic bladder neck can be unequivocally identified or excluded. Hypertrophy of a dyssynergic bladder neck mechanism itself is a late event and many bladder necks that are causing severe outflow obstruction do not appear abnormal in any way – so much so that having observed them endoscopically one feels the need to double-check the patient's identity with that of the pressure flow record before proceeding to endoscopic surgery.

The endoscopic appearances of hypertrophy of the bladder neck and bladder wall trabeculation are certainly not diagnostic of bladder neck obstruction; global hypertrophy is more often the result of unobstructed unstable detrusor dysfunction and such a secondary hypertrophy of a synergic bladder neck does not compromise its opening mechanism or result in obstruction. (Fig. 6.2) (Turner-Warwick et al. 1973a, b).

Unfortunately, the erroneous ablation of a normally functioning bladder neck sphincter, undertaken as a result of its hypertrophic appearance, is still all too common. Because a synergic bladder neck sphincter is opened

Selective bladder neck relaxation by endoscopic diathermy incision

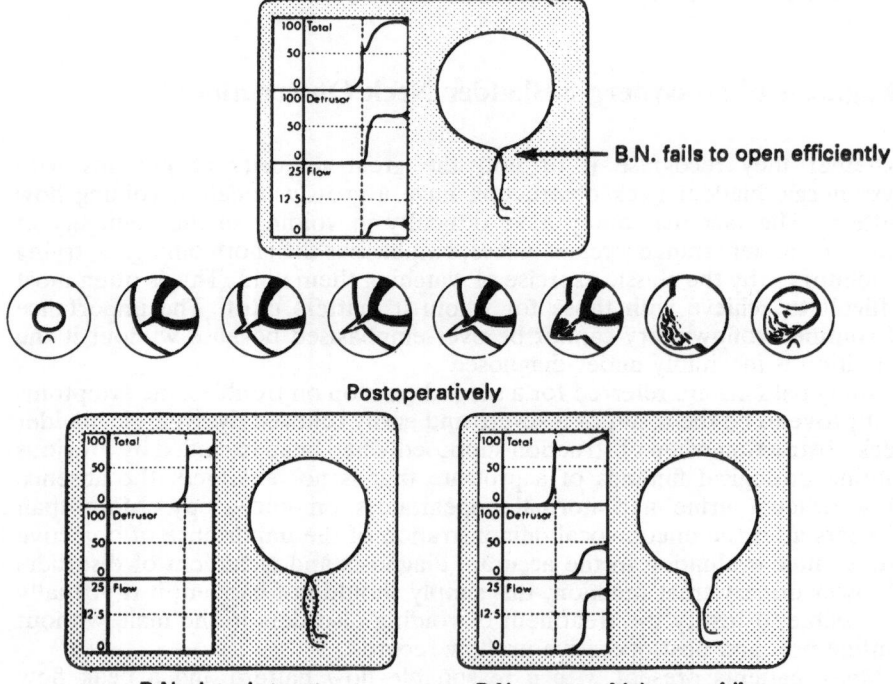

Fig. 6.2. The video-pressure-flow appearances of dyssynergic bladder neck obstruction before and after its relief by a single full-thickness endoscopic incision from bladder base to verumontanum (Turner-Warwick et al. 1973b)

and rendered incompetent by a detrusor contraction, its erroneous ablation does not compromise the continence of a patient with unstable detrusor behaviour because this is essentially dependent upon the distal sphincter mechanism. However, the erroneous ablation of a competent bladder neck that is hypertrophied as a result of a posterior bulbar stricture may be disastrous if a definitive repair is consequently contraindicated because it is bordering upon the only residual sphincter mechanism (Turner-Warwick et al. 1973b).

Thus, in summary, the diagnosis of dyssynergic bladder neck obstruction depends upon: (a) objective evidence of outflow obstruction by uroflowmetry, pressure-flow studies, or a significant residual urine; and (b) evidence that the thus proven outflow obstruction is located at the internal meatus. Although incontrovertible evidence of this is provided by voiding cystourethrography, in practice in the adult the diagnosis of an obstructive bladder neck mechanism is usually confirmed deductively, having excluded a distal stricture and prostatic enlargement endoscopically; this is because obstructive distal sphincter dyssynergia is exceedingly rare in the adult in the absence of an overt neuropathy (Turner-Warwick, 1979).

Indications for the Treatment of Dyssynergic Bladder Neck Obstruction

A proven dyssynergic bladder neck obstruction does not necessarily require treatment. This depends upon the extent of the trouble that it is causing, the degree of obstruction, the exclusion of pre-existing damage to the distal sphincter mechanism upon which continence will depend and the importance of ejaculation. Every case requires individual consideration. The decision is often simplified by a strong indication such as recurrent infection or episodes of retention; it is also facilitated if the prospect of a possible failure of ejaculation is unimportant to the patient.

Many patients with moderate obstruction are reassured by the identification of the cause of their problem and prefer to live with their symptoms and to postpone definitive treatment until their family is established. Medication with alpha blocking agents is sometimes used as a confirmatory diagnostic test and for short-term treatment, but side effects are common, particularly in the adult, and this drug is specifically contraindicated when postural hypotension might be critical, in occupations such as scaffolding workers, or augmented, such as aircrew.

Effective Relaxation of the Dyssynergic Bladder Neck by Endoscopic Incision

Dyssynergic bladder neck obstruction is definitively and reliably treated by transecting the full thickness of its ring with an endoscopic knife-electrode. A single full-thickness incision in one position is quite sufficient unless there is a coincidental element of prostatic enlargement (Fig. 6.2) (Turner-Warwick, 1970, 1979; Turner-Warwick et al. 1973b). The incision should extend from the bladder base down to the level of the verumontanum and as the cut, initially a V-shaped cleft, is deepened progressively, it springs open to a U-shape defect, the appearance of which suggests that several loopfuls of tissue have been removed. The incision is further deepened until minute interstitial fat globules are revealed between the latticework of the residual prostatic capsule fibres by pinpoints of reflected light. Haemostasis is achieved by electrocoagulation using the flat of the knife-electrode. The functional results of simple endoscopic relaxation of a dyssynergic bladder neck obstruction are both urodynamically reliable and relatively uncomplicated compared with treatment by loop resection.

There has been no case of recurrent dyssynergic obstruction or secondary bladder neck contracture in our series of more than 200 cases. The incidence of a diminished volume of ejaculate has been in the region of 10% and in less than 5% it has been absent altogether. However, if necessary, the ejaculate can be retrieved from the posterior urethra by post-coital self-catheterisation washout for artificial insemination. Videocystourethrography after incisional relaxation usually shows the bladder neck to be closed while the detrusor is at rest during stable bladder filling but it opens widely in association with a voiding detrusor contraction giving the appearance that an extensive loop resection has been performed (Turner-Warwick, 1979). Partial-thickness incisions are somewhat less reliable and generally inadvisable unless a patient requiring urgent treatment particularly wishes to reduce further the small incidence of ejaculation failure, in which case he must accept the possibility of the need to repeat the relaxation procedure.

Because the thickness of dyssynergic bladder neck is so variable, the precise depth of a partial incision cannot be judged accurately and thus it is necessary to accept an arbitrary limit such as the point at which the V-shaped cleft first opens into a U-shape; however, from this point the thickness of the residual bladder neck mechanism that remains uncut varies considerably and, of course, the potential of its residual dyssynergic occlusion is quite unpredictable.

Thus it is difficult to justify the treatment of dyssynergic bladder neck obstruction by loop resection; there are no advantages but there are the following potential complications involved in removing lumps of dyssynergic bladder neck muscle, particularly when this does not involve transection of the full thickness of the bladder neck ring at any point: (a) more blood vessels are exposed which inevitable carries an increased risk of secondary bleeding; (b) the first loop cut resects nearly 50% of the urothelial lining of the bladder neck and subsequent loopfuls increase the area of the urothelial defect and the potential for secondary scar formation; (c) the functional occlusion of the bladder neck is almost invariably destroyed by an effective loop resection so that the incidence of ejaculation failure is relatively high; (d) the incidence of secondary bladder neck contracture after the loop resection of a dyssynergic mechanism is significant. Unless the full thickness of the dyssynergic bladder neck ring is completely transected at at least one point, the residual dyssynergic occlusion created by its residual thickness, which is not apparent at the time of resection, continues to create an occlusion post-operatively. Because it never opens widely, it heals in a contracted state with extensive scar formation associated with excessive resected tissue deficiency.

Thus most functionally orientated urologists who understand the dysfunctional nature of obstruction by the bladder neck mechanism have thankfully abandoned this old method of treating it.

The Relationship of Prostatic Enlargement to the Normal Bladder Neck Mechanism

McNeal (1972) has shown that the origin of the so-called "lateral" and "middle" lobes do not represent areas of the normal prostate but develop by hypertrophy of small paraurethral glands; they naturally tend to enlarge into the lumen of the upper prostatic urethra. Initially a small enlargement is of no urodynamic significance; later, however, there are wide variations in size of a "prostatic enlargement" and the degree of outlet obstruction associated with it. Remarkably little consideration seems to have been given to the reason for this but it must in fact relate to the confines of the surrounding bladder neck and prostatic "capsule" (Turner-Warwick, 1979).

The bladder neck mechanism is integral with the so-called "prostatic capsule" which is formed by the expansion of the normal prostatic tissue by the grossly hypertrophic paraurethral gland's nodules which are conveniently, but erroneously, referred to by surgeons as "adenomata".

The enlarging "lobes" naturally expand into the prostatic urethra and, presumably because the normal bladder neck mechanism funnels widely open during a voiding detrusor contraction, they are normally free to extend upwards through the internal meatus into the base of the bladder, widely expanding the bladder neck mechanism and the upper prostatic capsule (Turner-Warwick, 1983). Thus, the lateral and middle lobes come to form the margins of the new "triangulated" internal meatus. Occasionally an enormous enlargement of over 100 g of hypertrophic prostatic tissue causes a minimal outlet obstruction, presumably because it escapes almost completely from the confines of the prostatic tissue to half-fill the bladder.

The Relationship of Prostatic Enlargement to the Dyssynergic Bladder Neck Mechanism

The functional and mechanical situation is quite different when the hypertrophic elements of the prostate enlarge below a tight bladder neck capsule, especially when the bladder neck mechanism is dyssynergic, because this not only remains closed between voiding but closes even tighter during voiding contractions. Furthermore, the bulk of the secondary hypertrophy of the bladder and bladder neck associated with outlet obstruction results from a deposition of interstitial collagen (vide supra) and, while this does not significantly affect its functional behaviour, it probably increases its resistance to expansion. Under these circumstances the "lateral lobes" expand into the mid-prostatic urethra but, failing to expand the bladder neck and its integral capsular ring, they become "trapped" in the restricted space below it so that a relatively small enlargement causes a significant obstruction and furthermore, augments any pre-existing bladder outlet obstruction caused by a dyssynergic bladder neck (Fig. 6.3) (Turner-Warwick et al. 1973b).

The characteristic endoscopic appearance of this situation is a relatively small enlargement of the lateral lobes meeting in the midline with a ring-shaped bladder neck mechanism above. In such cases no middle lobe is seen; this originates from a group of paraurethral glands in the midline posteriorly just above the verumontanum and when it enlarges in relation to a tight bladder neck mechanism, it tends to burrow outwards to expand behind it under the trigone (Fig. 6.4).

However, while the endoscopic appearances of an intra-urethral prostatic enlargement beneath a bladder neck ring are quite characteristic of a "double" obstruction, they are not diagnostic for it, unless a significant bladder outlet obstruction has been proven urodynamically. Identical endoscopic appearances are seen in the early stages of prostatic enlargement in patients who have no outflow obstruction whatsoever because their normally functioning bladder neck, which has not yet been expanded by the enlarging prostate, funnels widely open during a voiding detrusor contraction. This emphasises

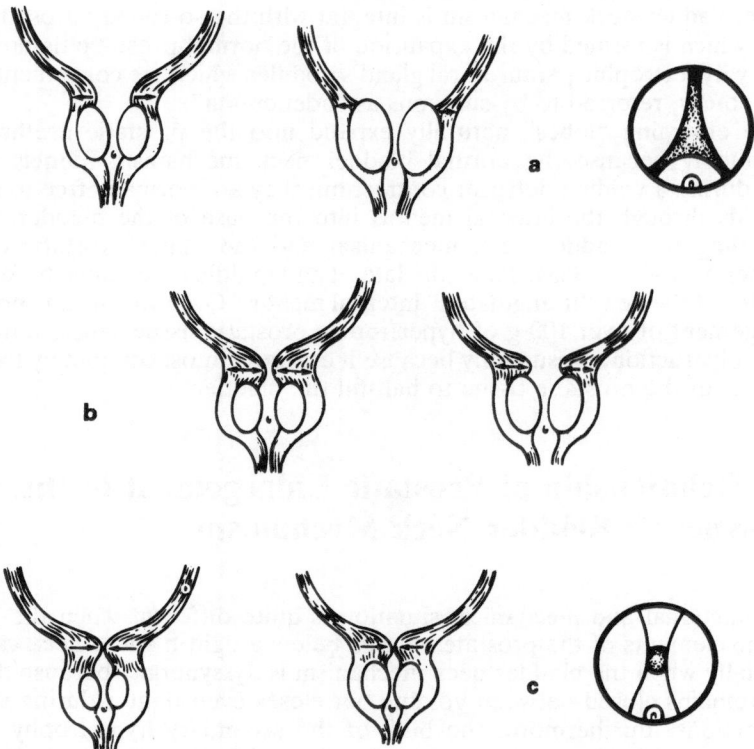

Fig. 6.3. **a** When the bladder neck opens normally the lateral and middle "lobes" expand widely as they enlarge upwards into the base of the bladder: the internal meatus is formed by prostatic tissue and appears triangulated. **b** A dyssynergic bladder neck never opens widely and positively closes during detrusor contraction so that a relatively small enlargement of the prostatic "lobes" trapped beneath a ring-shaped bladder neck causes a disproportionate obstruction: "double obstruction" (Turner-Warwick, 1970). **c** Equivocal degrees of bladder neck opening are not uncommon and result in intermediate appearances of the internal meatus; however, this does not invalidate the significance of "double obstruction".

once again the fact that the cystourethroscope is not a valid urodynamic instrument and that it is impossible to evaluate, with any degree of accuracy, the functional behaviour of the bladder neck mechanism with it.

Double Obstruction: The Combination of Prostatic and Dyssynergic Bladder Neck Obstruction – The "Trapped Prostate"

In general, minor degrees of prostatic enlargement do not seem to create a significant outlet obstruction unless they are trapped below a tight ring-shaped

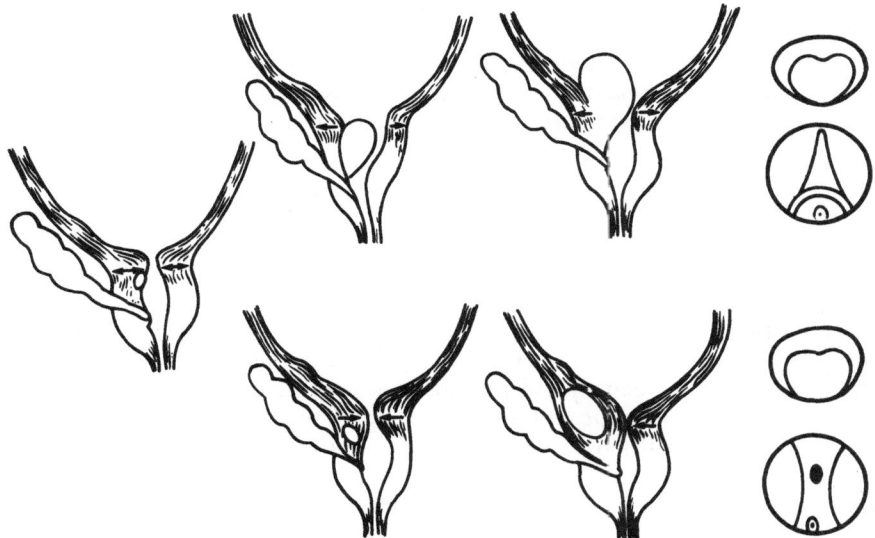

Fig. 6.4. When a "middle lobe" enlarges below a synergically opening bladder neck it expands upwards through it into the base of the bladder to create the posterior element of the triangulated internal meatus; when it enlarges below a dyssynergic bladder neck it tends to burrow under it into a subtrigonal position (Turner-Warwick, 1983).

bladder neck and much the commonest cause of this, outside areas of endemic schistosomiasis, is a dyssynergic mechanism.

Prostatic enlargement and dyssynergic bladder neck dysfunction are both common conditions so their coincidence is by no means uncommon; it should be suspected whenever a patient with a relatively minor degree of prostatic enlargement develops symptoms of bladder outlet obstruction (Turner-Warwick et al. 1973b).

In such cases the patient commonly gives a history of a recent onset of symptoms relating to the relatively short period of his prostatic enlargement, because he accepted his previous life-long slow flow as normal. The existence of double obstruction is often strikingly obvious after its relief because, while the patient with a simple prostatic obstruction is grateful for the restoration of his stream to its former state, patients with a double obstruction, like those with a simple dyssynergic bladder neck obstruction, often declare with delight that they have "never voided so well".

It follows that in most cases in which an outflow obstruction has been relieved by the resection of less than about 10 g of prostatic tissue, either the enlarged element has been incompletely resected or it was "trapped" by a tight bladder neck with the high probability of an additional element of dyssynergic obstruction (Turner-Warwick, 1979; Turner-Warwick and Whiteside, 1982).

Because there is a wide variation in the degree of dyssynergic obstruction associated with bladder neck dysfunction there are also gradations between the triangulated internal meatus associated with a simple trilobar prostatic enlargement on the one hand and the tight dyssynergic bladder neck ring that is unequivocally trapping the prostate on the other. Within the middle area, an enlargement of prostatic element may gradually stretch open and expand a moderately tight bladder neck (Fig. 6.5); however, these natural intermediates do not invalidate the practical value of the distinction between obstruction due to pure prostatic enlargement with those due to double obstruction.

Development of Secondary Bladder Neck Contracture after Loop Resection of a Double Obstruction

The mechanism of development of secondary bladder neck contracture after loop resection of a combination obstruction is precisely similar to that following loop resection of a simple dyssynergic bladder neck (Turner-Warwick, 1983). However, for conceptual reasons it is potentially commoner because the dyssynergic significance of the ring-shaped bladder neck is commonly unrecognised and although its margin is removed as an incidental to a resection that is primarily directed at the prostatic element, there is a considerable risk that a significant circumferential thickness of the bladder neck will remain; unless it is completely transected its continued dyssynergic contraction will result in secondary scarring contracture during the healing process (Fig. 6.6) Secondary bladder neck contracture rarely occurs after the endoscopic resection of a large prostate in which the normal bladder neck mechanism has been widely expanded; neither does it occur after even a circumferential partial thickness resection of a normal synergic bladder neck mechanism, the remnants of which continue to open widely during every voiding detrusor contraction throughout the healing period. Thus, it is fundamentally important to recognise the potential urodynamic significance of the endoscopic appearance of a ring-shaped bladder neck mechanism above an early prostatic enlargement and to treat it appropriately.

Treatment of Double Obstruction by Combined Endoscopic Incision and Loop Resection

The author's preferred procedure for resolving a double obstruction is to start with a full-thickness incision of the bladder neck ring in the 5, 7, 11, and 1 o'clock positions (Fig. 6.7). If, after this, the element of prostatic enlargement appears rather insignificant, it may not be necessary to proceed to its resection because the efficient relaxation of the bladder neck ring may have provided space for its enlargement (Fig. 6.7). Otherwise the initial full-thickness four-quadrant relaxation of the bladder neck ring seems to facilitate the complete loop resection of the prostatic element (Turner-Warwick and Whiteside, 1982).

Conservative Surgery of Double Obstruction

Naturally, double obstruction tends to present at an earlier age than pure prostatic enlargement so it is not unusual that a patient in his early fifties requires treatment when he has recently married or remarried and wishes to

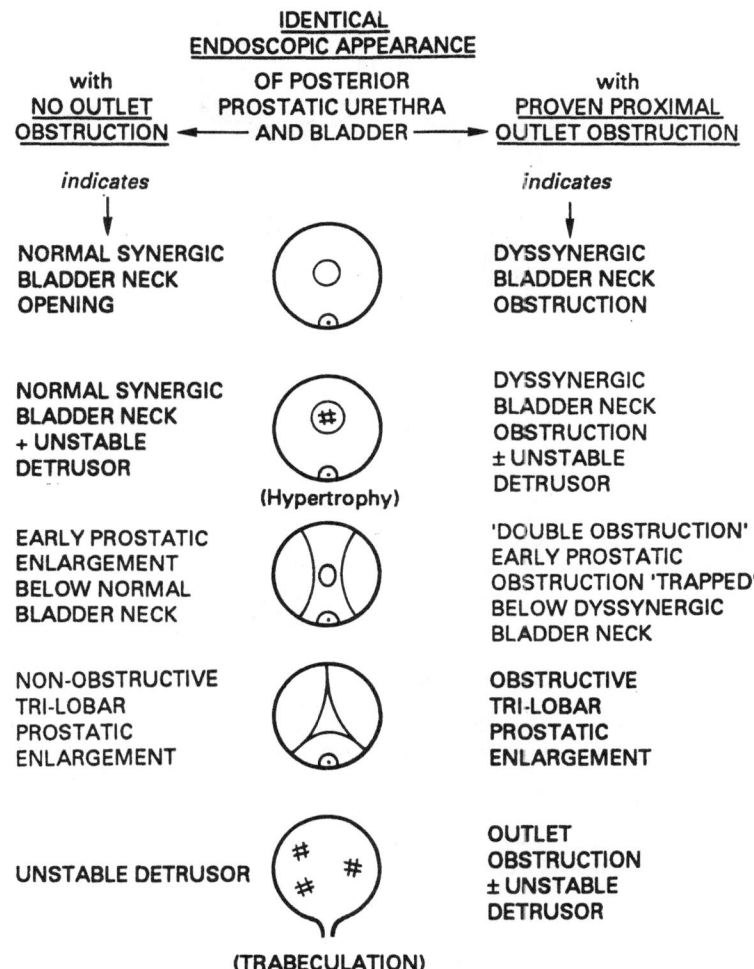

Fig. 6.5. The fallacies of "endoscopic guestimation" of obstruction. Each of the four basic endoscopic appearances of the proximal posterior urethra may or may not be associated with obstruction. *a* It is impossible to determine endoscopically whether a ring-shaped bladder neck mechanism is functionally normal, i.e., opens synergically during detrusor contraction, or whether it contracts dyssynergically. *b* Hypertrophy of the bladder neck associated with trabeculation does not necessarily indicate obstruction – it commonly results from non-obstructive unstable detrusor exercise. Global hypertrophy does not affect bladder neck function. *c* The endoscopic appearances of early prostatic enlargement beneath a ring-shaped bladder neck is only diagnostic of "double obstruction" due to a trapped prostate if outlet obstruction has been urodynamically proven – otherwise it is simply the normal appearance of early prostatic enlargement beneath a synergic bladder neck. *d* The degree of outlet obstruction is not proportionate to the size of the prostate. Gross intravesical enlargement may be associated with minimal obstruction, insufficient to create unstable detrusor behaviour. When a patient with an enlarged prostate presents with symptoms of unstable detrusor behaviour, failure to verify a diagnosis of outlet obstruction objectively may result in unavailing prostatic resections, dissatisfied patients and diminished urological reputations (Turner-Warwick, 1979).

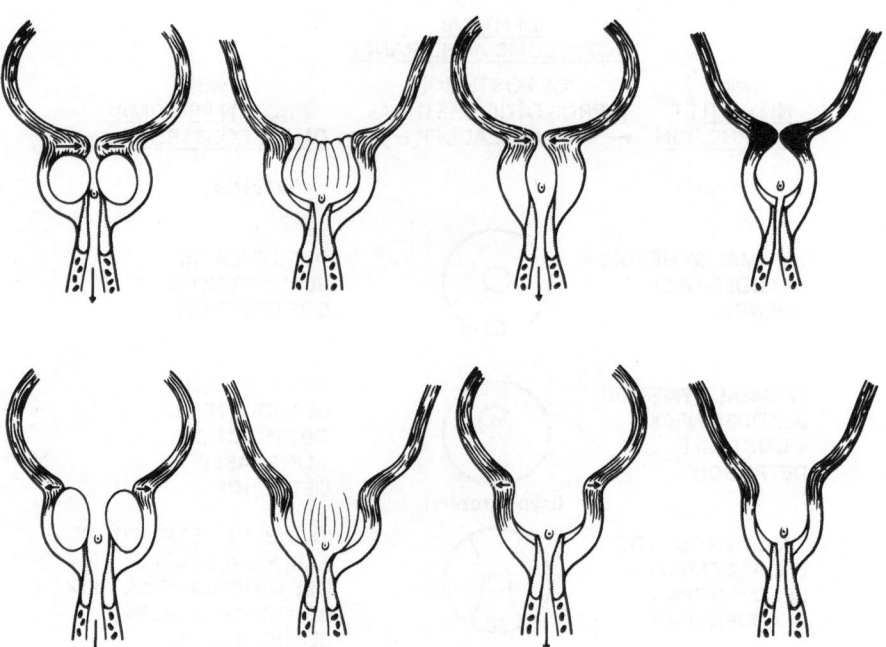

Fig. 6.6. In the case of proven outlet obstruction, failure to recognise the dyssynergic significance of the appearances of a circular bladder neck above a prostatic enlargement, and consequent failure to resect the full thickness of its ring in at least one position, is a common cause of secondary bladder neck contracture (Turner-Warwick, 1979; Turner-Warwick and Whiteside 1982). The uncut thickness of such a bladder neck continues to contract dyssynergically and tends to heal in a contracted state – the residual thickness of a partially resected normal bladder neck continues to open and heals open. Hence for simple urodynamic reasons, secondary bladder neck contracture almost never results from the resection of a triangulated prostatic internal meatus.

have children. While no definitive surgical treatment involving the bladder neck mechanism can guarantee the preservation of ejaculation, the effective loop resection of both obstructing elements virtually guarantees the failure of ejaculation. The temporising options that reduce this risk are:

1. The relaxation of the dyssynergic bladder neck ring at the 5 and 7 o'clock positions, without any resection of prostatic tissue or anterior incision. This is certainly the easiest option.

2. Resection of the prostatic element with maximal preservation of the bladder neck and the distal sphincter mechanisms. The accurate transurethral resection of the element of prostatic enlargement without compromising the function of the bladder neck mechanism is by no means as simple or as uncomplicated as it is sometimes thought to be. When preservation of either the bladder neck or the distal sphincter is particularly critical, for instance when a prostatectomy is required after the impairment of the function of the distal mechanism due to a pelvic fracture injury or to neuropathy, in the author's opinion this is probably best achieved by a conservative

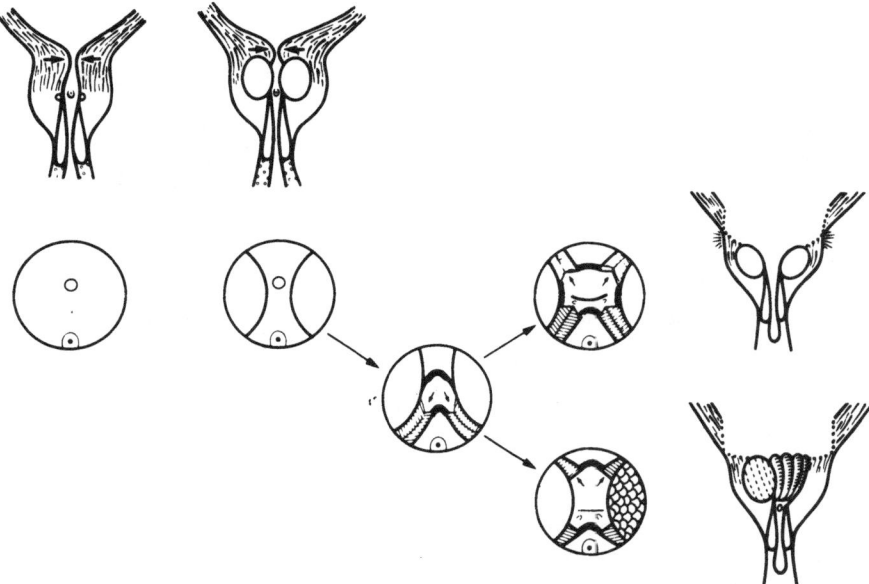

Fig. 6.7. Proven "double obstruction" can be simply treated by an initial endoscopic transection of the dyssynergic bladder neck element. Because secondary smooth muscle hypertrophy is associated with the extensive deposition of interstitial collagen (Gosling, 1980) a four-quadrant incision is advised to overcome secondary rigidity of the bladder neck ring – if procedure to a loop resection of prostatic tissue is also required, it is in fact facilitated by the initial incision (Turner-Warwick, 1979; Turner-Warwick and Whiteside, 1982).

transcapsular intra-urethral midprostatic dissection-reconstruction (Fig. 6.8); (Turner-Warwick, 1979).

Before undertaking a compromise conservative procedure, it is important that patients should understand that there is nothing experimental about a conservative approach; it is simply a question of a trial of a limited procedure to see whether it is sufficient. Subsequently, one can always proceed to a definitive procedure and, by the nature of both underlying conditions, it is likely that both the appropriate definitive procedures will indeed become necessary in the course of time.

The "Small Fibrous Prostate"

Strictly speaking, with the possible exception of specific conditions such as schistosomiasis, tuberculosis and carcinoma, there is no such entity as bladder outflow obstruction caused by a "small fibrous prostate". The term has been used as a synonym for Marion's disease or "sclerose du col"; however, this condition is simply the end result of a life-long dyssynergic bladder neck obstruction without a significant element of prostatic enlargement and the secondary collagen deposits seen in the histological sections is quite unrelated to the development of the obstruction.

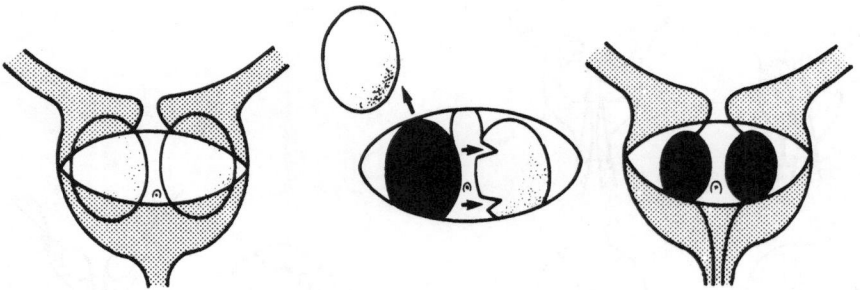

Fig. 6.8. Because the enlarging elements of the prostate arise in the mid posterior urethra from glands close to the verumontanum (colliculus) when maximum conservation of either the distal sphincter mechanism on the inner surface of the apex of the lateral lobe, or the bladder neck mechanism is required, it is best achieved by a meticulous intra-urethral dissection-enucleation through a transcapsular incision (Turner-Warwick, 1970; Turner-Warwick and Whiteside, 1982).

The situation most commonly referred to as a "small fibrous prostate" is that of double obstruction (Turner-Warwick et al. 1973b); resectionists have used the term somewhat phantasmagorically because of the tendency to develop secondary bladder neck contracture after a routine loop resection and enucleationists used it when they found difficulty in enucleating the small element of prostatic enlargement.

Summary: The Three Appearances of the Proximal Posterior Urethra and their Appropriate Treatment in Proven Outflow Obstruction

In summary, endoscopic examination of the proximal posterior urethra will generally reveal one of the three appearances each of which may or may not be associated with obstruction. When obstruction is urodynamically proven, the principles of the appropriate treatment of each is different:

1. A ring-shaped bladder neck with no prostatic enlargement indicates, in the absence of schistosomiasis, a dyssynergic dysfunction which is more appropriately treated by endoscopic incision than by loop resection.

2. A triangulated internal meatus, the margins of which are created by a large bulk of hypertrophic prostatic tissue. The resolution of this requires a formal loop resection or an enucleation procedure. The use of an endoscopic prostatotomy incision is manifestly inappropriate because there is no tendency for the cleft of such an incision into the solid tissue to open out into a U-shaped channel.

3. A relatively small intra-urethral prostatic enlargement with a proximal ring-shaped internal meatus: double obstruction. An initial bilateral full-thickness incision of the bladder neck element of this, down to the level of the

verumontanum, may be all that it is required to relieve the obstruction but if not, significant residual intrusion of prostatic tissue is treated definitively by an additional loop resection. To suppose that the effect of this endoscopic incision is the result of incising the prostate and to refer to this a "prostatotomy" is conceptually erroneous and this has tarnished the reputation of the excellent procedure of bladder neck relaxation.

Conclusion

The development of methods of objective urodynamic evaluation of bladder outflow obstruction in the male has led to a fundamental revision of many functional concepts relating to symptomatology, radiographic findings, endo-scopic appearances and, consequently, to treatment.

There can be no doubt that the fundamental basis of appropriate treatment of male outflow obstruction is uroflowmetry; without this, inevitably, prostatic obstruction is over-diagnosed, dyssynergic bladder neck obstruction is under-diagnosed and, furthermore, a surgeon may over-estimate the reliability of his obstruction relieving procedures.

It is highly questionable whether surgical treatment for male bladder out-flow obstruction is justifiable without at least pre-and post-operative uroflow records; the cystourethroscope is certainly an unacceptable substitute for a flow meter. The evidence of need for this relatively inexpensive basic equipment is overwhelming; furthermore, it is most certainly cost-effective in terms of patient care and the avoidance of unnecessary operations.

Simple videocystourethrography is also important to the urodynamic evalu-ation of many patients and although it is still sometimes under-used, this radiographic facility is in fact readily available to every practising urologist in the UK. Facilities for pressure-flow studies should be available in appropriate centres and synchronous video-pressure studies are essential in urodynamic referral units, but they are more often needed for the evaluation of post-prostatectomy problems than for pre-operative evaluation.

References

Abrams, P., Torrens, M. 1979. Clinical urodynamics. Urol. Clin. North Am. 6:71–79, 103–109

Arnold, E.P. 1980. Bladder outlet obstruction in the male: a urological analysis of the detrusor response. PhD thesis, London University

Bates, C.P., Whiteside, C.G., Turner-Warwick, R. 1970. Synchronous cine pressure-flow cystourethrography. Br. J. Urol. 42:714–723

Bates, C.P., Arnold, E.P., Griffiths, D.G. 1973. The progressive dyssynergic contraction of the bladder neck. Br. J. Urol. 45:58–59

Brown, A.G., Turner-Warwick, R. 1979. A urodynamic evaluation of urinary incontinence in the female and its treatment. Urol. Clin. North Am. 6:31–38

Farrar, D., Turner-Warwick, R. 1979. Outflow obstruction in the female. Urol. Clin. North Am. 6:217–227

Gosling, J.A., Dixon, J.S., Lendon, R.G., 1977. The automatic innervation of the human male and female bladder neck and proximal urethra. J. Urol. 118:302–305

Kirby, R.S., Fowler, C., Milroy, E.J.G., Bannister, R., Turner-Warwick, R., 1983. Vesico-urethral dysfunction in the Shy Drager Syndrome. Proceedings of the 13th annual meeting of the International Continence Society, Aachen

McNeal, J.E. 1972. The prostate and prostatic urethra: a morphological synthesis. J. Urol. 107:1008–1016

Smith, J. 1966. The measurement and significance of urinary flow. Br. J. Urol. 30:701–705

Tanagho, E.A. 1978. The anatomy and physiology of micturition. Clin. Obstet. Gynaecol. 5:3–25

Thomas, D. 1979. Neurogenic bladder dysfunction. Urol. Clin. North Am. 6:237–253

Turner-Warwick, R., Handley-Ashken, M. 1967. The functional results of partial, subtotal and total cystoplasty. Br. J. Urol. 39:3–12

Turner-Warwick, R. 1970. Clinical problems associated with urodynamic abnormalities. In: Urodynamics. Lutzyer, W., Melchior, H., eds. Berlin, Heidelberg, New York, Springer, pp 237–263

Turner-Warwick, R., et al. 1973a. A urodynamic view of prostatic obstruction and the results of prostatectomy. Br. Urol, 45:631–645

Turner-Warwick, R., Whiteside, C.G., Worth, P.H.L., Milroy, E.J.G., Bates, C.P. 1973b. A urodynamic review of clinical problems associated with bladder neck dysfunction and its treatment by endoscopic incision: transtrigonal posterior prostatectomy. Br. J. Urol. 45:44–59

Turner-Warwick, R. 1979. Observations on the functions and dysfunction of the sphincter and detrusor mechanisms. Urol. Clin. North Am. 6:13–30

Turner-Warwick, R., Whiteside, C.G., Milroy, E.J.G., Pengelly, A.W., Thompson, D.T. 1979. The intravenous urodynamogram. Br. J. Urol. 15:15–19

Turner-Warwick, R., Whiteside, C.G. 1982. Urodynamic studies and their effect on management. In: Scientific foundations of urology, 2nd edn. Chisholm, G.D., Williams, D.I., eds. London, Heinemann, pp 442–457

Turner-Warwick, R. 1983. The relationship of prostatic enlargement to the distal sphincter mechanism, the bladder neck mechanism and dyssynergic bladder neck obstruction. In: Benign prostatic hypertrophy. Hinman, F., Chisholm, G., eds. Berlin, Heidelberg, New York, Springer, pp 809–828

Turner-Warwick, R., Pitfield, J. 1984. Urodynamic evaluation. In: Outpatient urologic surgery. Kaye, K.W., Bronson, J.G., eds. New York, Lea and Febiger

Chapter 7

The Investigation of Benign Prostatic Hyperplasia

J.G Noble and C.R. Chapple

The clinical evaluation of patients suffering with benign prostatic hyperplasia relies upon the interpretation of clinical symptoms aided by the appropriate application of objective tests. The bladder is often said to be an "unreliable witness" not only because of the considerable overlap of symptom complexes but also as a result of subjective bias (Turner-Warwick et al. 1973). The value of symptom scoring remains the subject of ongoing debate at present.

The pathophysiological changes that occur secondary to prostatic hyperplasia have been discussed in the previous chapter but the following summary reviews the objective investigations that have been developed to quantify the functional response of the urinary tract.

The Bladder

Outflow obstruction secondary to benign prostatic hyperplasia (BPH) produces marked histological and functional changes in the human bladder (see Chapter 4). Bladder emptying becomes inefficient resulting in increased post-micturition urine residuals predisposing to urinary tract infections. It is at this juncture that the patient usually seeks medical advice either because of recurrent urinary tract infections or troublesome symptoms of detrusor instability, i.e. frequency, nocturia, urgency and urge incontinence.

Approximately one third of patients with symptomatic BPH do not develop secondary detrusor instability and may only notice the less debilitating "obstructive" symptoms of outflow obstruction, i.e. hesitancy, decreased urinary stream, post-micturition dribbling and incomplete bladder emptying. These are often not sufficiently severe to prompt medical advice and the patient may first present in acute urinary retention.

In a group of patients the clinical picture of chronic urinary retention occurs. The detrusor remains stable and fails to hypertrophy in response to outflow obstruction. The suggestion that there is an underlying sensory rather than motor dysfunction is an attractive hypothesis which as yet has not been proved by functional investigation (Turner-Warwick et al. 1979, 1973; Abrams et al. 1978; Ball et al. 1981). An alternative hypothesis is

that these patients represent a separate clinical subgroup and that in fact
the underlying pathology may be a life-long detrusor sphincter dyssynergia
rather than BPH.

Standard Investigations

Each patient, who on clinical grounds is suspected as suffering with urinary
problems secondary to BPH should undergo screening investigations to assess
renal function, urinary infection and the possibility of associated urinary tract
dysfunction either mimicking or coexisting with the suspected abnormality.
These investigations should include basic urinalysis (blood, protein, ketones
and sugar), urinary microscopy and culture and biochemical analysis for serum
urea, electrolytes and creatinine. A full blood count is not usually required
although it is often performed at the first visit of the patient especially if the
need for subsequent surgical intervention is expected on clinical grounds.

Upper Tract Assessment

Conventional investigation of the upper urinary tract in these patients has been
undertaken in the past by intravenous urography (IVU). It has in recent years
been recognised that routine investigation of the upper tracts is unnecessary in
the majority of cases and should be confined to those patients with symptoms
suggesting a potential upper tract abnormality or where another investigation
such as biochemistry reveals an abnormality.

The IVU reliably demonstrates renal cortical substance, upper tract dilatation (hydronephrosis or hydroureter) and prostatic enlargement by "hooking"
of the lower ureters due to upward displacement of the bladder base and/or
by a "prostatic impression" on the bladder films. These may also demonstrate
a thickened bladder wall with trabeculation and/or diverticula and a post-
micturition residual. However interpretation of some of these radiological
features is limited and functional correlates can not be made. For instance,
the presence of upper tract dilatation does not necessarily confirm upper tract
obstruction and bladder trabeculation per se does not confirm the presence
of obstruction. Functional assessment should rely totally on the application
of isotope renography (Webb, 1990).

In order to provide a better functional assessment the intravenous
urodynamogram (IVUD) evolved in which the "bladder" films are delayed
until the patient is adequately rehydrated. A film is then taken with the
bladder full and the patient voids whilst a recording of his flow rate is
taken. (see Uroflowmetry below). Many men find it difficult to void
during the test, especially after a period of dehydration as advised in
many departments performing IVU, and when voiding is achieved there
is frequently a significant delay before the "after micturition" film is taken.
The IVUD provides extra information about bladder capacity, urinary flow

rate and post-micturition residual as compared to the conventional IVU (Turner-Warwick et al. 1979).

Whilst IVU has been the mainstay of upper tract assessment for many years, recognition that ultrasonography provides a cheaper and less invasive method of investigation has led to its widespread use in the place of IVU. Urography requires the use of ionising radiation and contrast medium, both of which carry a small risk to the patient. Although, following IVU less than 5% of patients develop minor side effects, 0.1% develop major complications with the mortality rate following the intravenous administration of ionic contrast media falling between 1 in 40 000 and 1 in 750 000 (Ansell et al. 1980; Shehadi and Toniolo 1980; Hartman et al. 1982).

Ultrasonography provides sectional images of the kidney but in normal people the pelvicalyceal system is not well demonstrated in the absence of obstruction. Occasionally the collecting system is visualised if the patient has had a high fluid intake leading to a diuresis or in anatomical variants such as a large major calix or extrarenal pelvis. At the centre of the kidney "sinus echoes" are seen due to renal sinus fat. In the case of a distended system a multiloculated fluid collection is seen within the sinus which is composed of a larger, centrally lying renal pelvis communicating with smaller, peripherally lying calyces. The normal ureter is not seen during ultrasound screening and even when the ureter becomes distended it is often poorly visualised especially in the middle third because of overlying bowel gas. Like IVU, although ultrasonography can reliably demonstrate the presence of distension of the upper urinary tracts it does not provide functional evidence of chronic obstruction (Lyons et al. 1988; Davies, 1988; Ellenbogen et al. 1978). Indeed, in a small proportion of chronic obstruction cases, dilatation of the pelvicalyceal system doesn't occur.

Nevertheless, with careful scanning technique and interpretation, ultrasonography is a very sensitive detector of upper tract distension associated with BPH. Misinterpretation can occur, however, if the fluid collections within the kidney do not apparently communicate, when a diagnosis of renal cysts may be made, or when the renal pelvis contains solid matter such as blood or pus. False positive interpretation most commonly occurs as a result of mild dilatation of the collecting system in the absence of obstruction or due to the visualisation of normal intrarenal vessels, usually veins, and has been reported to occur in up to 26% of cases (Webb et al. 1984). The use of duplex Doppler ultrasound clearly shows venous or arterial waveforms arising from the central fluid collection in such patients and potential exists for the differentiation between obstructed and non-obstructed upper tract dilatation by changes in intrarenal vessel resistance utilising this technique (Scola et al. 1989; Platt et al. 1989).

Investigation of Bladder Function

It is vital that any patient undergoing investigation for BPH should have a functional assessment of the bladder. This evaluation utilises the scientific principles of "urodynamics". The degree to which a patient is investigated and the complexity of the urodynamic tests employed obviously depends upon the nature of the outflow obstruction and in particular, the presence of coexistent disease processes, e.g. neurological dysfunction that may alter lower urinary tract function, or a past history of surgery. Urodynamic testing is not without its limitations and the potential for misinterpretation of results undoubtedly exists. Ideally the patient should reproduce his "normal" voiding pattern during the investigation in an environment created with the minimum of embarrassment to him in mind. Patients should be questioned as to how representative voiding during the examination is to their normal pattern thus helping to establish the credibility of the urodynamic data obtained.

Urodynamic investigation can involve a number of complementary techniques which vary in complexity and range from simple documentation of frequency and volume of voided urine to detailed neurophysiological studies. Essentially the bladder has two functions: to store and to empty, and accurate assessment should include an evaluation of both.

Frequency–Volume Chart

The value of this relatively simple evaluation of bladder function is often overlooked. The patient is asked to record information about the number and time intervals between voidings over a defined period, e.g. 48 hours. The volume of each void is recorded and the total 24-hour urine output calculated. Four types of frequency–volume chart have been described:

- *Type 1*. Patients exhibit normal volumes and normal 24-hour urine output (i.e. without evidence of frequency or nocturia).
- *Type 2*. Normal voided volumes are produced but the 24-hour urine output is increased. (This suggests normal bladder function but symptoms result from polyuria, either habitual or secondary to diabetes or chronic renal insufficiency.)
- *Type 3*. Small single volumes recorded during day and night indicating urgency which may be either sensory or motor in origin. This is commonly seen in patients with outflow obstruction due to BPH either due to incomplete bladder emptying and/or secondary instability.
- *Type 4*. A large morning volume is recorded with variable small volumes during the day without nocturia. This is often associated with normal bladder function with a psychological aetiology.

This assessment can be modified by asking the patient to hold on to his maximum capacity before each void thus giving objective information as to the functional bladder capacity as compared with the cystometric bladder capacity determined during artificial bladder filling at cystometry.

Pad Testing

Urinary incontinence can complicate outflow obstruction secondary to BPH but is uncommon except in those patients with chronic retention bladders and "overflow incontinence". Objective evaluation of the degree of incontinence can be extremely difficult but the information may play a vital role in deciding the relative indication for operation, treatment, etc. in unfit patients. The International Continence Society (ICS) has established a number of guidelines to monitor incontinence during the patient's normal activities and although variation in results often occurs, the clinician is able to gain a more objective assessment of the problem.

Uroflowmetry

This is the simplest and often most useful test of bladder function, usually being the only requirement in the investigation of up to 50% of patients with BPH. "Flow rate" is defined as the volume of urine voided per unit time and is expressed in millilitres per second. The most modern flow meters allow these parameters to be recorded along with the flow pattern and because the flow rate is dependent upon both bladder function and outflow resistance a normal flow rate should indicate reasonable function of both. However, it must be emphasised that in the early stages of outflow obstruction, compensatory bladder hypertrophy can overcome outflow resistance producing normal flow rates by increased voiding detrusor pressures.

The flow rate may be measured utilising the following methods:

1. *Rotating disc method*: The voided urine is directed onto a rotating disc and the amount landing on the disc produces a proportionate increase in its inertia. By measuring changes in the power required to keep the disc rotating at a constant rate the flow rate can be calculated.

2. *Electronic dipstick method*: A dipstick is placed in a chamber and the capacitance of the dipstick is measured. The urine is voided into the chamber and as the fluid accumulates the capacitance of the dipstick changes. Thus the rate of change of capacitance is recorded giving a calculation of the flow rate.

3. *Gravimetric method*: The weight or alternatively the hydrostatic pressure of the urine at the base of the collecting chamber is measured and the flow rate thus calculated.

There are a number of uroflowmetry parameters that can be recorded but the ones of major importance to the clinician are maximum flow rate, voided volume and the flow pattern. The definitions of the various parameters are as follows:

- *Flow time*. Time over which the measurable flow occurs
- *Time to maximum flow*. Time elapsed from the onset of flow to the maximum flow
- *Maximum flow rate*. The maximal rate of flow
- *Voided volume*. The total volume expelled via the urethra
- *Average flow rate*. The voided volume divided by the flow time
- *Voiding time*. The total duration of micturition
- *Flow pattern*. This may be described as continuous, interrupted, prolonged, etc.

Although uroflowmetry is a convenient and accurate method of assessing lower urinary tract function, the interpretation of results in some instances may be misleading. Not only must the patient void in an environment which is not unduly embarrassing but he must also void with an adequately full bladder. Ideally flow measurement should be taken at flow volumes of greater than 200 ml and readings at voided volumes of less than this should be treated with caution. The flow rate will also vary relative to the volume voided. At the other extreme volumes of greater than 500 ml may also be accompanied by low flow rates which may reflect overstretching of the detrusor fibres (Siroky et al. 1979). There is a variation in flow rate with the age (and sex) of the patient and it must be remembered that straining at voiding is likely to significantly alter the flow rate.

The normal flow pattern exhibits a rapid rise to the maximum flow rate and this level should be attained within one third of the voiding time. In addition 45% of the voided volume should be evacuated before the maximum flow rate has been reached. Once maximum flow has been achieved the flow decreases more slowly so that the normal flow pattern is not symmetrical. In normal patients the average flow rate should be approximately half of the maximum flow rate.

If the bladder outflow is obstructed the patient will show a prolonged flow pattern with low maximum and average flow rates. In more advanced cases he will try to increase his voiding efficiency by abdominal straining which produces a characteristic interrupted flow pattern.

It is evident, therefore, that the flow rate can provide useful information suggesting whether a patient has outflow obstruction and a particular flow pattern may suggest the possible underlying pathology. The flow rate can be misleading if there has been detrusor compensation producing normal flow rates with high voiding detrusor pressures or alternatively if large post-micturition residues are being left. The flow rate may not be diminished in the early stages of BPH until the effective urethral calibre has diminished to below 10 Ch and occasionally irregularities occur due to collecting funnel artifacts or variations in direction of the urinary stream.

Overall uroflowmetry is an adequate investigation alone in over 50% of patients with BPH but where doubt remains following flow rate assessment or in more complex cases, e.g. neurological disease, post-surgery, etc. then more detailed assessment may be required.

Ultrasound Cystodynamogram (USCD)

Uroflowmetry may be combined with pre- and post-voiding bladder ultrasound and thus give additional information regarding functional bladder capacity and post-micturition residuals. This gives a more accurate assessment of lower urinary tract function than uroflowmetry alone and is easy to perform without the need for ionising radiation.

Cystometry

Cystometry is the method by which changes in bladder pressure are recorded progressively during bladder filling and subsequent voiding and is usually employed in equivocal or more complex cases where the diagnosis of benign prostatic hypertrophy is uncertain. During voiding a synchronous flow rate is measured and thus cystometry can give accurate information about detrusor activity, sensation, capacity and compliance.

The initial evaluation involves obtaining a free flow rate from the patient. The urethra is then anaesthetised using 1% lignocaine gel and a 1 mm diameter plastic pressure catheter is inserted into the bladder per urethram along with a small Nelaton filling catheter using a clean, aseptic technique. The pressure catheter is filled with normal saline and is connected to a pressure transducer such that intravesical pressure variations are transmitted via the saline within the catheter to the transducer where conversion to an electrical signal occurs. This signal is then converted into calibrated pressure readings within the integrated urodynamic system. The intravesical pressure measured by this system, however, has two components: pressure generated from the detrusor muscle activity (the detrusor pressure), and the abdominal pressure acting on the bladder. In studying the activity of the bladder it is the detrusor component of the intravesical pressure which is important and consequently it is necessary to measure the abdominal pressure simultaneously and subtract this from the intravesical pressure during the evaluation. In order to record the abdominal pressure the patient lies in the left lateral position and a 2 mm saline filled pressure catheter is introduced into the rectum. The end of this catheter is protected from blockage by a finger stall and a slit is cut in the side of this to prevent artefactual recording caused by tamponade. This line is connected to a similar pressure transducer connected to the integrated urodynamic apparatus. The lines are then flushed with saline to exclude any air bubbles within the system and the patient is asked to cough. This should record an increase in abdominal and thus intravesical pressure but correct subtraction should leave the detrusor pressure unchanged. All the pressure readings are then "zeroed" and bladder filling is then initiated at a predetermined rate via the filling catheter. In the absence of neuropathy we routinely perform "fast-fill" cystometry (100 ml/sec). Gas cystometry should not be used – as the medium involved, by virtue of its physical properties, will provide inaccurate results in the presence of environmental changes in temperature.

The normal adult bladder capacity averages between 400 and 750 ml and during filling it is widely held that the detrusor pressure should not rise above 15 cm H_2O. However the International Continence Society no longer recognises a specific value for the pressure rise as being essential to the diagnosis of detrusor instability (Abrams et al. 1988). The normal cystogram can be divided into four stages. During the first stage there is an initial rise in detrusor pressure to achieve the resting level. During the second stage pressure increases by very little, reflecting the vesicoelastic properties of the bladder wall. This property of smooth muscle is referred to as "tonus" or "receptive relaxation" and increases bladder compliance thereby allowing urine to be stored at low pressures. Patients often perceive the first sensation of bladder filling at about 150 ml and this point should be recorded because alterations in this value may indicate dysfunction in bladder sensation. As the bladder reaches its capacity the elastic properties of the bladder wall are stretched to their limit and there is a gradual rise in detrusor pressure in the absence of voluntary contraction. This stage is limited, however, by the overwhelming desire to pass urine and leads into the voiding stage when voluntary detrusor contraction is initiated. The detrusor pressure rises steeply to values of between 40 and 60 cm of H_2O and voiding commences with flow rates of up to 30–40 ml/sec.

The classical picture of detrusor instability is demonstrated by systolic waves of detrusor activity during filling which may or may not be associated with incontinence depending on the force of the contraction relative to the outflow resistance. The compliance of the bladder indicates the change in volume for a given change in detrusor pressure and the bladder is said to be "hypocompliant" if there is a steady linear rise in detrusor pressure above 15 cm H_2O. Whether this represents true detrusor instability is a matter of some controversy and as yet remains to be classified. The concept of a "urethral resistance factor" has been recognised to be too simplistic because the urethra does not generally behave like a rigid tube. However direct pressure flow plots can give an indication of the type of voiding dysfunction, readily distinguishing between "high pressure–low flow" obstructed voiding and detrusor underactivity.

Following micturition the residual volume is carefully measured and forms an integral part of the urodynamic assessment but its value must be interpreted with care, especially where there is associated vesicoureteric reflux or bladder diverticulae.

Videocystometrography is a more detailed urodynamic study in which conventional cystometry is combined with cystourethrography and is especially useful in evaluating patients where the site of bladder outflow obstruction is not clear on other investigation. During filling one may demonstrate bladder trabeculation and/or diverticula, vesicoureteric reflux or more unusual bladder configurations associated with neurological disease, e.g. "fir tree bladder". On reaching maximum bladder capacity the filling catheter is removed and the patient moved to the erect position for the voiding study. During voiding the patient is continually screened to demonstrate fluoroscopically the site of outflow obstruction and a "stop test" is performed. The stop test should result in voluntary contraction of the external sphincter with milk back of contrast from the prostatic urethra into the bladder. In cases of bladder neck dyssynergia the contrast is trapped in the posterior urethra (see Chapter 13). Detrusor pressure recorded at the time of the stop test gives a value of the isometric pressure of detrusor contraction (P_{ISO}) the significance of which is controversial.

Patients presenting with the clinical features of uncomplicated BPH will show high-pressure low-flow urodynamics with evidence of obstruction at the level of the posterior urethra on fluoroscopy. Occasionally reflux of contrast may be seen into the ejaculatory ducts and seminal vesicles.

Urethral Pressure Profile

The principle of the urethral pressure profile (UPP) is based on idealised concepts which represent the ability of the urethra to prevent the leakage of urine. There are various methods of obtaining urethral pressure readings which involve either measurements at one point over a defined time period or at several points along the urethra consecutively forming a urethral pressure profile. Urethral pressure profilometry has been advocated for use in the urodynamic evaluation of patients to provide detailed information on prostatic length and intraprostatic urethral pressure. It is inexpensive and quick to perform when used in conjunction with existing urodynamic equipment and has been reported to be of value in the diagnosis of bladder outlet obstruction in the male patient (Abrams, 1976).

Surprisingly, there have been no studies comparing the actual urethral length measured during endoscopy or on detailed radiological investigation with the functional prostatic length obtained from UPP. We therefore carried out a study to provide an objective assessment of the potential value of this technique by comparing the results for functional profile length and maximum intra-urethral closure pressure with urethral length measured endoscopically and with prostatic size and length measured on computed tomography (CT) scanning. In addition, the relationship between prostatic size and the amount of adenoma resected at operation was examined. The functional profile length was also calculated using the modification proposed as being more accurate by Kitada and Ishisawa (1981) namely; "the length from the most proximal pressure increase above bladder pressure to the position where the urethral pressure exceeds prostatic peak pressure". The functional profile length was documented, as was the maximum urethral closure pressure at the bladder neck, within the prostate and at the distal sphincter mechanism.

There was a poor correlation between pre-operative prostatic length and amount resected in the operating theatre. The results obtained with urethral pressure profilometry correlated poorly with those obtained using the other techniques and cannot therefore be relied upon in routine clinical practice. Although there was good correlation between the length of the prostate and prostatic size, assessed by pre-operative CT, this correlated poorly with the amount of tissue resected at operation.

It must therefore be concluded that the results of UPP are unfortunately not sufficiently accurate to be useful in routine clinical practice. We do not therefore utilise UPP in our unit in the investigation of BPH.

Benign or Malignant Prostatic Disease?

Clinical evaluation by rectal examination has increasingly been recognised to provide a poor assessment of prostate size and pathology. Whilst a frankly malignant gland will feel hard, indurated and may be fixed to the anterior rectal wall, it is not unusual, however, for a gland to feel slightly nodular raising the suspicion that a malignant change has occurred. In addition, subclinical prostatic malignancy is extremely common.

Patients with a suspicious-feeling prostate and/or a raised prostate specific antigen (PSA) level should be referred for further investigation. This takes the form of transrectal ultrasound (TRUS) with guided biopsy of sonographically suspicious lesions. TRUS may also be useful in staging a prostatic carcinoma or in differentiating other pathology, e.g. chronic prostatitis.

Occasionally a case occurs where despite benign appearances on clinical and TRUS evaluation persistent elevated PSA levels are obtained. Under these circumstances we recommend multiple quadrantic biopsies of the prostate gland under ultrasound guidance. Despite these screening measures there is still a significant risk of prostatic malignancy remaining undetected and such patients should be followed up with repeat PSA levels. The recent introduction of the concept of PSA density – thereby relating the PSA level to the size of the prostate gland as assessed by TRUS – should be helpful in allowing the determination those cases where the raised PSA is in fact attributable to the size of the gland alone.

References

Abrams, P.H. 1976. Sphincterometry in the diagnosis of male bladder outflow obstruction. J. Urol. 116:489–492

Abrams, P.H., Blaivas, J.G., Stanton, S.L., Andersen, J.T. 1978. The standardisation of terminology of lower urinary tract function. Scand. J. Urol. Nephrol. (suppl.) 114:5–19

Ansell, G, Tweedie, M.C., West, C.R., Evans, P., Couch, L. 1980. The current status of reactions to intravenous contrast media. Invest. Radiol. 15:S32–39

Ball, A.J., Feneley, R.C.L., Abrams, P.H. 1981. The natural history of untreated "prostatism". Br. J. Urol. 53:613–616

Davies, P. 1988. Obstructive uropathy. Br. Med. J. 297:68

Ellenbogen, P.H., Scheible, F.W., Talner, L.B., Leopold, G.R. 1978. Sensitivity of greyscale ultrasound in detecting urinary tract obstruction. A.J.R. 130:731–733

Hartman, G.W., Hattery, R.R., Witten, D.M., Williamson, B. 1982. Mortality during excretory urography. A.J.R. 139:919–922

Kitada, S., Ishisawa, N. 1981. Urethral pressure profilometry in the pre-operative assessment for prostatectomy. J. Urol. 126:89–91

Lyons, K., Matthews, P., Evans, C. 1988. Obstructive uropathy without dilatation: a potential diagnostic pitfall. Br. Med. J. 296:1517–1518

Platt, J.F., Rubin, J.M., Ellis, J.H. 1989. Distinction between obstructive and non-obstructive pyelocaliectasis with duplex Doppler sonography. A.J.R. 153:997–1000

Scola, F.H., Cronan, J.J., Schepps, B.B. 1989. Grade 1 hydronephrosis: pulsed doppler US evaluation. Radiology 171:519–520

Shehadi, W.H., Toniolo, G. 1980. Adverse reactions to contrast media: a report from the committee on safety of contrast media of the International Society of Radiology. Radiology 137:299–302

Siroky, M.B., Olsson, C.A., Krane, R.J. 1979. The flow rate nomogram. J. Urol. 122:665–668

Turner-Warwick, R.T., Whiteside, C.G., Arnold, E.P., et al., 1973. A urodynamic view of prostate obstruction and the results of prostatectomy. Br. J. Urol. 45:632–645

Turner-Warwick, R.T., Whiteside, C.G., Milroy, E.J.G., Pengelly, A.W., Thompson, D.T. 1979. The intravenous urodynamogram. Br. J. Urol. 51:15–18

Webb, J.A., Reznek, R.H., White, F.E., Cattell, W.R., Fry, I.K., Baker, L.R. 1984. Can ultrasound and computed tomography replace high dose urography in patients with impaired renal function? Q. J. Med. 53:411–425

Webb, J.A. 1990. Ultrasonography in the diagnosis of renal obstruction. Br. Med. J. 301:944–946

Chapter 8

The Complications of Prostatectomy

J.W.H. Evans and N. MacCartney

> Any operation carries with it the risk of complications.
> *Harold Ellis and Sir Roy Calne (1983)*

Introduction

An operation can only be considered "routine" when the patient has recovered from surgery and been relieved of the symptoms. A complication is any adverse event which prevents or delays this outcome. After transurethral prostatectomy (TURP) 75% of patients satisfy these criteria at 1 year post-operatively (Neal et al. 1989). With patients' expectations rising, the explosion of litigation, limited availability of medical resources, and the advent of competition in hospital practice, the prevention of complications will have an increased priority in surgical decision making.

The implementation of audit programmes, with routine gathering of information concerning all aspects of surgical care, will provide the means to assess and compare the outcome of surgical procedures objectively, using hard data and effective statistical analysis. If applied as intended, the aim of surgical audit is an improvement in the safety and efficacy of any procedure to which it is applied. Prostatic surgery constitutes 24% of the total workload and 38% of the major surgery performed by urologists (Holtgrewe et al. 1989) and should not be spared rigorous examination if we are to manage our patients and resources effectively.

There are several points concerning the nature of surgery for prostatic outflow obstruction which need to be considered before embarking on a discussion of its complications. At present TURP is the gold standard procedure although it is by no means a minor operation, nor is it the only treatment option available (Chisholm, 1990). Open prostatectomy still has a role to play (Neal, 1990) and minimally invasive techniques which minimise the physiological trespass associated with prostatic surgery are being assessed (Chapple et al. 1990; Lindner et al. 1987; McLoughlin and Williams, 1990). The question of which technique is appropriate in an individual patient is answered largely by personal preference of the operator.

Benign prostatic hypertrophy is a disease of men in their middle and late years. This age group has a high incidence of intercurrent medical problems, particularly cardiological, respiratory and cerebrovascular – if a general surgeon is a physician who operates, then the prostatic surgeon may be considered to be a geriatrician who operates. Careful pre-operative assessment of the whole patient is vital and the presence of intercurrent medical disease, particularly coronary insufficiency or arrhythmia, should result in careful consideration as to the indications to operate, which operation to perform and which anaesthetic technique should be employed.

This discussion of the complications of prostatic surgery takes the subject of anaesthesia in the elderly male patient first and then proceeds to consider complications of prostatectomy, both open and transurethral. Since 90%–95% of prostatectomies are performed transurethrally, the discussion will concentrate on that procedure. The chapter finishes with an examination of physiological disturbances peculiar to TURP and not seen after other procedures commonly performed in elderly men. These disturbances include fluid overload, hypothermia and cardiovascular responses.

ANAESTHETIC COMPLICATIONS IN THE ELDERLY MALE

TURP can be performed using a variety of anaesthetic techniques; general anaesthesia is preferred in the UK, although regional anaesthesia is safe, effective and in wide use, especially in the USA. The reason for this bias is a mixture of patient preference and expectation together with departmental routine.

Risks of Surgery and Anaesthesia

Overall Risks of Mortality During Anaesthesia and Surgery

Anaesthesia and surgery have a mortality which increases with age (Marx et al. 1973). Overall physical status as determined using physical status scoring systems has been shown to be a good predictor of risk of death following surgery in patients over 80 years of age (Djokovic and Hedley-Whyte, 1979). However, others have not found the use of such systems to be of benefit (Dripps et al. 1963; Goldmann et al. 1977).

Many studies have attempted to define a clear and precise indication of the risk of anaesthesia and surgery, especially in the elderly patient. For example between 1951 and 1960, elective hernia repair in the over 60-year-old carried a 1.8% mortality (Williams and Hale, 1966). Between 1975 and 1980, elective hernia repair in patients over 70 years of age carried a zero mortality (Tingwald and Cooperman, 1982).

Whatever surgical procedure is performed, "intuition suggests that the less the physiological trespass the lower will be the extent of the morbidity and mortality" (Krechel, 1989). This dictum is illustrated by the observation that the myocardial reinfarction rate following local anaesthesia for ophthalmic procedures is zero, whereas general or major regional anaesthesia for non-ophthalmic surgery carried a reinfarction rate of 6.1% (Steen et al. 1978).

Risk of Cardiac Arrest During Surgery

The overall risk of cardiac arrest for all operations is between 0.06% and 0.078% (Cohen et al. 1986). The incidence of death from cardiac arrest caused solely by anaesthesia is 0.009% (Keenan and Boyen, 1985), the usual causes including overdose of anaesthetic agents, inadequate ventilation, airway problems, oesophageal intubation, ventilator disconnection, long periods of hypotension and drugs (Keenan and Boyen, 1985; Tiret et al. 1986; Sorensen et al. 1984).

Risk of Myocardial Infarction During Surgery

The risk of perioperative myocardial infarction for all operations is 0.13% in patients without pre-operative cardiac disease (Tarhan et al. 1972; Steen et al. 1978). The risk of myocardial infarction in patients undergoing TURP between 1965 and 1971 has been reported as 0.8% (Melchior et al. 1974). Investigation of patients over 80 years of age demonstrates post-operative myocardial infarction in 2.1% (Wyatt et al. 1989). Patients over the age of 80 have a naturally high incidence of coronary artery disease and consequently a higher incidence of myocardial infarction is to be expected.

Studies of patients undergoing surgery between 0 and 6 months after a myocardial infarction, demonstrate pre-operative optimalisation and an aggressive invasive approach to haemodynamic monitoring with prompt treatment of any haemodynamic aberration reduces the risk of post-operative reinfarction from 6.1%–7.7% down to 1.9% (Tarhan et al. 1972; Steen et al. 1978; Rao et al. 1983a). This is good evidence that minimising the physiological disturbances incurred by surgery reduces cardiac stress.

In patients with coronary artery disease there is a fine balance between myocardial oxygen demand and delivery. Peroperative myocardial ischaemia will result if myocardial oxygen use exceeds the capacity of the coronary circulation. Left ventricular afterload is the main determinant of cardiac work (Braunwald, 1971). Effective coronary perfusion pressure, coronary vascular tone, regional vascular distribution and oxygen extraction are all important in determining myocardial oxygenation. Anaesthetic drugs, regimens and surgical trauma all affect cardiac function and the delicate balance of myocardial oxygen supply and demand. The anaesthetic management of the patient with cardiac disease is consequently a highly specialised field.

Risks of General Anaesthesia in the Elderly Male

The complications of general anaesthesia are best considered according to body systems.

Central Nervous System

A confusional state is common after anaesthesia in the elderly. The usual cause of brain dysfunction in the post-operative period is cerebral hypoxia; however, a fall in core temperature of 0.7–1 °C (Coleshaw et al. 1983) may be sufficient to cause confusion. Cerebral hypoxia causes death from brain stem hypoxia in its worst form. More frequently, especially in the elderly patient, marked confusion, disorientation and hallucination in the recovery room or in the first 24–48 hours is seen. There are three mechanisms, decreased oxygen availability, increased oxygen use and specific drug effects.

Decreased oxygen availability may be due to hypoxia with normal cerebral perfusion or decreased cerebral perfusion with normal oxygen saturation. Hypoxia may also be caused by hypothermia which shifts the oxygen–haemoglobin curve to the left. The increased use of pulse oximeters and improved anaesthetic equipment standards should reduce the contribution made by human error. Cerebral perfusion pressure is important in elderly patients who may have compromised cerebral vasculature and is determined by the difference between the mean arterial and cerebral venous pressures. Hypotension, increased venous pressure or increased intracerebral pressure can all reduce cerebral perfusion. Clearly hypotension should be avoided and especial care taken in heart failure. Effects related to drugs are usually seen in the recovery period and range from frank psychosis to mild disorientation. All these possibilities need to be considered in the patient with an acute post-operative confusional state; an immediate blood gas analysis, oxygen treatment and judicious use of benzodiazepines should be instituted. The patient and his relatives require reassurance once hypoxic brain damage is eliminated as the cause.

Awareness during surgery is due to insufficient anaesthetic agent. Sympathetic overactivity (dilated pupils, sweating, tachycardia and hypertension) indicates that increased anaesthetic is required.

Cardiovascular System

Changes in heart rate, rhythm, contractility and valvular function cause cardiac problems. A heart rate of over 100 or less than 50 is considered abnormal. Tachycardia, resulting in shortened diastolic filling time of the coronary circulation, can precipitate ischaemia. Sinus tachycardia may result from inadequate anaesthesia, anxiety, cardiac disease and drug effect (pancuronium, atropine, isoflurane). Bradycardia, resulting from increased vagal tone or drug effects (suxamethonium, halothane, enflurane, high-dose opioids or neuromuscular blocking agents), requires treatment when organ perfusion becomes impaired. Arrhythmias occur in 4.3%–7.6% of all patients perioperatively (Cohen et al. 1986) and ECG monitoring is now a standard requirement. All arrhythmias reduce cardiac output and prompt treatment should be instituted for hypotension, ischaemia, ventricular fibrillation or asystole (O'Carroll, 1985). Sinoatrial node conduction disorders are common in anaesthetised patients. A wandering pacemaker or inferior displacement of the site of impulse generation may be seen with changes in the shape or site of the P-wave (Brown et al. 1985). Absence with nodal or junctional escape rhythm are also seen. The dysfunction produced is proportional to the loss of the atrial kick – poorly tolerated by some patients. Reducing the inspired concentration of inhalational agent will usually restore an ECG to normal, but treatment with atropine or other drugs may be required.

Excitatory arrhythmias may be caused by the sinu-atrial node and although premature atrial contractions are usually self-limiting they can result in supraventricular tachycardias in patients with pre-excitation syndromes (Wolff–Parkinson–White) with inadequate anaesthesia and mimic the signs of myocardial ischaemia. Chronic valvular lesions predispose to atrial flutter or fibrillation.

Heart block or conduction defects below the sinu-atrial node will have been detected pre-operatively and cardiological advice sought on pacing. Patients with a pacemaker should not be denied surgery but are at risk from the effects of radio-frequency interference from diathermy and consequent malfunction. Again full cardiological advice and knowledge of the type of pacemaker are essential.

Elderly patients are predisposed to premature ventricular contractions, sympathetic overdrive is the commonest cause. Ventricular arrhythmias are also more common, possibly due to deterioration in sinus pacemaker activity. Hypokalaemia increases the risk of ventricular tachycardia or fibrillation, especially in patients who are digitalised or who have myocardial ischaemia; acute hypokalaemia is particularly dangerous in this respect. Ventricular irritability can also be precipitated by myocardial ischaemia.

Valvular lesions may cause problems on induction, unrecognised aortic or mitral stenosis precipitating circulatory collapse. Bacterial endocarditis in patients with valvular lesions can be prevented by appropriate prophylaxis.

Respiratory System

Trauma to the lips, teeth or tongue may occur during anaesthetic manipulations. The airway is vulnerable to obstruction as in all anaesthesia. Intubation may be difficult and precautions must be taken to ensure that the endotracheal tube is correctly sited, inflated and correctly connected to the anaesthetic circuit and ventilator. Awareness of these dangers and appropriate care is required with continuous examination of the patient and close attention to monitoring equipment.

Respiratory function decreases with age as a result of decreased motor power, decreased elastic recoil, stiffening of the chest wall and decrease in the size of intervertebral spaces (Krechel, 1989). Impaired gas exchange and reduced ventilatory reserve are the main consequences and lead to reduced arterial oxygen tension. Sleep apnoea is common post-operatively and care must be exercised prescribing pain relief.

Complications of General Anaesthesia Specific to TURP

During TURP the patient is usually positioned with the legs elevated and abducted. The use of the lithotomy position is to be avoided, especially combined with Trendelenburg, because of the potential adverse effects on the cardiovascular, respiratory and central nervous systems (Sear and Holland, 1989). The cardiovascular system may be affected as a result of increased venous return causing excessive preload. Similarly hypotension may follow if the legs are lowered suddenly at the end of the procedure. Slight elevation of the legs with moderate Trendelenburg may protect against hypotension during regional anaesthesia.

Diaphragmatic movement may be restricted due to the weight of abdominal contents in the lithotomy position. Post-operative atelectasis is proportional to the degree of hip flexion and the length of surgery. Cerebral blood flow is decreased in the lithotomy position as a result of increased intracranial venous pressure and air embolism from open prostatic venous sinuses may occur. Oesophageal reflux is another problem associated with the lithotomy position. Nerve damage and pressure sores must not be forgotten.

All of these problems will be accentuated in patients who are obese or have chronic lung disease. The Lloyd-Davies position is to be preferred in all TURP patients because these risks are minimised.

Regional Anaesthesia

Regional anaesthesia is considered by many to be the anaesthetic technique of choice for TURP, especially in the medically compromised patient. It is not, however, without its own complications. Spinal anaesthesia consists of the injection of a small volume of local anaesthetic into the cerebrospinal fluid in the subarachnoid space. The injection is performed below the termination of the spinal cord at L1 to avoid damage. All sensation is blocked rapidly. Extradural anaesthesia involves the injection of a relatively large volume of local anaesthetic into the extradural space between the spinal dura and spinal periosteum.

The innervation of the lower urinary tract from the inferior hypogastric plexus, sympathetic T12–L3 and parasympathetic S2–S4 demands that spinal or extradural anaesthesia extends to the level of T10, providing anaesthesia up to the umbilicus.

Cardiovascular Effects

An inevitable consequence of sympathetic blockade is loss of arterial and venous tone to the lower limbs. A compensatory increase in vascular tone occurs in non-blocked areas. The arterial pressure can fall by 15% during spinal anaesthesia to T10 as a direct result of decreased peripheral resistance. Reduced venous return may cause a fall in stroke volume and cardiac output (Reiz and Mangano, 1989). The effects of lumbar spinal anaesthesia on the coronary circulation have been studied in patients with coronary artery disease. Coronary blood flow was reduced in direct proportion to afterload, the main peripheral determinant of myocardial oxygen usage (Hackel et al. 1956). Lumbar extradural anaesthesia, combined with volume loading, caused a reduction in cardiac and stroke volume indices and a reduced arterial pressure. This however, improved global and regional left ventricular function, as demonstrated by an increased left ventricular ejection fraction (Baron et al. 1987). Reducing impedance to left ventricular ejection improves left ventricular performance and will reduce cardiac work and myocardial oxygen demand.

During vascular, general or orthopaedic surgery, hypotension is corrected by Trendelenburg and fluid infusion. TURP is a very different haemodynamic situation because the patient's position will afford some protection against loss of venous and arterial tone as a cause of haemodynamic changes. The debate as to whether general anaesthesia or regional block is safer in the elderly patient continues. Proponents of regional anaesthesia state that the perioperative lability of blood pressure caused by general anaesthesia will cause greater morbidity, whereas those who favour general anaesthesia use the same argument to support the opposing view. Many authorities feel that TURP is safer under regional anaesthesia as the patient is awake and alert. However, a large study of over 2000 patients failed to demonstrate any difference in morbidity or mortality between general and regional anaesthesia (Melchior et al. 1974). One advantage of spinal anaesthesia may be that significantly less blood loss occurs (Abrams et al. 1982). In general, patients with severe cardiovascular disease are not normally given regional anaesthesia because of their reduced compensatory capacity and increased susceptibility to hypotension.

Respiratory System

Regional anaesthesia is the technique of choice in patients with severe intercurrent respiratory disease because the adverse respiratory effects of general anaesthesia are avoided. However, the patient must be able to lie in an acceptable position, without coughing, for the duration of the procedure. Respiratory complications may also be avoided by the reduced opiate requirements.

Other Complications

Regional anaesthesia can cause other complications, the most dangerous of which is infection, resulting in meningitis. Trauma to the spinal cord, intravascular injection of anaesthetic agent and toxicity can also result. The most common but fortunately minor problem is post-spinal headache.

Summary

In summary, all anaesthesia is potentially hazardous, especially in the elderly. The risk of death due to anaesthesia has fallen from over 600 per million operations in 1950, to less than 40 per million in 1973 as a result of technical and pharmacological advances in anaesthesia (Office of Health Economics, 1976). Medical risks in general show an exponential decay and the level of risk decreases at a decreasing rate as a "minimum threshold" is approached. The significance of this pattern is that there comes a point when further reductions in the risk of any procedure are much harder to achieve and effectively the minimum attainable risk is reached. The concept that very old or unfit patients should not be operated upon is contentious for, although this will not subject them to the risk of operation, most of these patients would benefit from surgery.

COMPLICATIONS OF PROSTATECTOMY

Mortality of Prostatectomy

Mortality of Open Prostatectomy

Early urologists appreciated the hazards of their operations which, due to primitive anaesthesia and surgical techniques combined with lack of antibiotics, resulted in a high mortality. The literature from 1890 to 1910 has many papers referring to the conservative treatment of prostatic obstruction. However, as the safety of anaesthesia and surgery improved, so did the popularity of open prostatectomy. By the 1920s papers were being published of large series of open and perineal prostatectomy with zero mortality. However, these low mortalities were not representative of the true picture: the mortality in general hospitals in the 1920s was 19.5% reducing to 12% at a teaching centre (Thompson-Walker, 1930; Riches and Muir, 1933). More recently the average mortality rate of open prostatectomy was 2.5% (Turner and Belt, 1957; Beck and Gaudin, 1970; O'Connor et al. 1963).

A more recent series reported a 2% mortality at 1 month after open prostatectomy; this was related to cardiorespiratory status with fit patients having a mortality of 1%, moderate risk 1.2% and high risk patients 6.5%; age was also important, patients under 70 years of age had a 1.9% mortality which rose to 4% in patients over 80 (Sach and Marshall, 1977). Roos and Ramsay (1987) reported on deaths within 42 days of surgery and found a mortality rate of 1.5% after TURP, 2.1% after suprapubic prostatectomy and

0.9% after retropubic prostatectomy. The best current hospital mortality rate is thought to be in the order of 1% (Neal, 1990).

Mortality of TURP

TURP has justifiably earned an excellent reputation because of its low hospital mortality which has fallen over the last 28 years from 2.5% in 1962, to 1.3% in 1974 and to between 0.5% and 0.23% in specialist units in 1989 (Holtgrewe and Valk, 1962; Melchior et al. 1974; Kohlmert and Norlen, 1989; Mebust et al. 1989). In the district general hospital the mortality is currently 1% (Mudd et al. 1990). Improvements in anaesthesia and the trend towards specialised units with 95% of TURPs now being performed by a urologist are both factors which have contributed (Neal, 1990).

The causes of post-operative death, defined as death occurring within 30 days of surgery, are sepsis, myocardial infarction, peptic ulceration, pulmonary embolism, cerebrovascular accident, pneumonia, haemorrhage, acute renal failure, ruptured aortic aneurysm and mesenteric artery thrombosis (Holtgrewe and Valk, 1962; Melchior et al. 1974; Mebust et al. 1989).

There are several factors which significantly increase the risk of death. Chilton et al. (1978) reported 10 deaths in 1004 TURPs, 9 of these occurred in patients aged over 81 or with recent myocardial infarction, stroke, pneumonectomy, abdominoperineal resection or with a pacemaker. Sach and Marshall (1977) reported a 10% mortality from TURP in high-risk patients and an 8% mortality in men aged over 80. Wyatt et al. (1989) looked specifically at prostatectomy in the over 80-year-old and reported a 2.1% immediate mortality due to myocardial infarction, interestingly in low-risk patients on the evening of operation.

While these figures are reassuring, a number of recent studies have focused on long-term survival. In the United States a cohort study based on a 20% sample of TURPs performed on the Medicare population showed that the 3.5 month death rate following TURP is 2.8% in university hospitals, ranging to 10.8% in one small hospital, the overall 3.5 month mortality being 3.7% (Wenneburg et al. 1987). A large retrospective study has identified a 2.5 times increased risk of death from myocardial infarction 5 years after TURP as opposed to open prostatectomy. The increased death rate remained significant after controlling for age and comorbidity (Roos et al. 1989).

Morbidity of TURP

The morbidity rate following TURP is 18% and has not altered significantly in the last 15 years (Melchior et al. 1974; Mebust et al. 1989). Complications can be classified as peroperative, early post-operative, intermediate and late.

Peroperative complications include complications related to the operation itself such as urethral damage, bladder perforation, prostatic capsule perforation, extravasation of irrigation fluid, transfusion of irrigation fluid, haemorrhage, sphincter damage, nerve damage and risks to the surgeon such as hepatitis B or human immuno-virus transmission. The medical status of the patient may increase the risks of major peroperative cardiovascular complications.

Early post-operative complications (0–24 hours) in the recovery room and ward, include problems such as pain, haemorrhage, clot retention, septicaemia, hypothermia, confusion, the TUR syndrome, myocardial infarction, cardiac arrhythmias, heart failure and cardiac arrest.

Post-operative complications (after 1–5 days) may occur in the form of infections both of the urine and epididymis and strict management of the drainage system is required. The irrigation can be discontinued once the urine is the colour of rosé wine and the catheter removed after a further 24 hours. Failure to void is the most serious complication and affects up to 6.5% of cases. The overall incidence of complications in the most recent study was failure to void (6.5%), haemorrhage requiring transfusion (6.4%), clot retention (3.9%), infection (2.3%), TUR syndrome (2%), myocardial arrhythmia (1.1%) and extravasation (0.9%)(Mebust et al. 1989).

The first few (0–8) weeks after discharge can be very distressing and uncomfortable. Fifteen per cent of patients report difficulty in voiding due to blood clots and 9% had to be recatheterised. Urinary tract infection is seen in 7% and a total of 24% consulted their general practitioner within 3 months of prostatectomy (Fowler et al. 1988). Many patients report dysuria due to operative trauma or urinary tract infection. There may be severe and persistent frequency and urgency with incontinence. A most alarming problem can occur when the prostatic eschar separates after 10–12 days, often causing the passage of large fragments of clot in the urine which is uncomfortable and occasionally precipitates a substantial haemorrhage and clot retention, 2.3% of patients are rehospitalised with this problem (Roos and Ramsay, 1987). It is not surprising that most urologists review their patients after 6–8 weeks when all the trouble has settled down, usually due to an efficient general practitioner, and the patient is so pleased to be feeling better that he forgets the discomfort and misery of the first few weeks.

Long-Term Morbidity

TURP carries a high risk of reoperation compared to open surgery and the incidence of stricture formation is also high (Roos and Ramsay, 1987). The reoperation rate 8 years after TURP is 12%–15.5% compared to 1.8%–4.5% for open prostatectomy (Roos et al. 1989). There is a high incidence of cystoscopy after TURP, possibly an indication of persistent and unrelieved symptoms.

Incontinence after TURP may be the consequence of peroperative damage to the distal sphincter mechanism, detrusor failure with overflow or may be the result of unstable detrusor contractions. Detrusor failure and overflow should be apparent on physical examination and require a period of free drainage by catheter.

If the bladder is emptying then detrusor instability is a likely cause. The bladder may be unstable because of the high resistance to flow pre-operatively or as a result of irritation from the healing operation site but infection must be excluded.

A weak sphincter may respond to drills such as stopping and starting the stream several times during micturition. If the patient complains that the urine just runs away from him when he stands, then serious sphincter damage may have occurred.

If symptoms persist despite bladder training and there is no evidence of infection, then further investigation is indicated. All patients who complain of persistent frequency, urgency, or incontinence after TURP should be offered full investigation in the form of videocystometrography followed by careful cystoscopy by an experienced surgeon. Further management depends on the findings. It must be emphasised that there is no place for a repeated resection unless indicated after the patient's lower urinary tract function has been fully investigated.

Impotence is a complication which can have serious medico-legal repercussions especially in the younger patient. This is an important consideration since 34% of sexually active patients notice a deterioration in sexual function and the incidence of retrograde ejaculation is 90% (Malone et al. 1988). Excessive diathermy near the nervi erigentes at the apex of the prostate should be avoided. The potency of every patient must be recorded pre-operatively and the patient warned that failure of erection can occur after prostatectomy. All patients must similarly be informed regarding retrograde ejaculation.

Peroperative Complications of TURP

Trauma

As in other rigid endoscopic procedures such as upper gastrointestinal endoscopy, the fact that the endoscope is not merely dangerous, but potentially lethal should never be forgotten. The patient's urethra can be traumatised in four ways: (1) during instrumentation by forced attempts to pass the resectoscope blindly; (2) a tight fitting sheath or excessive movement of the resectoscope during resection can denude the urethra of epithelium leading to stricture in the long term; (3) catheterisation at the end of the procedure is usually performed "blind" using a catheter introducer – while this may prevent misplacement of the catheter under the bladder neck, the dangers of introducers are well known; and (4) the irrigation catheter itself may cause urethral bed sores and lead to stricture formation.

The following measures are recommended to avoid trauma. Instrumentation of the lower urinary tract is best accomplished under direct vision at all times. A urethrotomy using an Otis urethrotome and blade, opened to 30 Fr has been found effective in reducing the incidence of post-TURP strictures (Schultz et al. 1989). Also the appropriate size of resectoscope should be selected for each patient, adequate lubrication ensured and the instruments handled gently at all times. The irrigating catheter should be removed as soon as the bleeding is minimal.

The bladder is at risk of perforation by the diathermy loop, especially when the bladder is almost empty. This may be caused by insertion of the resectoscope or inadvertently pressing the diathermy pedal when the loop is in contact with bladder mucosa. A further method of perforating the bladder is the siting of a suprapubic catheter immediately pre-operatively in the mistaken belief that this will aid bladder drainage. It certainly may do – into the anterior abdominal wall. Several litres of irrigating fluid may be extravasated in this manner. The point of technique is that flow along a 16 Fr catheter is relatively low even without blockage by prostatic chips or blood clot. Therefore the bladder distends and irrigation fluid is forced out of the bladder around the catheter. If peroperative suprapubic drainage is contemplated, the system should be specifically designed for the job it is expected to do: wide bored, rigid and on suction (Adair, 1972; Reuter and Jones, 1972; Yachia, 1988). Otherwise suprapubic catheters should be sited at the end of the procedure.

Perforation of the bladder or prostatic capsule will result in extravasation either into the peritoneal cavity or periprostatic tissues. The situation is usually detected when smaller volumes of fluid emerge on emptying the bladder than are expected. This type of fluid load may cause delayed falls in serum sodium with hypervolaemia because the fluid is extravascular and it takes time for diffusion of electrolytes and water to occur. The management of suspected vesical perforation is to proceed immediately to laparotomy, open drainage and repair. If major extravasation secondary to a capsular perforation is suspected, then retropubic drainage should be instituted.

After TURP the patient is entirely reliant on the distal sphincter mechanism for continence. This sphincter may be damaged if resection has been performed too far distally. This is prevented by assiduous attention to the landmark of the verumontanum and the technique of holding the resectoscope so as to anchor it in such a way as to prevent the loop from being withdrawn beyond the verumontanum. The surgeon in training should not perform any resection distal to this point even though in some cases residual apical tissue will cause persistent obstruction. Such tissue can always be resected at a later date.

The nervi erigentes run close to the apex of the prostate gland and may be damaged by excessive diathermy at the apex, resulting in impotence. Haemostasis in this area should be confined to obvious individual vessels.

Diathermy is a potent source of trauma to the patient and there is no defence against thermoelectrical burns in a medico-legal action. It is the duty of both the medical and nursing staff to ensure that the diathermy plate is correctly attached to the patient and that there are no other metal contacts providing an earth as severe burns can result.

Haemorrhage

TURP is a remarkable operation in that neither the surgeon nor anaesthetist has any quantitative information as to the amount of blood loss, preferring to rely on pulse and blood pressure for haemodynamic monitoring. Haemorrhage has been correlated to the amount of irrigant absorption, length of resection and weight of tissue resected. The mean blood loss ranges from 170 to 513 ml and there is a severely skewed distribution with massive haemorrhage occurring in very few patients and not necessarily those with the largest gland size (Rawstron and Walton, 1981; Heathcote and Dyer, 1986; Hahn et al. 1988). Major blood loss is a potent cause of cardiovascular stress. Between 5% and 25% of patients require blood transfusion (Mebust et al. 1989; Perkins and Miller, 1969).

Elderly patients with a poor cardiorespiratory reserve tolerate hypovolaemia extremely poorly. Clinical signs of hypovolaemia, tachycardia and hypotension, may only appear after a substantial haemorrhage in a patient who is in the Lloyd-Davies position possibly with some Trendelenburg and who may already be vasconstricted. Massive bleeding will impair vision and render identification of anatomical landmarks difficult. The anaesthetist should be informed and resection must stop at once. The surgeon should concentrate on haemostasis and the anaesthetist on volume replacement. However, prolonged moderate blood loss is a more frequent occurrence. A resection using 15 l of irrigant which contains 0.5 g/dl of haemoglobin represents a haemoglobin loss of 75 g or a blood loss of 580 ml if the pre-operative Hb is 13 g/dl. If we remember that a starved patient may be depleted of 500 ml of fluid as a consequence of being nil by mouth for 6 hours then the loss of a further 500 ml demands action.

Despite these dangers, haemorrhage is not routinely measured during TURP. There is a simple method of measuring blood loss which uses readily available equipment at no extra cost with an accuracy of ±100 ml. This is to take an aliquot of the collected irrigating fluid and run it through a haemoximeter, usually found in the intensive care unit. The figure obtained will be between 0.1 and 1.5 g/dl. While this represents the extreme of range of the haemoximeter, an immediate estimate of haemorrhage can be obtained as follows:

([Hb]irrigation fluid × volume of irrigation fluid × 1000)/pre-operative [Hb]

This estimation is recommended for all patients undergoing TURP. The equipment to perform it is readily available at no expense and the information obtained invaluable in detecting those patients who may require volume replacement or transfusion.

Several methods of reducing blood loss have been studied. The use of cooled irrigation solution at 2°C has been reported to reduce per- and post-operative blood loss when compared to room temperature irrigation solution (Robson and Sales, 1966; Serrao et al. 1976; Kulatilake et al. 1981). This is not a uniform finding and other workers report no benefit (Cockett et al. 1961). The use of cooled irrigation solution increases the risk of hypothermia (vide infra) and cold resectoscopes and tubing are difficult and uncomfortable to handle. On the other hand, the use of warmed irrigation solutions does not appear to increase blood loss, reduces the risk of hypothermia and lowers the incidence of post-operative shivering (Heathcote and Dyer, 1986). Our view is that potential benefit from cooled irrigation solution is outweighed by the risks to the patient and discomfort to both patient and operator.

The use of drugs, particularly ethamsylate, to reduce haemorrhage does not appear to be effective (Lyth and Booth, 1990). Mention must be made of the tendency for patients who are taking aspirin to bleed more both in the perioperative and post-operative period due to the effect on platelet aggregation and vascular endothelium (Watson et al. 1990). The use of mini-dose heparin as prophylaxis against deep venous thrombosis may increase haemorrhage but the evidence is not convincing. Its use remains controversial given the operative position, which should aid venous blood flow from the legs, and early mobilisation.

Irrigation Fluid Loading and the TUR Syndrome

An additional risk peculiar to endoscopic surgery, is excessive transfusion or extravasation of irrigation solution. This complication, highly specific to TURP, remains the subject of much debate and its pathophysiology is highly complex. The reported incidence ranges from 0.9% to 7% (Melchior et al. 1974; Rhymer, 1985; Mebust et al. 1989). The mortality associated with this complication depends on the severity but can be up to 50%.

History

TURP was first performed in 1926 and became popular during the 1930s. Sterile water was used to flush the chippings into the bladder and maintain a clear field of vision both by dilution and haemolysis of red blood cells. However, some patients were noted to suffer from haemolysis, associated with a spectrum of cardiovascular, neurological and renal disturbances including hypertension, bradycardia, hypotension, heart failure, pulmonary oedema, confusion, convulsions, coma and renal failure. This clinical picture was referred to as the TUR syndrome and carried a high mortality. Its physiological basis was initially felt to be rapid intravascular absorption of sterile water causing intravascular haemolysis (Creevy, 1947). The basis of renal failure was thought to be a lower nephron nephrosis caused by formation of acid haematin from haemoglobin in an acid urine which caused mechanical blockage of renal tubules. The cardiovascular effects were thought to be the result of peripheral vasoconstriction secondary to haemoglobinaemia. These effects were attributed to the use of water and an alternative irrigating medium was sought. The characteristics of an ideal solution were that it should be non-electrolytic, non-toxic locally and systemically, transparent and cheap (Nesbit and Glickman, 1948).

Nesbit investigated the use of glycine and found no haemolysis in 45 cases using 2.2% glycine and 200 cases using 1.1% glycine. However, the use of glycine and other solutions failed to abolish the TUR syndrome. Moreover, a study of 428 patients using water as irrigant, identified significant haemolysis in 27 patients, no cases of renal failure were seen and post-operative serum haemoglobin levels were well below toxicity (Stratte, 1960). This is strong evidence that haemolysis plays little if any role in the TUR syndrome.

Harrison et al. (1956) produced the first detailed discussion of the cause and effects of the TUR syndrome in patients where an alternative to water was used. He hypothesised that dilutional hyponatraemia was responsible and that expansion of the blood volume by intravasation of electrolyte-poor fluid resulted in water intoxication. Subsequent shift of fluid from the extra-cellular space to the intracellular space caused cellular overhydration and cerebral oedema gave rise to the hypotension, bradycardia and neurological symptoms.

Animal studies in the dog demonstrated that infusion of double the plasma volume of water produced symptoms of water intoxication, killed 40% of the animals but failed to produce hypotension or renal damage despite intravascular haemolysis; a similar volume of cytal did not cause water intoxication or shock despite causing a more profound hyponatraemia. This was explained by the different volume of distribution of cytal as opposed to water (Berg et al. 1962). Further work in the rat where non-electrolytic and electrolytic infusions were given, supported the concept that hyponatraemia and cerebral oedema as a result of overhydration were the cause of the TUR syndrome (Wakim, 1971).

Cellular overhydration and hypovolaemia will have profound effects on the cardiovascular, respiratory and central nervous systems causing bradycardia and hypotension (Still and Modell, 1973; Kirchenbaum, 1979; Osborne et al. 1980). This may occur in association with hypokalaemia, hypocalcaemia, hypomagnesaemia and elevated serum bicarbonate (Malone and Dunn, 1986). Wide QRS complexes with ST depression may be observed on the electrocardiograph (Osborne et al. 1980; Rao, 1987). Pulmonary alveolar and interstitial oedema also follow volume loading and fluid shifts. Cerebral oedema could contribute to the bradycardia and hypotension while causing confusion and coma (Harrison et al. 1956; Still and Modell, 1973; Bird at al. 1982).

Other workers have focused on differences between intravascular injection and extravasation of irrigation fluid. An elegant study using a double isotope technique indicated that 29% of the fluid entered the circulation while 71% was extravasated (Oester and Madsen, 1969). A large quantity of non-electrolytic fluid in the extravascular compartment might cause movement of sodium from the intravascular space into the extravascular space while water moved in the opposite direction leading to a hypo-osmolar intravascular space (Zucker and Bull, 1984).

Other workers have suggested glycine or the products of its metabolism as a cause of symptoms after TURP (Hoyt et al. 1958). Glycine is metabolised by the liver either to oxalate or by deamination to ammonia. Hyperoxaluria may represent a hazard to the renal tubules (Fitzpatrick et al. 1981). Hyperammonaemia may cause an encephalopathy which contributes to the TUR syndrome (Hoekstra et al. 1983; Shepard et al. 1987).

Pathophysiology

The TUR syndrome is now accepted to occur as the physiological consequence of the transfusion and extravasation of large quantities of irrigating solution. The term "transfusion" is used because it is more physiologically correct: the patient does not lie on the operating table absorbing irrigation fluid, it is pumped into him at pressure. "Irrigation fluid load" describes the total amount transfused and extravasated because that is exactly what it is, a load which the patient could well do without.

The average fluid load during TURP is between 668 and 896 ml with a range of 40 ml to 2.28 l. Approximately 27% is transfused directly into the circulation and 73% is extravasated; needless to say these proportions vary. More than 1 l is absorbed in 40% of cases (Norlen et al. 1986; Oester and Madsen,

1969). The amount of fluid absorbed has been related to surgical technique, in particular, pressure in the prostatic fossa, the duration of resection and the weight of the resected tissue (Madsen and Naber, 1973; Iglesias et al. 1975; Logie et al. 1980; Gow et al. 1982; Rao et al. 1983b). For these reasons most urologists limit the duration of TURP to a maximum of 1 hour.

Fluid loading will produce physiological effects which are related to the quantity, constituents, rate and route of administration. Quantities of over 2l in 1 hour are required to produce symptoms and > 3.5 l produces coma (Ghanem and Ward, 1990). Most surgeons use either 1.5% glycine solution, sorbitol or mannitol, basing their choice on personal preference. These solutions have entirely different osmotic effects which are dependent upon the distribution, metabolism and excretion of the osmotically active component.

Glycine Infusion and Extravasation   Glycine is a non-essential amino acid which has a half-life of 85 minutes (Norlen et al. 1986). The physiological consequences of glycine infusion may be predicted as follows: an initial expansion of the plasma volume occurs causing dilutional isosmotic hyponatraemia, increased preload, filling pressures and arterial pressure; however, when the osmotically active component is metabolised, water is left in the vascular space and a hypo-osmolar situation results. The excess water redistributes to the extracellular and then the intracellular spaces causing a reduction in plasma volume, interstitial and cellular oedema. Hahn (1990) in a meticulous and definitive study of 12 patients, all of whom received a 1.5% glycine fluid load greater than 1 l, confirms this sequence of events. He reported two phases in the development of the TUR syndrome. The first phase consists of an increase in plasma volume with diffusion of sodium and potassium from the interstitial fluid into the circulation. This causes a rise in central venous pressure, plasma volume and mean arterial pressure (> 10 mm Hg) after 20 minutes. The second phase is produced by the diffusion of water from the plasma into the interstitial fluid with a sudden decrease in blood volume, central venous pressure, and arterial pressure. The initial hypertension was attributed to hypervolaemia and the fluid and electrolyte dynamics responsible for the puzzling feature of hypotension despite fluid overload and hyponatraemia is explained.

Extravasation into the periprostatic tissues will exert a less immediate effect because diffusion of fluid and electrolytes into and out of such a depot takes several hours. The glycine is not metabolised and therefore the osmotic activity is unchanged. The extravasated fluid may draw sodium in from the plasma volume and the fluid will slowly reach the intravascular space. This is demonstrated by the slow fall in serum sodium which occurs over 8 hours in patients with extravasation. These patients may be remarkably well in the immediate post-operative period but then deteriorate as sodium levels fall (Zucker and Bull, 1984).

Sorbitol and Dextrose (Metabolisable Sugars)   The osmotic effects of these solutions are similar to those of glycine as they are rapidly metabolised by the liver to fructose and glucose with a half-life of 21 minutes and 7% excreted in the urine. When large quantities are transfused the half-life increases indicating saturation of the metabolising enzyme system (Dimberg et al. 1987).

Because of the rapid metabolism of sorbitol, there is no advantage to be gained from its use. While hyperammonaemia is avoided, the catastrophic fluid and electrolyte shifts which cause hypovolaemia and cellular overhydration with glycine are just as likely to occur with sorbitol.

Mannitol   Mannitol is a non-metabolisable sugar which has therapeutic uses as an osmotic diuretic. It is excreted by the kidney and has a half-life of 163 minutes (Allgen et al. 1987). Mannitol is not metabolised but remains osmotically active in the circulating blood volume, therefore there is no hypo-osmolality associated with a mannitol fluid load. Severe hyponatraemia may result, but as there is no osmotic disturbance, cellular overhydration is obviated and the physiological consequences are minimal. The transfused mannitol will cause an osmotic diuresis and therefore the only potential clinical problems may be transient volume overload or if 5% mannitol is used the profound diuresis might cause hypovolaemia. Once the offending mannitol has been excreted the biochemical situation reverts to normal.

A case which illustrates the consequences of a mannitol load is reported by Kirchenbaum (1979). A patient underwent a resection where bleeding occurred and 40 l of 3% mannitol were used, 1l of normal saline and 2 units of blood were administered. The serum sodium fell to 99 mEq/l immediately post-operatively. However the patient displayed no clinical signs whatsoever and was alert, orientated and comfortable with normal serum osmolality. The author felt that 3% mannitol transiently increased extracellular fluid osmolality and caused a shift of water into the extracellular fluid space causing the profound hyponatraemia and stated that the presence of circulating hexose maintained serum osmolality. He also noted the early profound diuresis which prevented circulatory overload (Kirchenbaum, 1979).

Logie et al. (1980) reported on 39 patients undergoing TURP with 3% mannitol. Fluid overloading of from 4 to 7 l was detected in 6 patients, all of whom had a fall in blood pressure and bradycardia, but no fall in serum osmolality or other evidence of the TUR syndrome.

Cytal   Cytal contains sorbitol 2.7 g/100 ml and mannitol 0.54 g/100 ml. The combination of the two sugars is an attempt to treat fluid loading as it occurs, the sorbitol being metabolised and the mannitol causing an osmotic diuresis. However, 5 cases of cytal loading with a mean fluid load of 4.3 l were reported by Norris et al. (1973). All patients had symptoms and signs of hypo-osmolar hyponatraemia including chest pain, hypotension, restlessness, convulsions and cardiac arrhythmias. Two of the cases died despite the use of hypertonic saline solutions. These cases do not support the concept that a mixture of sorbitol and mannitol may reduce the dangers of fluid loading.

In summary, hypervolaemia followed by hypovolaemia is seen as an immediate consequence of intravascular fluid loading. Hyponatraemia secondary to dilution occurs. There is minimal initial change in osmolarity, but hypo-osmolarity may develop if the osmotically active component is metabolised. Hypovolaemia develops as a result of fluid shift from the intravascular volume. Interstitial and intracellular oedema follows.

Hypervolaemia and consequent circulatory overload may precipitate left ventricular failure and pulmonary oedema. Initially hypertension may be seen as filling pressures rise, however overdistension may affect ventricular function causing heart failure and hypotension.

Hyponatraemia may occur immediately or develop after several hours depending on whether the irrigation fluid load was transfused or extravasated. The hyponatraemia may be iso-osmolar or hypo-osmolar depending on the solute used. Of these two types of hyponatraemia, it is the hypo-osmolar which is most dangerous, causing interstitial and cellular oedema.

The Role of Glycine and its Metabolites

Glycine as an irrigant can exert its own effects via its breakdown products. It is metabolised by two pathways; it may be converted in the liver to glyoxalate then oxalate, which is excreted in the urine; or alternatively it can undergo deamination with the release of ammonia. Hyperoxaluria may cause renal failure by blocking the tubules if urine flow is reduced post-operatively. If large quantities of glycine need to be metabolised, a larger proportion may undergo deamination which could result in hyperammonaemia. Toxic levels of ammonia are above 350 μmol/l and levels of 850 μmol/l have been reported resulting in agitation, nausea, vomiting and coma. Raised levels of ammonia have been found in 46% of cases but the mean ammonia post-operative concentration was only 50–76 μmol/l, well below toxic levels (Hoekstra et al. 1983; Roesch et al. 1983). While serum ammonia levels do rise after TURP this rise is usually well below toxic levels. A recent study found that 8 out of 21 patients who had glycine irrigant had raised ammonia levels. Three of these exhibited signs of confusion, agitation, twitching and nausea, indeed 1 patient was comatose (Shepard et al. 1987).

When hyperammonaemia does occur the pathophysiology is related to the depressant properties of ammonia on the central nervous system. It causes increased production of the inhibitory neurotransmitter serotonin and decreases production of the excitatory neurotransmitters dopamine and noradrenaline, this imbalance leading to agitation, nausea, confusion and coma.

Prevention of Irrigation Fluid Transfusion

Operative Technique   Most patients have some degree of unnecessary fluid loading and much effort has been expended on attempts to reduce irrigation fluid loading. As fluid load is related to operative time and resected weight, many recommend that operating time should not exceed 1 hour. Once the potential for intravascular injection via open prostatic sinuses or extravasation via capsular perforations was appreciated, most operators limit resection after opening a sinus or perforating the capsule.

The Irrigation Tubing and Pressure Head   There is a consensus that hydrostatic pressure in the prostatic fossa is the cause of fluid loading (Rao, 1987). It has been elegantly demonstrated that a pressure head of 60 cm of water results in significantly less fluid loading than pressures of 70 and

90 cm of water (Madsen and Naber, 1974). Irrigation systems use gravity to provide the potential energy which generates flow between two points in a hydraulic system.

High flows of 400–1000 ml per minute are required to ensure clear vision during TURP. Due to the construction of commercial irrigating systems much energy is wasted overcoming losses due to "shock" in the tubing. This energy is lost when the tubing changes section. The tubing supplied is unnecessarily long. As a result of this the reservoir of fluid has to be elevated to a greater height above the patient if flow is to be sufficient. It has been demonstrated that adequate flow is possible at a pressure head of only 15 cm of water if a well-designed giving set is used (Rao et al. 1983b).

Intermittent and Continuous Flow Resection   Intermittent irrigation is the simplest and most popular technique of TURP. This comprises a filling stage during which resection proceeds and an emptying phase to empty the bladder when it becomes full. Studies have shown that the intravesical pressure, which follows prostatic fossa pressure closely, remained at less than 5 cm of water until the bladder reached 80% capacity. Then the pressure rose rapidly until it equalled the pressure head available. At this point the pressure equalises in the system and flow stops. This final 20% of filling is the danger area where fluid is forced into open vessels or extravasated (Rao et al. 1983b). It is erroneously stated that when flow is zero, vision deteriorates at once. While this is the case when the reservoir empties, the situation which arises when the bladder is full and the reservoir is not empty is different and highly dangerous. Although flow is zero, the pressure in the prostatic fossa is equivalent to the pressure head. Venous bleeding will be minimal and provided there are no arteries bleeding, vision remains clear and resection or haemostasis continues with high local pressures which drive fluid into open veins or through capsular perforations. It is important to be alert to this possibility and empty the bladder before it fills completely.

Continuous flow resectoscopes have been developed in an attempt to drain the bladder continuously and keep intravesical pressure low; however, they have not reduced the amount of fluid absorbed (Flechner and Williams, 1982; Stephenson et al. 1980). This failure is accounted for by the fact that these instruments do not provide efficient bladder drainage and during resection bladder pressure rises slowly to 30–40 cm of water where it remains for the duration of the procedure. This represents a prolonged intermediate pressure whereas the intermittent technique gives an intermittently high pressure (Rao et al. 1983b).

It is easy to understand why the continuous flow resectoscopes do not work. The reason lies in the position of the exit channel perforations on the resectoscope sheath. During resection the resectoscope should not perform in-and-out movements, therefore these exit perforations lie distally in the region of the sphincter mechanism. When suction is applied, the urethral mucosa is sucked onto and occludes the perforations. This produces an excess of inflow and raises the intravesical pressure. Resection can continue because flow is not halted completely. A possible solution is to place the openings of the exit channel at the tip of the sheath or beak. Meanwhile, the only advantage of continuous flow resection is that no time is wasted emptying the bladder.

Intravesical pressure can be monitored using a pressure line passed suprapubically or through the resectoscope. If the surgeon knows when the intravesical pressure is rising he can interrupt resection and empty the bladder. The fluid volumes entering and leaving the bladder can also be measured.

Specially designed systems can be used to provide suprapubic bladder drainage (Adair, 1972; Reuter and Jones, 1974; Yachia, 1988). These systems have not proven popular because of the time taken to set them up, the tendency to block and the fact that this effectively results in a bladder perforation before the resection has started. It should be emphasised again that a size 16 Foley catheter will not provide adequate flow to keep the bladder empty and should not be used for peroperative suprapubic drainage.

Early Detection of Fluid Load Irrigation fluid loading may therefore be difficult to prevent due to local conditions resulting from the requirement for a clear field of vision. An alternative approach is to accept that some fluid load is inevitable and that while in most patients, the quantity is insufficient to cause clinical problems, some patients will suffer a large transfusion which is entirely idiosyncratic and unpredictable. Therefore an effective strategy may be to detect the presence of fluid loading at an early stage. This will allow the operation to be stopped, preventing the development of full-blown TUR syndrome.

A gravimetric system consisting of transducers placed under the operating table is under assessment at the Middlesex Hospital. This system gives a continuous readout of the patients weight change which is accurate to 50 g. Initial results indicate that this simple non-invasive method of assessing total fluid balance is of great clinical value in the early detection of irrigation fluid loading, enabling resuscitation to be instituted at an early stage and possibly preventing the development of the full-blown TUR syndrome.

Another method suggested for routine use is the addition of alcohol to the irrigation solution and the performance of regular "breathalyser" tests. This method certainly works, but it is not ideal to add alcohol to what may already be a complicated pharmacological cocktail. Serial measurement of serum sodium has also been advocated (Watkins-Pitchford et al. 1984)

Invasive monitoring of central venous, atrial and pulmonary artery pressures to look for haemodynamic effects of fluid loading is highly invasive and inappropriate for fit patients undergoing routine TURP.

Diagnosis and Management of the TUR Syndrome

The management of the TUR syndrome is firstly to recognise that fluid loading has occurred. A high index of suspicion is required because delayed recovery from anaesthesia is often the first indication of fluid loading.

Clinical Picture The awake patient may complain of a prickling or burning sensation in the hands or neck, nausea, chest pains, visual disturbances and shortness of breath prior to confusion, agitation and eventual coma. The signs are an initial increase in blood pressure followed by bradycardia and hypotension. Cerebral irritability, confusion, coma or convulsion may be seen. If the TUR syndrome is suspected, the operation must be stopped and biochemical analysis performed. A serum sodium of less than 125 mmol/l combined with the clinical features above is diagnostic. Changes in osmolality are dependent upon the constituents of the irrigation fluid and are predictable. Special assays for the constituents of the irrigation fluid are not usually available.

Treatment   There is no consensus for the treatment of the TUR syndrome. The aim of treatment must be to correct the physiological and homeostatic imbalance. Mild cases may be managed by fluid restriction, close observation and waiting for spontaneous diuresis. Homeostatic mechanisms usually return the serum biochemistry to normal within 24 hours.

Severe cases of water intoxication with hypo-osmolar hyponatraemia, cellular overhydration and cerebral oedema, with serum sodium < 120 mmol/l, hypocalcaemia, hypomagnesaemia and profound clinical signs, demand intervention (Osborne et al. 1980). Recommended treatment regimes have included the use of frusemide to induce a diuresis (Osborne et al. 1980). Mannitol in 10% or 20% solutions has been recommended as an osmotic diuretic; it is also a treatment for cerebral oedema (Allen et al. 1981). Sodium bicarbonate, 100 ml of 8.4% solution is potentially hazardous because it can exacerbate alkalosis and hypocalcaemia (Malone et al. 1986). Hypertonic saline solutions, 500 ml of 1.8% solution or 200 ml of 5% solution infused over 20 minutes are the most popular methods with rapid responses seen (Swaminathan and Tormey, 1981; Roesch et al. 1983; Ghanem and Ward, 1990). Care should be exercised in intervention aimed at correction of hyponatraemia due to the risk of exacerbating volume overload and the development of central pontine myelinolysis which is associated with over rapid correction of hyponatraemia (Norris et al. 1973; Laureno and Karp, 1988; Sterns et al. 1989). The usual course of events is for a large diuresis to occur and the electrolytes to return to normal.

The steps to take after recognition of the TUR syndrome are firstly to stop surgery and send blood for sodium estimation. If the clinical picture is of a severe overload, the patient should be transferred to the intensive care unit. The complex situation of hypovolaemic shock with volume overload and hyponatraemia can then be managed with full cardiovascular support including invasive haemodynamic monitoring using a pulmonary artery catheter, intravenous calcium, inotropic therapy and plasma volume expanders. Hyponatraemia must be corrected slowly in order to avoid cerebral pontine myelinolysis. Controlled hyperventilation may help reduce cerebral oedema. The use of diuretics or hypertonic saline solutions is not essential provided that full cardiovascular support is implemented (Singer et al. 1990).

Risks to the Surgeon

The surgeon is at risk from conjunctival contamination by droplets. Because of the risk of hepatitis B and the new spectre of HIV infection, it has been recommended that surgeons wear eye protection or use video-TUR (Davies and Harrison, 1991; O'Boyle, 1990).

Prophylactic Measures in Prostatectomy Patients

Much debate surrounds the use of prophylaxis against both septicaemia and deep venous thrombosis. While there is no doubt that patients with valvular heart disease, any prosthetic implant or similar indication should have antibiotic prophylaxis for any anaesthetic or urological procedure, the question remains as to whether all TURP patients should have antibiotic prophylaxis. The fact that septic complications were the commonest cause of death in the most recent major survey (Mebust et al. 1989) indicates that this question demands to be taken seriously. The incidence of septicaemia is between 1% and 4% (Robinson et al. 1980; Shah et al. 1981) and the mortality is 20% in the over 65-year-old. It is surprising that only 10% of British urologists use antibiotic prophylaxis routinely (Wilson and Lewi, 1985). Prophylaxis has been shown to reduce the incidence of post-operative bacteriuria, urinary tract infections and septicaemia (Shearman et al. 1988). In this last study, 5 of 55 developed septicaemia in the placebo group whereas in the treatment group only 1 out of 55 suffered septicaemia.

Whatever the incidence of septic complications, it only takes 1 patient to die from septic complications for the antibiotic and prophylaxis policy of a unit to be placed firmly under the spotlight at audit meetings. A sensible local prophylaxis policy should be agreed with the help of a microbiologist. There will be much argument over what the best policy is; the current policy of this unit is to use three doses of gentamicin and ampicillin, the first dose given intravenously on induction of anaesthesia. Single dose oral prophylaxis is an attractive alternative.

The use of prophylaxis against deep venous thrombosis (DVT) and pulmonary embolism is another contentious issue. General surgical patients over the age of 55 all receive subcutaneous heparin or anti-thromboembolism stockings or both. Urologists are concerned that blood loss may be increased if heparin is used; however, there is no convincing evidence for this. Anti-embolism stockings carry no such risk and can be used as routine. In addition, patients with additional risk factors such as a previous history or family history of DVT should probably have low-dose heparin dependent upon individual risk factors.

The Recovery Room and Ward

Situations which arise in the recovery room include clot retention, pain, hypothermia, confusion or hypotension. Clot retention is manifest by failure of irrigation and lower abdominal discomfort. It is usually relieved by bladder washout, but if haemorrhage is profuse and continuous, traction on the catheter may help. If this fails, resuscitation should be instituted and the patient returned to theatre for haemostasis, should endoscopic measures fail, then open operation is indicated to control bleeding.

Pain control is usually achieved with opiates. Hypothermia can contribute to discomfort. Opiates will relieve the pain and prevent shivering which is a severe cardiorespiratory stress. Hypothermia is best corrected slowly using a space blanket. The management of confusional state has been considered previously.

Post-operative hypotension and collapse may be caused by haemorrhage, myocardial infarction, TUR syndrome or septicaemia. Diagnosis is dependent on history, particularly intraoperative events and notice should be taken of the duration of surgery as this is related to fluid transfusion and haemorrhage. Clinical signs may be unhelpful in making a diagnosis but immediate measures are to ensure adequate oxygen supply and circulation. Blood should be drawn for serum electrolytes, haemoglobin, blood cultures and blood gas estimation, an electrocardiograph will indicate myocardial ischaemia. If simple measures fail to produce an improvement then the patient should be transferred to an intensive care unit where full cardiorespiratory control can be established and further management undertaken with full reference to the results of invasive monitoring.

Other Physiological Disturbances Caused by TURP

Thermodynamics, Hypothermia and TURP

The possibility that hypothermia consequent upon TURP may be responsible for adverse effects has not received sufficient attention. Indeed hypothermia may be responsible for a number of the disturbances seen in the TUR syndrome which have previously been attributed to hypo-osmolarity, hyponatraemia or more recently hyperammonaemia. The addition of the physiological catastrophe of hypothermia to these disturbances may contribute to the high mortality seen. A review of thermoregulation and the systemic effects of hypothermia will be followed by a discussion of the relationship between TURP and hypothermia.

Thermoregulation

The human is homeothermic and thermoregulates to maintain an optimal core temperature for respiration, gas exchange, enzyme action, and electrophysiological processes. There is a homeostatic balance between heat production and loss. Heat production may be obligatory from metabolic processes or facultative. Facultative heat production may be derived from shivering or non-shivering thermogenesis. Heat loss is by conduction, convection, radiation and sweating. 75% of heat loss is from exposed surfaces and 25% is divided between sweating and the respiratory tract. Man has been referred to as a tropical animal and requires an ambient air temperature of 28°C to maintain body temperature in an unclothed state.

Thermoregulation is impaired in the elderly (Collins et al. 1977). This is exacerbated by both general and regional anaesthesia (Jenkins et al. 1983). Elderly patients have been found to have lower core temperatures both on arrival in theatre and post-operatively than a younger control group (Vaughan et al. 1981).

During general anaesthesia, body heat energy is distributed away from the body core to the periphery. This occurs because the usual mechanisms of protecting the core temperature are in abeyance. The temperature of the operating theatre is 21–23ºC and this is the most important factor relative to body temperature during general surgery (Morris and Wilkey, 1970; Morris, 1971 a,b; Roizen et al. 1980). The administration of cold fluids and high flow dry anaesthetic gases also cause heat loss. During laparotomy heat loss occurs at a rate of 40–50 kJ/hr. Therefore elderly patients undergoing surgery are entirely at the mercy of their environment and are at risk from developing hypothermia.

Hypothermia is defined as a core temperature of less than 35 ºC although some anaesthetists feel that the definition should be extended to less than 36 ºC (Carli, 1990). There are effects upon every system. The physiological definition of hypothermia is "the condition of a temperature-regulating animal when the core temperature is more than one standard deviation below the mean core temperature of the species in resting conditions in a thermoneutral environment" (Bligh and Johnson, 1973).

Systemic Effects of Low Core Temperatures

Cardiovascular Effects   In the unanaesthetised patient, hypothermia is known to affect myocardial performance because of effects upon myocardial conduction, contractility and excitability; the consequences are bradycardia, fall in stroke volume and decreased cardiac output; disturbances of electrical activity result in arrhythmias; there is also a marked rise in systemic vascular resistance and left ventricular afterload (Carli, 1989; Reuler, 1978).

The anaesthetised patient is unable to generate heat by shivering but vasoconstriction does occur and filling pressures may be misleading. The rise in afterload secondary to vasoconstriction increases demand on the heart. The incidence of deep vein thrombosis and pulmonary embolism is higher when surgery is performed at cold ambient temperatures (Lunn, 1969).

Disturbances in perfusion lead to tissue ischaemia and metabolic acidosis. The oxyhaemoglobin dissociation curve is shifted to the left, further impairing oxygen delivery.

Respiratory Effects   A fall in temperature reduces the rate and depth of respiration and shifts the oxyhaemoglobin dissociation curve to the left, affecting oxygen uptake in the lungs and delivery to the tissues.

Effects on the Central Nervous System   A fall in core temperature of 0.7° C is sufficient to cause impaired memory registration and reasoning with confusional state (Coleshaw et al. 1983). Cerebral blood flow falls by 7% per degree fall in body temperature as a result of decreased cardiac output and increased cerebrovascular resistance (Carli, 1989).

Renal Effects   Cold diuresis results because of reduced oxidative tubular reabsorption leading to sodium and water loss, hypovolaemia can result from both renal losses and the effect of a fluid shift to the extracellular space (Reuler, 1978).

Haematological Effects   The haematocrit can be increased by 7% and viscosity and platelets by 25% following a fall in body temperature of 0.4 °C (Keatinge et al. 1984). The risk of deep venous thrombosis has already been mentioned.

Pharmacokinetic Effects   The pharmacology of anaesthetic and adjuvant drugs is affected profoundly. The MAC of inhaled agents decreases with temperature and the half-life of intravenous drugs may be prolonged. These factors predispose to relative anaesthetic overdose and delayed awakening.

Rewarming   The physiological insult of hypothermia continues with the rewarming phase. Shivering may increase oxygen consumption by between 300% to 800% (Horvath et al. 1956; Benzinger 1969). Shivering increases oxygen demand and lactic acid production significantly. There may be no adverse effects in a patient with a normal haemoglobin, no large pulmonary shunt and who is able to increase cardiac output and ventilation adequately; however, the increased minute ventilation and cardiac output plus hypoxaemia may be tolerated poorly by patients with a limited cardiac reserve or a decreased ventilatory capacity. Hypoxia, delayed awakening and myocardial infarction can occur (Johnstone and Vaughan, 1988).

Thermodynamics and TURP

The similarity between the effects seen during the TUR syndrome and those caused by hypothermia is remarkable. The core temperature falls at a rate of 1–1.5 °C per hour during TURP especially if cooled irrigating solution is used (Allen, 1973). Reductions of up to 6 °C have been reported (Rawstron and Walton, 1981; Allen, 1973; Carpenter, 1984). These rapid falls in core temperature indicate that body heat is lost substantially faster during TURP than during other operations. Heat is lost 32 times faster into water than into air, and the obvious cause is the routine use of room temperature, or worse, cooled irrigation fluid.

The simple precautions of warming the irrigation fluid to 38 °C, a warming mattress and a humidifying filter in the anaesthetic circuit reduced the loss in core temperature to 0.3 °C and rendered the patient isothermic in terms of total body heat. Peroperative core temperature changes during control procedures in age-matched men (hernia repair and testicular exploration) and standard TURP using ambient temperature irrigant are displayed in Fig. 8.1. Measures to avoid reductions in core temperature are sensible precautions in elderly patients and are recommended as routine.

Acute Haemodynamics of TURP

There is little data available on peroperative cardiovascular performance during routine TURP. Dilution techniques performed before and after

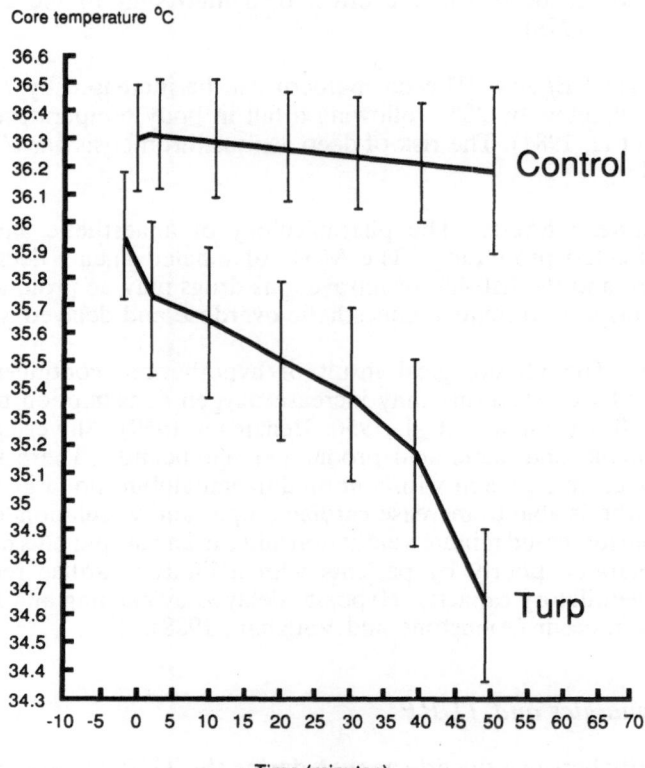

Fig. 8.1. The changes in peroperative core temperature seen following TURP as contrasted with control procedures (± SE).

TURP in an unselected group of 30 patients showed a fall in cardiac output of 17% after surgery (Mebust et al. 1970). A study of patients with intercurrent cardiac disease sufficient to merit a Swan-Ganz catheter identified unpredictable haemodynamic responses, particularly an elevated pulmonary artery wedge pressure (> 21 mmHg) in 4 cases and marked changes in systemic vascular resistance in 7 cases (De Angelis et al. 1982). Pulmonary artery catheterisation is inappropriate in a study of healthy patients undergoing routine TURP. A pilot study of haemodynamic response to TURP using oesophageal Doppler ultrasound to measure blood flow in the descending thoracic aorta has confirmed that unexpected haemodynamic responses occur during routine TURP (Evans et al. 1991). Cardiac output fell as a result of bradycardia and decreased stroke volume, no significant changes could be identified during control procedures (Fig. 8.2). The mean fall was 29% (range 20%–43%). The systemic vascular resistance rose; the mean rise was 47% (range 10%–72%). These changes were not related to irrigation fluid load, haemorrhage, operating time or the surgeon. They could not be detected by measurement of heart rate and blood pressure alone and are remarkably similar to those seen during hypothermia. A rise

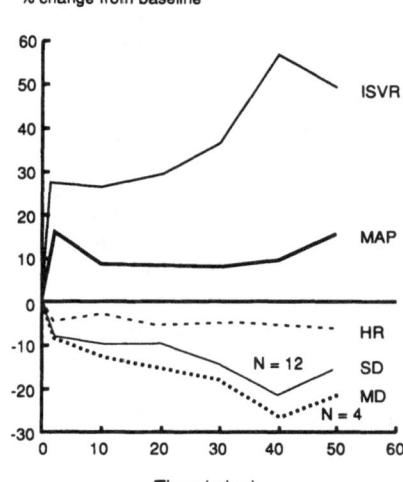

Fig. 8.2. Graphs demonstrating the haemodynamic responses during control procedures as contrasted with those seen during transurethral resection of the prostate looking at the parameters: mean arterial pressure (MAP); stroke distance (volume) (SD); heart rate (HR); minute distance (cardiac output) (MD); index of systemic vascular resistance (ISVR).

in systemic vascular resistance indicates increased left ventricular afterload and cardiac work, this will in turn increase myocardial oxygen demand and should coronary perfusion be unequal to increased oxygen demand, ischaemic damage could result.

Preliminary results indicate that these haemodynamic responses are prevented when an isothermic technique of TURP is used which stops heat loss and stabilises the core temperature. A fall in core temperature could increase afterload as a result of neurovascular response or increases in whole blood viscosity (Evans, unpublished data).

Conclusion

TURP remains the treatment of choice for prostatic bladder outflow obstruction (Chisholm, 1990). It appears to have a slightly lower hospital mortality than open prostatectomy and the shorter inpatient stay and convalescence with rapid return to active life give it the edge over open surgery in terms of patient acceptability and health care economics. However, there is an increased reoperation rate of 2% per year and an increased risk of myocardial infarction compared to open surgery. The mortality of TURP rises in unfit patients and in patients aged over 80 years, this has stimulated interest in alternative methods of treatment such as stenting, laser and microwave;

however, the initial enthusiasm for new methods will have to bear the test of time and the scrutiny of properly designed clinical trials before their role is defined.

Open prostatectomy remains a valid option in the younger, fitter patient with a big prostate gland which may take over 1 hour to resect. This patient has to be served by his operation for longer and open surgery has a significantly lower reoperation rate.

TURP remains the gold standard procedure, affording excellent results in the hands of the experienced operator. It is not, however, an operation to be undertaken lightly and there are still many questions which need to be resolved, particularly which irrigation solution is safest. I would suggest 3% mannitol on the evidence presented in this chapter. Which technique of TURP is safest, intermittent resection, continuous flow resection or suprapubic drainage? Which anaesthetic technique is safest? How best to prevent heat loss and thermal stresses? Despite these questions and the threat posed by new techniques, particularly in phase ultrasound which can deliver accurate tissue damage and new pharmacological treatments which do reduce gland size, it is likely that TURP will continue to outperform its competitors for many years.

References

Abrams, P.H.P., Shah, P.J., Bryning, K., Gaches, C.G.C., Ashken, M.H., Green N.A. 1982. Blood loss during transurethral resection of the prostate. Anaesthesia 37:71–73

Adair, E.L. 1972. Suprapubic shunt. J. Urol. 108:449

Allen, P.R., Hughes, R.G., Goldie, D.J., Kennedy, R.H. 1981. Fluid absorption during transurethral resection. Br. Med. J. 282:740

Allen, T.D. 1973. Body temperature changes during prostatic resection as related to the temperature of the irrigation solution. J. Urol. 110:433–435

Allgen, L.G., Norlen, H., Kolmert, T., Berg, K. 1987. Absorption and elimination of mannitol solution when used as an isotonic irrigating agent in connection with transurethral resection of the prostate. Scand. J. Urol. Nephrol. 21:177–184

Baron, J.F., Coriat, P., Mundler, O., Fauchet, M., Bousseau, D., Vicars, P. 1987. Left ventricular global and regional function during lumber epidural anaesthesia in patients with angina pectoris. Influence of volume loading. Anaesthesiology 66:621

Beck, A.D., Gaudin, H.J. 1970. The Hryntschak prostatectomy. I. A review of 1346 cases. J. Urol. 103:637–640

Benzinger, T.H. 1969. Heat regulation: homeostasis of central temperature in man. Physiol. Rev. 49:671–759

Berg, G., Fedor, E.J., Fisher, B. 1962. Physiologic observations related to the transurethral resection reaction. J. Urol. 87:596–600

Bird, D., Slade, N., Fenely, R.C. 1982. Intravascular complication of transurethral resection of the prostate gland. Br. J. Urol. 54:564–565

Bligh, J., Johnson, K.G. 1973. Glossary of terms for thermal physiology. J. App. Physiol. 35:941–961

Braunwald, E. 1971. Control of myocardial oxygen consumption. Physiologic and clinical considerations. Am. J. Cardiol. 27:416–432

Brown, B.R. Jr., Blitt, C.D., Vaughan R.W.. 1985. Anaesthesia complications. In: Clinical anaesthesiology. St Louis, Mosby, pp 317–331

Carli, F. 1990. Metabolic disturbances of hypothermia. Baillière's Clin. Anaesthesiol. 3(2):405–421

Carpenter, A.A. 1984. Hypothermia during transurethral resection of prostate. Urology 23:122–124

Chapple C.R., Milroy E.J.G., Rickards D. 1990. A permanently implanted urethral stent for prostate obstruction in the unfit patient; preliminary report. Br. J. Urol. 66:58–65

Chilton, C.P., Morgan, R.J., England, H.R., Paris, A.M.I., Blandy, J.P. 1978. A critical evaluation of the results of transurethral resection of the prostate. Br. J. Urol. 50:542–546

Chisholm, G.D. 1990. Benign prostatic hyperplasia: the best treatment. Br. Med. J. 299:215–216

Cockett, A.T.K., Schultz, J., Franks, D. 1961. Use of refrigerated solutions during transurethral surgery. J. Urol. 85:632–635

Cohen, M.M., Duncan, P.G., Pope, W.D.B., Wolkenstein C. 1986. A survey of 112 000 anaesthetics at one teaching hospital (1975–1983). Can. Anaesth. Soc. J. 33:22–31

Coleshaw, S.R.K., Van Someren, R.N.M., Wolff, A.H., et al. 1983. Impaired memory registration and speed of rewarming caused by low body temperature. J. Appl. Physiol. 27:209–212

Collins, K.J., Dore, C., Exton-Smith, A.N., et al. (1977) Accidental hypothermia and impaired temperature homeostasis in the elderly. Br. Med. J. i:353–356

Creevy, C.D. 1947. Haemolytic reactions during transurethral resection. J. Urol. 58:125–131

Davies, J.H., Harrison, G.S.M. 1991. Should urologists wear spectacles for transurethral resection of the prostate? Br. J. Urol. 67:182–183

De Angelis, L., Chang, P., Kaplan, J.H., et al. 1982. Hemodynamic changes during prostatectomy in cardiac patients. Crit. Care. Med. 10:38–40

Dimberg, M., Allgen, L.G., Norlen, H., Kolmer, T. 1987. Experience with 2.5% sorbitol solution as an irrigating fluid in transurethral resection of the prostate. Scand. J. Urol. Nephrol. 21:169–176

Djokovic, J.L., Hedley-Whyte, J. 1979. Prediction of outcome of surgery and anesthesia in patients over 80. J.A.M.A. 242:2301–2306

Dripps, R.D., Lamont, A., Eckenhoff J.E., 1963. New classification of physical status. Anaesthesiology 24:111

Ellis, H.R., Calne, Sir R.C. 1983. Complications of surgery. In: Lecture notes in general Surgery. Oxford, Blackwell Scientific Publications, p 19

Evans, J.W.H., Singer, M., Chapple, C.R., MacCartney N., Coppinger, S.W.V., Milroy, E.J.G. 1991. Haemodynamic evidence for cardiac stress during transurethral prostatectomy: preliminary communication. Br. J. Urol. 67:376–380

Fitzpatrick, J.M., Kasidas, G.P., Rose, G.A. 1981. Hyperoxaluria following glycine irrigation for transurethral prostatectomy. Br J. Urol 53:250–252

Flechner, S.M., Williams, R.D. 1982. Continuous flow and conventional resectoscope methods in transurethral prostatectomy: comparative study. J. Urol. 127:257–259

Fowler, S.J., Wennberg, J.E., Timothy, R.P., Barry, M.J., Mulley, A.G., Hanley, D. 1988. Symptom status and quality of life following prostatectomy. JAMA 259:3018–3022

Ghanem, A.N., Ward, J.P. 1990. Osmotic and metabolic sequelae of volumetric overload in relation to the TUR syndrome. Br. J. Urol. 66:71–78

Goldmann, L., Caldera, D.I., Nussbaum, S.R., et al. 1977. Multifactorial index of cardiac risk in non-cardiac surgical procedures. N. Engl. J. Med. 297:845

Gow, J.G., Blandy, J.P., Kinder, C.H., Lumb, G.N., Milroy, E.J.G., Ress, R.W.M. 1982. Report of the standing committee on urological instruments: irrigating cystoscopes. Br. J. Urol. 54:1–4

Hackel, D.B., Sancetta, S.M., Kleinerman, J. 1956. Effects of hypotension due to spinal anaesthesia on coronary blood flow and myocardial metabolism in man. Circulation 13:92

Hahn, R., Berlin, T., Lewenhaupt, A. 1988. Irrigating fluid absorption and blood loss during transurethral resection of the prostate studied with a regular interval monitoring method. Scand. J. Urol. Nephrol. 22:23–30

Hahn, R.G. 1990. Fluid and electrolyte dynamics during development of the TUR syndrome. Br. J. Urol. 66:79–84

Harrison, R.H., Boren, J.S., Robison, J.R. 1956. Dilutional hyponatraemic shock: another concept of the transurethral prostatic resection reaction. J. Urol. 75:95–110

Heathcote, P.S., Dyer, P.M. 1986. The effect of warm irrigation on blood loss during transurethral prostatectomy under spinal anaesthesia. Br. J. Urol. 58:669–671

Hoekstra, P.T., Khanosiki, R., McCamich, M.A., Bergen, W., Heetderks, D.R. 1983. Transurethral prostatic resection syndrome. A new perspective: encephalopathy with associated hyperammonaemia. J. Urol. 130:704–707

Holtgrewe, H.L., Valk, W.L. 1962. Factors influencing the mortality and morbidity of transurethral prostatectomy: a study of 2015 cases. J. Urol. 87:450–459

Holtgrewe, H.L., Mebust, W.K., Dowd, J.B., Cocket, A.T.K., Peters, P.C., Proctor, C. 1989. Transurethral prostatectomy: practice aspects of the dominant operation in American urology. J. Urol. 141:248–253

Horvath, S.M., Spurr, G.B., Hutt, B.K., Hamilton L.H. 1956. Metabolic cost of shivering. J. Appl. Physiol. 8:595–602

Hoyt, H.S., Goegel, J.L., Lee, H.I., Schoenbrod, J. 1958. Types of shock-like reaction during transurethral resection and relation of acute renal failure. J. Urol. 79:500–506

Iglesias, J.J., Sporer, A., Gellman, A.C., Seebode, J.T. 1975. New Iglesias resectoscope with continuous irrigation, simultaneous suction and low intravesical pressure. J. Urol. 114:929–933

Jenkins, J., Fox, J., Sharwood-Smith, 1983. Changes in body heat during transvesical prostatectomy. Anaesthesia 38:748–753

Johnstone, K.J., Vaughan, R.S. 1988. Delayed recovery from general anaesthesia. Anaesthesia 43:1024–1025

Keatinge, W.R., Coleshaw, S.R.K., Cotter, F., Mattock, M., Murphy, M., Chelliah, R., 1984. Increase in platelet and red cell counts, blood viscosity and arterial pressure during mild surface cooling factors in mortality from coronary and cerebral thrombosis in winter. Br. Med. J. 289:1405–1408

Keenan, R.L., Boynean, C.P. 1985. Cardiac arrest due to anaesthesia. J.A.M.A. 253:2373–2377

Kirchenbaum, M.A. 1979. Severe mannitol-induced hyponatraemia complicating transurethral resection of the prostate gland. J. Urol. 121:687–688

Kohlmert, T., Norlen, H. 1989. Transurethral resection of the prostate, a review of 1111 cases. Int. Urol. Nephrol. 21:47–55

Krechel, S.W., 1989. The elderly. In: General anaesthesia. Nimmo, W.S., Smith, G. eds. Oxford, Blackwell Scientific Publications, pp 933–950

Kulatilake, A.E., Roberts, P.N., Evans, D.F., Wright, J. 1981. The use of cooled irrigating solution during transurethral resection of the prostate. Br. J. Urol. 53:261–262

Laureno, R., Karp, B.I. 1988. Pontine and extrapontine myelinolysis following rapid correction of hyponatraemia. Lancet ii:1439–1440

Lindner, A., Golomb, J., Sigel, Y., Lev, A. 1987. Local hyperthermia of the prostate gland for the treatment of benign prostatic hyperplasia and urinary retention. Br. J. Urol. 60:567–571

Logie, J.R.C., Keenan, R.A., Whiting, P.H., Steyn, J.H. 1980. Fluid absorption during transurethral prostatectomy. Br. J. Urol. 52:526–528

Lunn, H.F. 1969. Observations on heat gain and loss in surgery. Guy's Hosp. Rep. 118:117–127

Lyth, D.R., Booth, C.M. 1990. Does ethamsylate reduce haemorrhage in transurethral prostatectomy? Br. J. Urol. 66:631–634

Madsen, P.O., Naber, K.G. 1974. The importance of pressure in the prostatic fossa and absorption of irrigating fluid during transurethral resection of the prostate. J. Urol. 109:447–452

Malone, P.R., Cook, A., Edmonson, R., Gill, M.W., Shearer, R.J. 1988. Prostatectomy: patients' perception and long-term follow-up. Br. J. Urol. 61:234–238

Malone, W., Dunn, M. 1986. The management of massive haemorrhage following transurethral resection of the prostate in the elderly. Br. J. Urol. 54:564–565

Marx, G.F., Matco, C.V., Orkin, L.R., 1973. Computer analysis of postanaesthetic deaths. Anaesthesiology 39:54–59

McLoughlin, J., Williams, G., 1990. Alternatives to prostatectomy. Br. J. Urol. 65:313–316

Mebust, W.K., Brady, T.W., Valk, W.L. 1970. Observations on cardiac output, blood volume, central venous pressure and electrolyte changes in patients undergoing transurethral prostatectomy. J. Urol. 103:632–636

Mebust, W.K., Holtgrew, H.L., Cocket, A.T.K., Peters, P.C., 1989. Transurethral prostatectomy: immediate and postoperative complications. A cooperative study of 13 participating institutions evaluating 3855 patients. J. Urol. 141:243–247

Melchior, J., Valk, W.L., Foret, J.D., Mebust, W.K. 1974. Transurethral prostatectomy; computerised analysis of 2223 consecutive cases. J. Urol. 112:634

Morris, R.H., Wilkey, B.R. 1970. The effects of ambient temperature on patient temperature during surgery not involving body cavities. Anaesthesiology 32:102–107

Morris, R.H. 1971a. Operating room temperature in anaesthetized paralysed patients. Arch. Surg. 102:95–97

Morris, R.H. 1971b. Influence of ambient temperature on patient temperature during intra-abdominal surgery. Ann. Surg. 173:230–233

Mudd, D.G., Deans, G.T., Lee, B.G. 1990. Prostatectomy in a district hospital. J.R. Coll. Surg. Edinb. 35:365–368

Neal, D.E., Ramsden, P.D., Sharples, L., et al. 1989. Outcome of elective prostatectomy. Br. Med. J. 299:762–767

Neal, D.E. 1990. Prostatectomy: an open or shut case (review). Br. J. Urol. 66:449–454

Nesbit, R.M., Glickman, S.I. 1948. The use of glycine solution as an irrigating medium during transurethral resection. J. Urol. 59:1212–1216

Norlen, H., Allgen, L., Vinan, E., Bedrelidou-Classon, G. 1986. Glycine solution as an irrigating solution during transurethral resection of the prostate. Scand. J. Urol. Nephrol. 20:19–26

Norris, H.T., Aasheim, G.M., Sherrard, D.J., Tremain, 1973. Symptomatology, pathophysiology and treatment of the transurethral resection of the prostate syndrome. Br. J. Urol. 45:420–427

O'Boyle, P.J. 1990. Video endoscopy, the remote operating technique. Br. J. Urol. 65:557–559

O'Carroll, T.M. 1985. Complications during anaesthesia. In: Textbook of anaesthesia. Smith, G., Aitkenhead, A.R., eds. Edinburgh, Churchill Livingstone, pp 176–189

O'Connor, V.J., Bulkley, G.J., Sokol, J.K. 1963. Low suprapubic prostatectomy: comparison of results with the standard operation in two comparable groups of 142 patients. J. Urol. 90:301–304

Oester, A., Madsen, P.O. 1969. Determination of absorption of irrigating solution during transurethral resection of the prostate gland by means of radio isotopes. J. Urol. 102:714–719

Office of Health Economics. 1976. Anaesthesia. Office of Health Economics, London

Osborne, D.E., Rao, P.N., Green, M.J., Barnard, R.J. 1980. Fluid absorption during transurethral resection. Br. Med. J. 281:1549–1550

Perkins, J.B., Miller, H.C. 1969. Blood loss during transurethral prostatectomy. J. Urol. 101:93–97

Rao, T.L.K., Jacobs, K.H., El-Etr, A.A. 1983a. Reinfarction following anaesthesia in patients with myocardial infarction. Anaesthesiology 59:449–505

Rao, P.N., Lister, B., Livesey, J.L., Barnard, R.J. 1983b. Are we using the right irrigating system? Br. J. Urol. 55:287–293

Rao, P.N., 1987. Fluid absorption during urological endoscopy. Br. J. Urol. 60:93–99

Rawstron, R.E., Walton, J.K. 1981. The effect of local hypothermia on blood loss during transurethral resection of the prostate. J. Urol. 53:258–260

Reiz, S., Mangano, D.T. 1989. Anaesthesia and cardiac disease. In: General anaesthesia. Nimmo, W.S., Smith, G. eds. Oxford, Blackwell Scientific Publications, pp 863–897

Reuler, J.B. 1978. Hypothermia: pathophysiology, clinical settings and management. Ann. Intern. Med. 89:519–527

Reuter, H.J., Jones, L.W. 1974. Physiologic low pressure irrigation for transurethral resection: suprapubic trocar drainage. J. Urol. 111:210–212

Rhymer, J.C., Bell, T.J., Perry, K.C., Ward, J.P. 1985. Hyponatraemia following transurethral resection of the prostate. Br. J. Urol. 57:450–452

Riches, E.W., Muir, E.G. 1933. Prostatectomy. Br. J. Surg. xx:366

Robinson, M.R.G., Cross, R.J., Shetty, M.B., Fittall, B. 1980. Bacteraemia and bacteriogenic shock in district hospital urological practice. Br. J. Urol. 52:10–14

Robson, C.J., Sales, J.L. 1966. The effect of local hypothermia on blood loss during transurethral resection of the prostate. J. Urol. 95:393–395

Roesch, R.P., Stoelting, R.K., Lingeman, J.E., Kahnosoki, R.J., Backes, D.J., Gephardt, S.A. 1983. Ammonia toxicity resulting from glycine absorption during a transurethral resection of prostate. Anaesthesiology 58:577–579

Roizen, M.F., Sohn, Y.J., L'Hommedieu, C.S., Wylie, E.J., Ota, M.K. 1980. Operating room temperatures prior to surgical draping. Anaesth. Analges. 59:852–855

Roos, N., Ramsay, E.W. 1987. A population-based study of prostatectomy: outcomes associated with differing surgical approaches. J. Urol. 137:1184–1188

Roos, N., Wenneburg, J.E., Fisher, E.S., et al. 1989. Mortality and reoperation after open and transurethral resection of the prostate for benign prostatic hyperplasia. N. Engl. J. Med. 320:1120–1124

Sach, R., Marshall V.R. 1977. Prostatectomy: its safety in an Australian teaching hospital. Br. J. Surg. 64:210–214

Schultz, A., Bay-Nielsen, H., Bilde, T., et al. 1989. Prevention of urethral stricture formation after transurethral resection of the prostate: a controlled randomised study of Otis urethrotomy versus urethral dilatation and the use of the polytetrafluoroethylene coated versus the uninsulated metal sheath. J. Urol. 141:73–75

Sear, J.W., Holland, D.E. 1989. Anaesthesia for patients with renal dysfunction. In: General anaesthesia. Nimmo, W.S., Smith, G. eds. Oxford, Blackwell Scientific Publications, pp 913–933

Serrao, A., Mallik, M.K., Jones, P.A., Hendry, W.F., Wickham, J.E.A. 1976. Hypothermic prostatic resection. Br. J. Urol. 48:685–687

Shah, P.J.R., Williams, G., Chaudry, M. 1981. Short-term antibiotic prophylaxis and prostatectomy. Br. J. Urol. 53:339–343

Shearman, C.P., Silverman, S.H., Johnson, M., et al. 1988. Single dose oral antibiotic cover for transurethral prostatectomy. Br. J. Urol 62:434–438

Shepard, R.L., Krause, S.E., Babayan, R.K., Siroky, M.B., 1987. The role of ammonia toxicity in the post-transurethral prostatectomy syndrome. Br. J. Urol. 60:349–351

Singer, M., Patel, M., Webb, A.R., Bullen, C. 1990. Management of the transurethral prostate resection syndrome: time for reappraisal? Crit. Care Med. 18:1478–1479

Sorensen, M., Engback, J., Viby-Mogensen, J., Guldager, H., Molke Jensen, F. 1984. Bradycardia and cardiac asystole following a single dose of suxamethonium. Acta Anaesthesiol. Scand. 28:232–235

Steen, P.A., Tinker, J.H., Tarhan, S., 1978. Myocardial reinfarction after anaesthesia and surgery. J.A.M.A. 239:2566–2570

Stephenson, T.P., Latto, P, Bradley, D, Hayward, M., Jones, A. 1980. Comparison between continuous flow and intermittent flow transurethral resection in 40 patients presenting with acute retention. Br. J. Urol. 52:523–525

Sterns, R.H., Thomas, D.J., Herndon, R.M., 1989. Brain dehydration and rapid neurologic deterioration after rapid correction of hyponatraemia. Kidney Int. 35:69

Still, J.A. Jr., Modell, J.H. 1973. Acute water intoxication during transurethral resection of the prostate, using glycine solution for irrigation. Anaesthsiology 38:98–99

Stratte, P.B. 1960. A safe irrigating medium in transurethral resection of the prostate gland. J. Urol. 83:721–723

Swaminathan, R., Tormey, W.P. 1981. Fluid absorption during transurethral prostatectomy. Br. Med. J. 282:317

Tarhan, S., Moffitt, E.A., Taylor, W.F., Giuliani, E.R. 1972. Myocardial infarction after general anaesthesia. J.A.M.A. 22:1451–1454

Thompson-Walker, Sir J. 1930. Lettsomian lectures. Br. Med. J. i:402,451,511

Tingwald, G.R., Cooperman, M. 1982. Inguinal and femoral hernia repair in geriatric patients. Surg. Gynecol. Obstet. 154:704–706

Tiret, L., Desmonts, J.M., Hatton, F., Vourch, G. 1986. Complications associated with anaesthesia: a prospective study in France. Can. Anaesth. Soc. J. 33:334–336

Turner, R.D., Belt, E. 1957. The result of 1694 consecutive simple peritoneal prostatectomies. J. Urol. 77:853–863

Vaughan, M.S., Vaughan, R.W., Cork, R.C. 1981. Postoperative hypothermia in adults: relationship of age, anaesthesia and shivering to rewarming. Anaesth. Analg. 33:1180–1186

Wakim, K.G. 1971. The pathophysiological basis for the clinical manifestations and complications of transurethral prostatic resection. J. Urol. 106:719–728

Watkins-Pitchford, J.M., Payne, S.R., Rennie, C.D., Riddle, P.R. 1984. Hyponatraemia during transurethral resection: its practical prevention. Br. J. Urol. 56:676–678

Watson, C.J.E., Deane, A.M., Doyle, P.T., Bullock, K.N. 1990. Identifiable factors in post-prostatectomy haemorrhage: the role of aspirin. Br. J. Urol. 66:85–87

Wenneburg, J.E., Roos, N., Sola, L., Schuri, A., Jaffe, R. 1987. Use of claims data systems to evaluate health care outcomes, mortality and reoperation after prostatectomy. J.A.M.A. 257:933–936

Williams, J.S., Hale, H.W. 1966. The advisability of inguinal herniorrhaphy in the elderly. Surg. Gynecol. Obstet. 122:100–104

Wilson, N.I.L., Lewi, H.J.E. 1985. Survey of antibiotic prophylaxis in British urological practice. Br. J. Urol. 57:478–482

Wyatt, M.G., Stower, M.J., Smith, P.J.B., Roberts, J.B.M. 1989. Prostatectomy in the over 80-year-old. Br. J. Urol. 64:417–419

Yachia, D. 1988. Low pressure transurethral resection of the prostate using a suprapubic trocar. Br. J. Urol. 62:494
Zucker, J.R., Bull, A.P. 1984. Independent plasma levels of sodium and glycine during transurethral resection of the prostate. Can. Anaesth. Soc. J. 31:303–307

Chapter 9

Prostate Stents

E.J.G. Milroy

Introduction

Recent anxieties about the risks of carrying out prostate surgery on elderly and unfit patients has generated considerable interest in a variety of recently developed urethral devices for holding open mechanically the prostatic urethra thereby avoiding the need for prostate surgery.

Problems caused by leaving foreign material in the urinary tract are well recognised. Catheters, indwelling stents of any type and sutures will inevitably become infected and encrust with phosphatic deposits when left in contact with urine. Newer materials will reduce these problems but have failed to prevent them completely. Once infection or encrustation have occurred it is always necessary to remove the implanted material to deal with the problem satisfactorily. These difficulties have meant that implanted material in the lower urinary tract can only be used as a temporary measure to drain urine or to relieve obstruction whilst awaiting more definitive treatment.

A major development was the finding that woven mesh stents manufactured of fine corrosion resistant "superalloy" wire would cover with normal urothelium if the wire was held against the wall of the urinary tract by the radial spring force of the device. Rapid covering with urothelium prevented contact of the wire with urine and thus avoided the complications of infection and encrustation (Milroyet al. 1988; Sarramon et al. 1989).

Prostate Stents

Temporary Stents

Fabian (1980) first described an indwelling urethral device to replace a permanent urethral catheter in the treatment of prostate obstruction. He called this a "partial catheter" or "urological spiral". The device consists of a closely coiled spiral of stainless steel wire narrow at the inner end to allow for its introduction into the urethra. At the outer end of the coil a single wire extends through the sphincter with another smaller coil lying just outside the distal sphincter mechanism. This permits adjustment in position and enables the stent to be removed without difficulty. If the stent is left for a prolonged period of time encrustation of the stent will occur because the close-coiled nature of the spiral does not allow urothelium to cover the device. The design of the coil also prevents the passage of a catheter or cystoscope while the stent remains in position. In spite of these difficulties the stent works well as a temporary device (Vincente et al. 1989) and is now marketed by Porges as the Urospiral[R] (Fig. 9.1).

A Danish company (Engineers & Doctors) has recently developed a modification of the Fabian spiral. This is known as the Prostakath[R] and consists of a very similar design to the Urospiral but is gold-plated to reduce the risk of encrustation (Fig. 9.2). The device can be introduced without difficulty using a detachable catheter and local anaesthetic with transrectal ultrasound control. Good results have been obtained with the use of this device particularly in patients with acute urinary retention unfit for surgery (Nordling et al. 1988). Problems of encrustation and infection will inevitably occur if this device is left in place because there is no possibility of the wires covering with urothelium. Although the gold plating may reduce the encrustation and prolong useful life of the device it can still only be used for temporary relief of obstruction unless it is changed regularly. Harrison and DeSouza (1990) reported their experience with the stent in 30 unfit patients. Most of these presented with urinary retention and successful relief of obstruction was achieved in 80% with acute retention. A report of the urodynamic evaluation of 8 patients using this device was made by Nielson et al. (1989). They found that the stent resulted in unobstructed voiding in the majority of their patients. All authors have found problems in patients with chronic retention and severely reduced detrusor function. A number of patients also continue to suffer irritative symptoms of frequency and urgency while the device is in place.

Both the Urospiral and the Prostakath are made in various lengths; the diameter of each device is fixed and has no intrinsic means of fixing itself within the prostatic urethra. This accounts for the occasional difficulties with these temporary stents moving proximally into the bladder or distally into the sphincter mechanism causing urinary incontinence. Attempts to catheterise patients with stents may also cause displacement of the stent.

The Urospiral and the Prostakath can be inserted using a variety of different techniques. Ultrasound or radiological guidance may be used, or the stents may be inserted under direct endoscopic vision. In most reports the stents had been inserted without difficulty under local anaesthetic, an obvious advantage in the elderly and unfit population.

Nissenkorn (1989; Nissenkorn and Richter, 1990) recently described a new intra-urethral stent which consists of a short double Malecot 16F catheter which can be introduced into the prostatic urethra of patients with acute urinary retention (Fig. 9.3). The short length of catheter lies within the prostatic urethra with the inner Malecot end within the bladder at the bladder neck and the outer end of the catheter, with its second smaller Malecot retention device, lying just distal to the verumontanum. The catheter is made in 45, 55 and 60 mm lengths and can be introduced into the prostatic

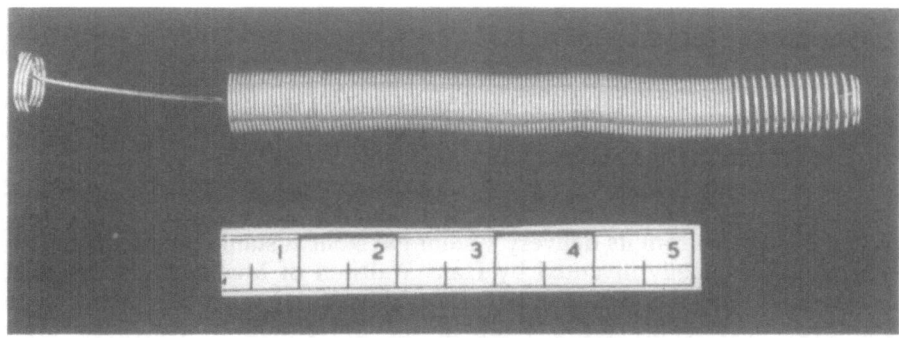

Fig. 9.1. Porges Urospiral^R.

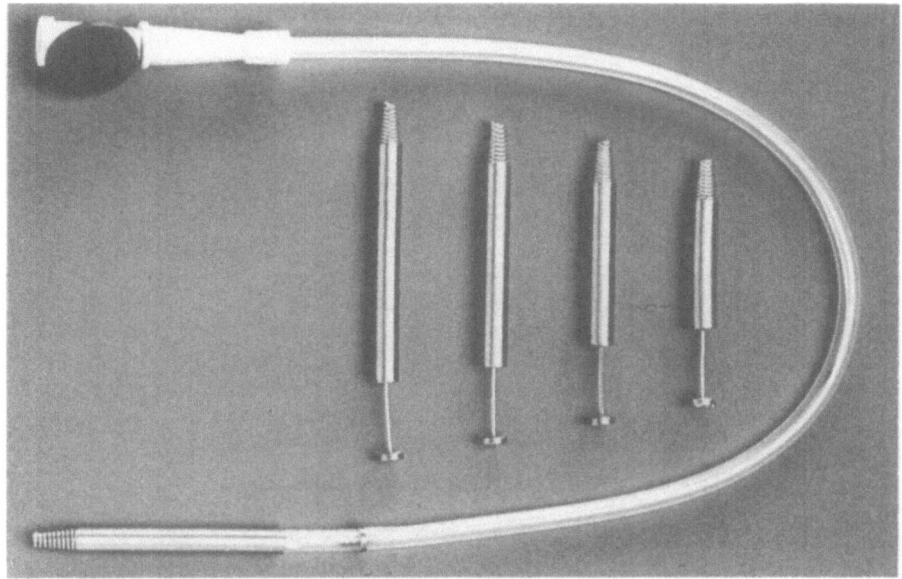

Fig. 9.2. Prostakath^R urethral stent: Engineers & Doctors.

urethra under local anaesthetic through a cystoscope sheath, the length of the prostatic urethra having been measured endoscopically or by transrectal ultrasound. A nylon suture is threaded through the distal end of the device and emerges from the urethra. This can be used to remove the device if necessary. If the stent is to be left in place the nylon can be cut short and left lying in the anterior urethra. The device is only intended for temporary relief of obstruction although it has been left in place for up to 18 weeks without complication. The catheter is marketed by Angiomed Ltd. All 14 patients described by Nissenkorn were able to void after insertion of this device and were continent although three devices had to be removed because of severe frequency and urgency.

Permanent Stents

We first used the Urolume Wallstent 4 years ago for the treatment of recurrent bulbar urethral strictures. It proved so successful that we then started using it in patients with prostatic obstruction (Chapple et al. 1990).

The Urolume Wallstent is a woven tubular mesh of corrosion resistant superalloy wire manufactured in various lengths and diameters (Fig. 9.4). When expanded from its delivery system the stent is stable but flexible. This device was originally invented by Hans Wallsten of Medinvent, Lausanne, Switzerland, and was first designed for endovascular use where it has been employed successfully for 6 years in the prevention of .restenosis after transluminal angioplasty (Sigwart et al. 1987). It is now manufactured and marketed by American Medical Systems, Minnesota, USA.

We first used a modification of the device developed for endovascular use. This consisted of a small diameter (9F) delivery catheter on which a

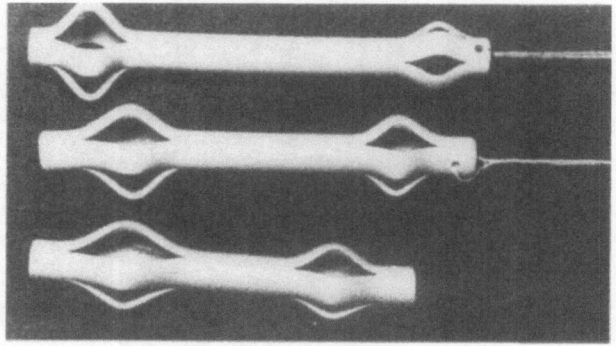

Fig. 9.3. Nissenkorn catheter: Angiomed.

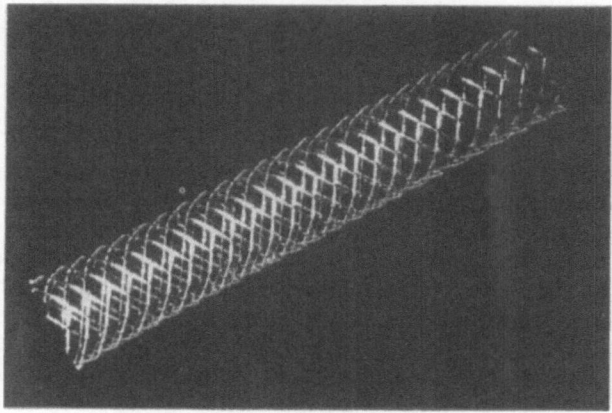

Fig. 9.4. Urolume^R urethral Wallstent^R: American Medical Systems.

doubled-over plastic membrane held the stent in a compressed and elongated form. The double membrane system could be pressurised to 3 atmospheres after which the outer layer of membrane was progressively withdrawn to allow the stent to expand once it had been positioned within the prostate cavity or previously dilated urethral stricture. The expansile force of the mesh then held it in position preventing any possibility of displacement and allowing urothelium to grow over the implanted material while holding open the urethra. Because of difficulties with the considerable shortening of the stent as it expanded from its small diameter delivery catheter, resulting in inaccurate positioning of the stent, we developed, with Hans Wallsten, a new delivery system for the stent. This consists of an endoscopic delivery tool developed specifically for the urologist (Fig. 9.5). With this device the stent emerges as the outer retaining sheath is pulled back. Because the endoscopic system is much larger than the original small diameter delivery catheter far less shortening of the stent takes place as it expands into its final position. A standard 0° telescope fits down the centre of the device and may be moved longitudinally allowing the full length of the stent to be observed as it opens. This ensures that both ends of the stent are positioned correctly (Fig. 9.6). The device includes a locking mechanism to prevent final deployment of the stent until it has been correctly positioned. Until the lock is released the stent can be recovered into the delivery system by advancing the outer sheath back over the stent. The device can then be repositioned before the stent is opened once more and deployed finally. The outer sheath of the new delivery system measures 21F.

The internal diameter of the Urolume stent is large enough to permit endoscopic surgery or catheterisation if necessary, although these are not advisable until the stent has epithelialised. The stents used for prostate obstruction have all been 14 mm diameter (43F) in lengths of 20 or 30 mm. These dimensions are measured with the stent unconstrained and exerting no radial force. When used in the prostatic urethra the diameter will be somewhat smaller than this as the stent will then exert a radial force against the prostatic urethra. In this situation the length of the stent is of course correspondingly greater.

Experimental Work

The first experimental work on the Urolume Wallstent in the blood vessels of experimental animals was carried out by Professor Sarramon, in Toulouse, France. He demonstrated rapid covering of the stent with normal endothelium and in collaboration with Professor Sarramon we then carried out studies using the same stent in the normal posterior urethra of a number of male dogs. Stents 4.5 mm diameter, 10 mm length were placed in the dogs' urethras using the original small diameter delivery catheter. The stents were introduced to lie in the bulbar part of the urethra proximal to the os penis. Urethras were examined at between 2 and 12 months after implantation and scanning electron microscopy showed excellent covering of the stent with very little surrounding inflammation or fibrosis (Milroy et al. 1988; Sarramon et al. 1989).

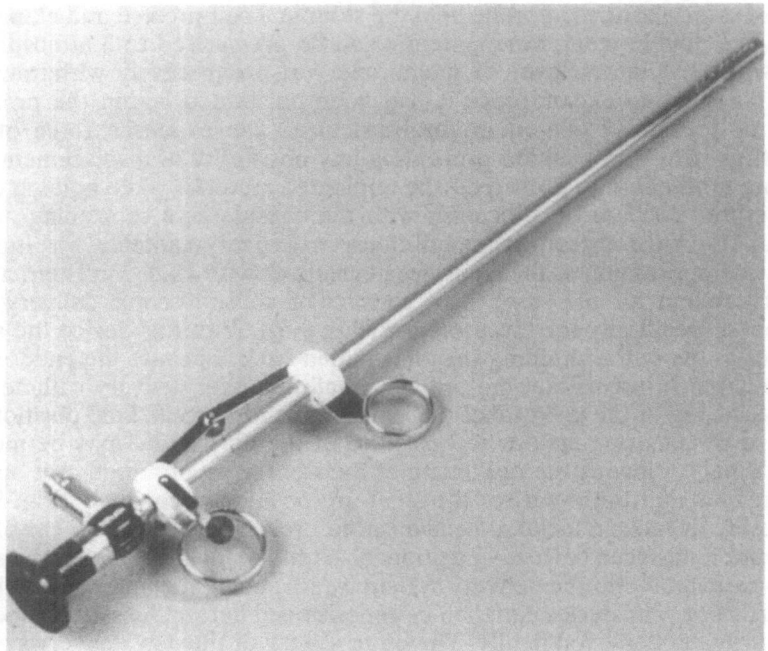

Fig. 9.5. New introducer for Wallstent[R].

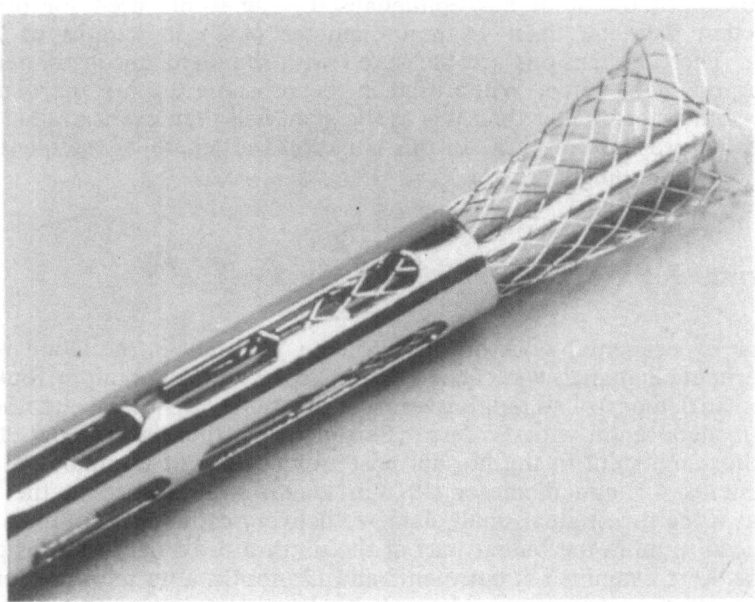

Fig. 9.6. Close úp view of stent within sheath of introducer. Note telescope within lumen of stent.

Clinical Experience

Prostate Obstruction

We have developed two techniques for inserting the Urolume Wallstent into the prostatic urethra. These stents have all been inserted using local urethral lignocaine with additional intravenous short-acting benzodiazepine as necessary because of the mainly elderly and unfit population being treated. With some patients we have used a spinal or epidural anaesthetic.

Ultrasound-Guided Technique

The first technique used transrectal ultrasound guidance with the stent loaded on the original small diameter catheter delivery system. The patient lies in the left lateral position and after local urethral anaesthesia a careful cystourethroscopy is carried out using a flexible cystoscope. Following this a transrectal ultrasound probe is inserted and the length of the prostate is measured. The Urolume stent on the catheter system is then threaded over a guide wire into the bladder. The compressing double membrane system is pressurised to 3 atmospheres with normal saline and the outer layer of the membrane is then peeled back to open approximately one third of the stent (Fig. 9.7). The whole device is then gently withdrawn using ultrasound guidance until the inner margin of the stent lies exactly at the bladder neck. The membrane can then be fully withdrawn allowing the stent to be released into the prostatic urethra. In a few cases where the prostatic urethra is longer than the largest 3 cm stent a second overlapping stent can be inserted. The position of the stent can be checked with the flexible cystoscope if necessary. Occasionally the stent fails to expand completely from the catheter delivery system (Fig. 9.8) and in these patients a 12 mm diameter dilating balloon catheter can be passed over the guide wire and inflated within the lumen of the stent.

The main difficulty with this stent delivery system is that we have found the considerable shortening that takes place from the small diameter delivery catheter up to the final expanded size of the stent results in such shortening of the stent that exact positioning within the prostatic urethra is difficult. It is vitally important that no wires are left remaining within the bladder as this will prevent the stent covering with urothelium and will allow encrustation to take place. At the distal end of the prostatic urethra any encroachment of the stent on the distal sphincter mechanism will of course cause urinary incontinence.

The ultrasound guidance system of stent delivery remains a useful technique for patients whose immobility or other medical conditions prevent them being put in the lithotomy position which is necessary for the more accurate endoscopic delivery technique which we now use for all Urolume stent insertions using the new stent delivery system (Fig. 9.5).

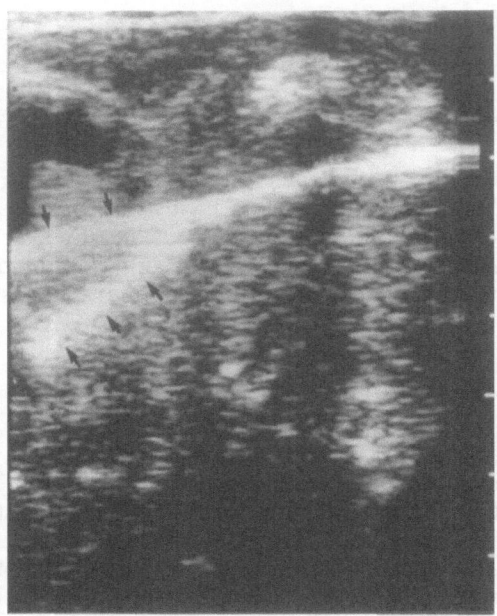

Fig. 9.7. Transrectal ultrasound showing partially open stent at bladder neck. Arrows mark stent.

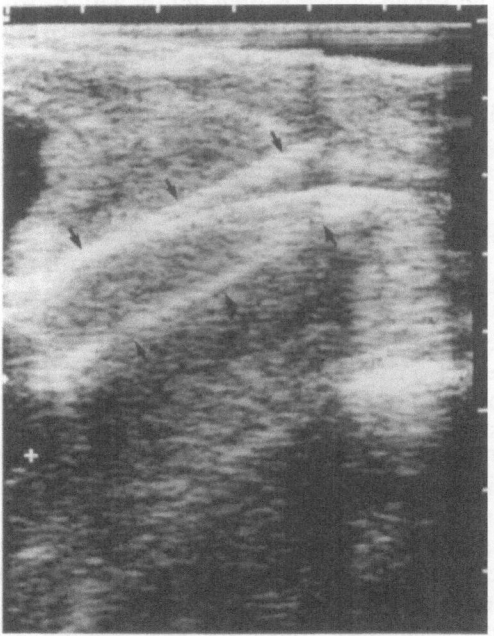

Fig. 9.8. Stent now fully released. Arrows mark stent.

Endoscopic Technique

Because of the difficulties with the ultrasound-guided technique we now use the new endoscopic delivery system for all prostate stent insertions. With this device more accurate positioning of the stent can be ensured (Figs. 9.5, 9.6).

Urethral lignocaine anaesthesia and intravenous sedation are given and the patient is placed in the extended lithotomy position. A careful cystoscopy is carried out in order to check for any bladder abnormality and also to check on the length of the prostatic urethra which has previously been measured using transrectal ultrasound. This pre-operative ultrasound scan is also used to confirm the digital diagnosis of a benign prostate. If any suspicious areas are found ultrasound-guided biopsies are taken before proceeding to stent insertion. Prostatic length is measured endoscopically either with a calibrated cystoscope sheath or a calibrated ureteric catheter. This is easier if a balloon occlusion calibrated ureteric catheter is used with the balloon inflated just inside the bladder neck to prevent movement during the measurement.

Having selected an appropriate length stent in its endoscopic delivery system – the stents are supplied preloaded and sterile packed by the manufacturer – this is then introduced into the prostatic urethra under direct vision using a standard 0° telescope. The first safety lock, which prevents premature opening of the stent as the device is passed down the urethra, is then removed and the stent is deployed within the prostatic urethra under direct vision by pulling back the outer sheath from the stent allowing it to expand. Once the sheath has been pulled back as far as the second safety lock the position of the stent is checked by moving the telescope along the full length of the stent within the prostatic urethra. The verumontanum and the position of the distal sphincter mechanism can be observed through the slots cut in the outer covering sheath for this purpose. If the position of the stent is not correct the outer sheath can be pushed back over the device which will then close inside the sheath allowing repositioning if necessary. The inner end of the stent should lie exactly at the bladder neck and the outer distal margin of the stent should cover fully the lateral lobes of the prostate. Once this final position is confirmed the final safety lock is removed and the outer sheath fully retracted to allow the stent to spring open into its final position. Before removing the delivery system it is very important to check that the three stent-retaining clasps have been fully released from the wires of the stent. This can be determined by direct observation of the distal end of the stent while gently rotating the delivery system. If it is found that one or other of the clamps is still attached to the wires gentle manipulation will free it without difficulty. Before withdrawing the delivery system the three clamping jaws should be withdrawn into the covering sheath for at least the length of the safety clip in order to prevent any damage to the distal urethra as the device is removed from the urethra. If necessary once these grasping jaws have been withdrawn into the sheath and the safety clip reapplied the delivery system can be introduced down the length of the stent to check its position (Fig. 9.9). If it is necessary to carry out a cystoscopy at this stage great care must be taken not to damage the wires of the distal end of the stent with the beak of the cystoscope as it passes through the sphincter mechanism.

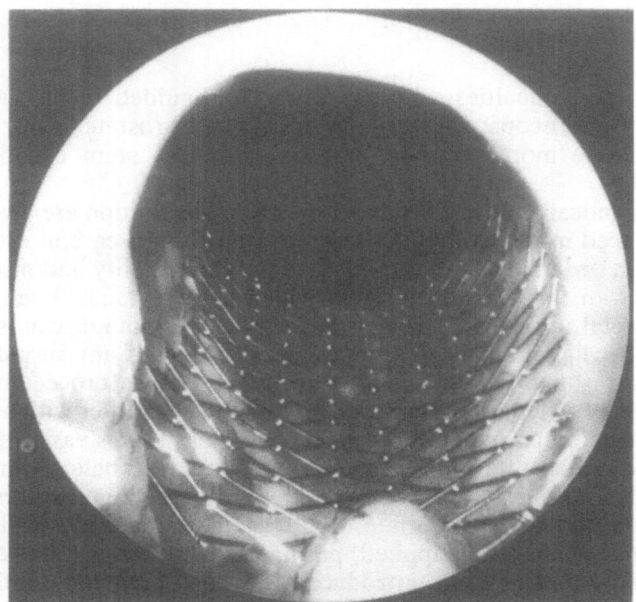

Fig. 9.9.   Prostate stent immediately after insertion.

Results

We have now treated 45 patients with prostate obstruction using the Urolume Wallstent of whom 32 presented with acute retention (Table 9.1). Forty-two patients are fully satisfied with the stent and are passing urine normally with significantly reduced reduced residual urines. Where possible full urodynamic videocystograms have been carried out before stent insertion and at 3–6 months post-operatively. Post-operative studies have not been possible in a number of these patients because of the severe medical problems which prevented prostate surgery when they first presented. Some idea of the general condition of these patients can be gained from Table 9.2.

As with all other types of urethral stents we have found that most patients suffer frequency urgency and occasional urge incontinence following stent insertion, presumably because of the mechanical irritation of the

Table 9.1.   Presenting features of prostate patients treated with Urolume Stent

45 patients	32 acute retention
(39 benign	7 chronic retention
6 malignant)	3 severe symptoms
	3 prostate symptoms /Parkinson's
	disease symptoms (therapeutic trial)

Mean age 74.8 (range 49–95) years.

Table 9.2. American Society of Anesthesiology grades of patients treated

ASA grade	Patient fitness status	No. patients
1	Healthy	2
2	Mild systemic disease	5
3	Severe disease	15
4	Threat to life	23
5	Moribund	0

prostatic urethra caused by these devices. We have found that using the Urolume Wallstent these symptoms settle, presumably as the stent covers with epithelium, over a period of 1–2 months. Only 2 patients, both of whom have severe detrusor instability, still have persistent symptoms of frequency and urgency. Six patients failed to pass urine immediately after stent insertion and required suprapubic catheterisation. It is important that no urethral catheter is passed in these patients for the first month to avoid the risk of damaging the stent. Providing care is taken no damage should result from catheterisation or cystoscopy once epithelial covering is underway. Voiding commenced in all these patients without difficulty during the next 2 or 3 days and all suprapubic catheters (except one inserted pre-operatively for chronic retention and advanced prostate cancer) were removed by 6 weeks. These stents seemed to cause remarkably few other symptoms and no patient has experienced pain other than the dysuria associated with a urinary infection in 3 patients after insertion of the stent. All of these settled with a standard course of antibiotics and healing of the stent was not affected. Any pre-existing urinary infection was treated vigorously before stent insertion and all procedures were covered with broad spectrum antibiotics for the perioperative period.

Whenever possible we have carried out regular cystoscopies on these patients under local anaesthetic to check on healing of the stent. As detailed above a number of our patients were unfit or unwilling to undergo these procedures because of failing health. The stent covers with urothelium in a similar fashion to that we have observed in urethral strictures. There is a considerable hyperplastic reaction (Fig. 9.10) which seems to last longer in prostate stents than in those used for urethral strictures but which settles between 12 and 18 months after stent insertion (Fig. 9.11). We have seen no encrustation of stents within the prostatic urethra although a number of our earlier patients in whom some of the wire mesh was left lying within the bladder, proximal to the bladder neck, have developed fine encrustation on the wire after a period of 6 to 12 months. None of these has yet caused symptoms or needed removing.

Stent Removal

Five stents have had to be removed subsequent to deployment. Two of these were removed at the time of surgery because of poor position, one

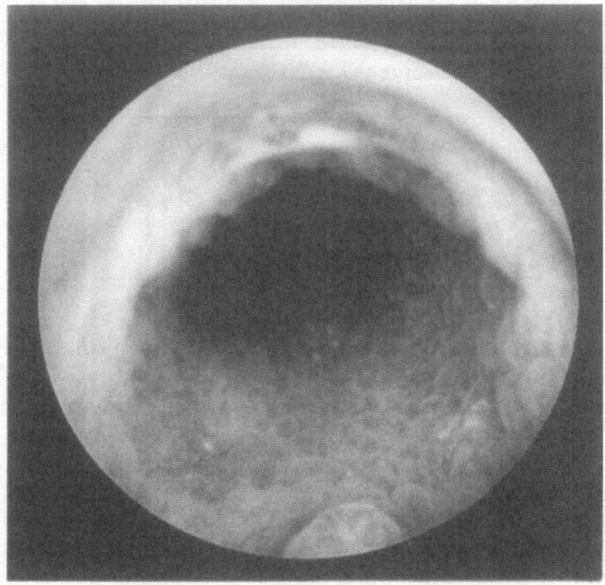

Fig. 9.10. Endoscopic appearance of prostate stent covered with hyperplastic urothelium 5 months after insertion. Patient has no symptoms.

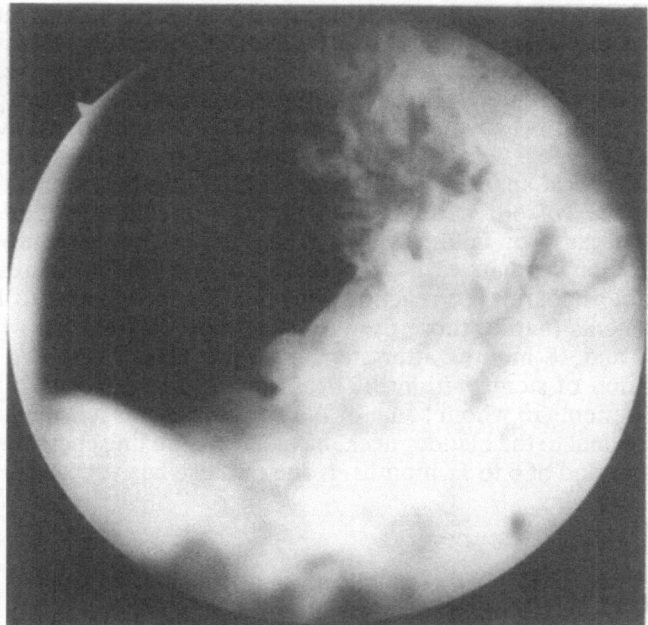

Fig. 9.11. Appearance of prostate stent 1 year after insertion. Stent covered; little hyperplasia remaining.

was removed after 1 week, and one after 1 month because the stent was encroaching onto the distal sphincter mechanism causing a degree of urinary incontinence. All these stents were removed easily by grasping the stent at the bladder neck and pushing it into the bladder using standard grasping forceps. The stent can then be pulled into a large resectoscope sheath or simply pulled out through the urethra. As the stent is pulled it lengthens and narrows causing remarkably little damage to the distal urethra as it is pulled out. One stent was removed 11 months after implantation at the request of the patient because of persistence of severe detrusor instability. The hyperplastic lining epithelium was resected endoscopically without difficulty and the stent pushed into the bladder and removed as described above. This patient did not improve but he has, perhaps understandably, declined further treatment.

Several patients have noticed a minor degree of intermittent haematuria for the first 3 to 6 months and one of these presented with clot retention 3 months after implantation. This was treated with suprapubic catheterisation and spontaneous voiding recommenced 48 hours later with no further bleeding or other symptoms.

No patient has reported any change in potency as a result of stent insertion although the majority of these patients were elderly and suffering from severe chest and heart disease preventing normal sexual intercourse. Most of those patients having regular sexual intercourse report retrograde ejaculation, although it is interesting that two state that normal ejaculation has been maintained. The mean age of these patients is 74.8 years (49–95 years) with a mean follow-up of 10.6 months (range 4–18 months).

Other Permanent Prostate Stents

At the present time there is only one other stent suitable for the permanent treatment of prostate obstruction; this stent is manufactured by Advanced Surgical Intervention Inc., San Clemente, California. This stent consists of a titanium fixed mesh design loaded on a prostate balloon dilatation system which can be deployed using either radiography, ultrasound, or direct endoscopic control. The balloon is positioned within the prostatic urethra and as it expands the balloon forces open the titanium mesh into the prostate. Once the stent has expanded the balloon is deflated and removed. Unlike the Urolume Wallstent this device has no intrinsic spring radial force, the diameter being fixed by inflation of the 12 mm diameter balloon to approximately 32F. The rigid structure of the mesh is quite different from that of the Urolume Wallstent woven wire mesh structure – the ASI stent is an open framework of malleable titanium, the cross-section area of the frame being considerably larger than the fine wire used in the construction of the Wallstent. The ASI stent (Fig. 9.12) certainly seems to work well in clinical trials in patients with acute retention and early results have confirmed that it covers with epithelium.

There are a number of other companies in the process of trying to perfect endoscopically delivered prostate stents but at the present time

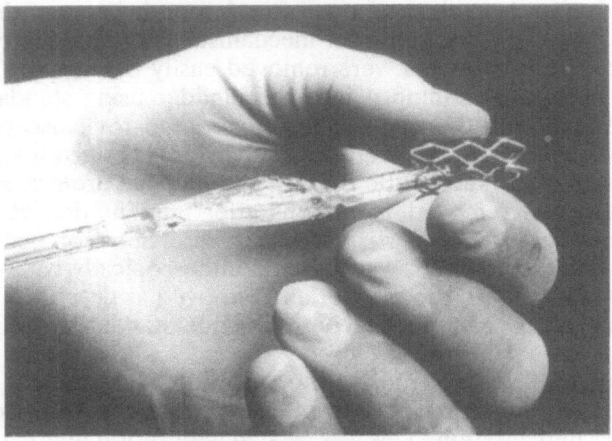

Fig. 9.12. ASI stent with balloon catheter.

only the Urolume Wallstent and the ASI stent are available for clinical trials.

Indications for Prostate Stents

Recent anxieties about the risks of prostate surgery have stimulated great interest in the medical profession and amongst a well-informed general public in alternative treatments for prostate obstruction. It is important that urologists with their interests, knowledge and experience in prostate disease remain at the forefront of these new developments and involve themselves in the necessary clinical studies.

In the elderly and unfit patient, for whom prostate surgery would be a major risk and in whom pharmacological treatment might cause unacceptable side effects, some form of prostate stenting to relieve acute retention or severe prostate symptoms offers an excellent alternative providing the treatment can be carried out rapidly and uses local anaesthesia (Chapple et al. 1990; Williams et al. 1989), included in this group may be patients who for one reason or another refuse prostate surgery or other forms of treatment. Until other new treatments are fully assessed and evaluated there will remain in many parts of the world long waiting lists for prostate surgery, these patients are particularly suited to the various temporary prostate stents which are in general less expensive than the permanent stents.

We have also used the Urolume Wallstent as a theraputic trial in 3 patients with Parkinson's disease whose urinary symptoms are difficult to distinguish symptomatically and urodynamically between those caused by prostate obstruction and those caused by Parkinson's disease. Insertion of a prostate stent relieved prostate obstruction in our 3 patients and as both the symptoms and urodynamic results improved the stents were left in place. If there is no improvement the stent can easily be removed.

Other Indications for Urethral Stents

We have now used the Urolume Wallstent in over 60 patients with recurrent bulbar urethral strictures. Although further follow-up is needed, at 3 years the results remain very good for the vast majority of these patients and there is no doubt that this device will continue to make a major contribution to the treatment of difficult strictures (Milroy et al. 1989a,b).

We have also used the same Urolume Wallstent for the treatment of patients with traumatic high cervical spinal injuries causing tetraplegia and dyssynergic sphincters. All these patients have had high-pressure voiding and were unsuitable for intermittent catheterisation. Stents were inserted using the same device as that used for urethral strictures and prostate obstruction and the procedure was notable for its simplicity and lack of complications. Although some difficulties have been experienced in these patients after stent insertion it does seem that this is an excellent alternative to endoscopic sphincterotomy (Shaw et al. 1990).

The stent is also being used successfully for the treatment of biliary strictures (Dick et al. 1989) and in a number of cases of tracheal and oesophageal obstruction. The hyperplastic reaction seen when the stent is first inserted, particularly in experimental models, has prevented widespread use of the Urolume Wallstent in ureteric obstruction. Clinical trials are, however, continuing in carefully selected patients with ureteric obstruction and early results are promising.

Future Developments

There is no doubt that the concept of a mechanical device to hold open the obstructed prostate will continue to play an important role in the elderly unfit patient. Permanently implanted devices which cover with epithelium may well find an important role in a far larger group of patients.

There are still problems with the delivery systems. A far larger range of sizes of stents is necessary and ensuring accurate positioning remains a vital requirement. Changes in the design and structure of the stents may improve the ease of delivery and may also help to reduce the early symptoms of irritation when the stents are first implanted. Similar changes may also help to improve the speed of epithelial covering and reduce the hyperplastic reaction. Careful positioning and rapid epithelial covering remain vitally important to prevent the inevitable encrustation and infection which will otherwise occur with any foreign material left in contact with urine.

The long-term stability of the permanent stent within the urethra cannot of course be determined because of the short time these stents have been in use. The alloy used in the Urolume Wallstent is well tried and tested and is know to be well tolerated within the body. After a period of 20 to 30 years corrosion and fragmentation of any metallic device may occur in body fluids. This of course will hardly be a problem in the elderly patient with a limited life expectancy. As the prostate and urethral stents are covered by a thin layer of urothelium in contact with urine it is unlikely that any accumulation of corrosion products would occur and fragmentation of the wires after this period of time is unlikely to cause any problems. Other metals and alloys would still be liable to corrosion and fragmentation and there is therefore interest in coated alloys, and non-metallic stents for these patients.

Conclusion

Temporary prostate stents inserted under local anaesthetic offer a useful alternative for the short-term relief of urinary retention and prostate symptoms in patients with limited life expectancy or awaiting prostate surgery. Because of problems with encrustation and infection they cannot be left in place for a long period of time without changing the stent. Permanent prostate stents which are known to cover with epithelium whilst holding open the prostatic urethra will, if long-term results confirm the early successes with these devices, offer a simple and effective alternative to prostate surgery for many patients.

References

Chapple, C.R., Milroy, E.J.G., Rickards, D. 1990. Permanently implanted urethral stent for prostatic obstruction in the unfit patient: preliminary report. Br. J. Urol. 66:58–65

Dick, R., Gillams, A., Dooley, J.S., Hobbs, K.E.F. 1989. Stainless steel mesh stents for biliary strictures. J. Interventional Radiol. 4:95–98

Fabian, K.M. 1980. Der Intraprostatische "Partielle Katheter" (Urologische Spirale). Urologe A. 19:236–238

Harrison, N.W., DeSouza, J.V. 1990. Prostate stenting for outflow obstruction. Br. J. Urol. 65:192–196

Milroy, E.J.G., Chapple, C.R., Cooper., J.E., et al. 1988. A new treatment for urethral strictures. Lancet i:1424–1427

Milroy, E.J.G., Chapple, C.R., Eldin, A., Wallsten, H. 1989a. A new stent for the treatment of urethral strictures. Br. J. Urol. 63:392–396

Milroy, E.J.G., Chapple, C.R., Eldin, A., Wallsten, H. 1989b. A new treatment for urethral strictures: a permanently implanted urethral stent. J. Urol. 141:1120–1122

Nielson, K.K., Kromann-Andersen, B., Nordling, J. 1989. Relationship between detrusor pressure and urinary flow rate in males with an intra-urethral prostatic spiral. Br. J. Urol. 64:275–279

Nissenkorn, I. 1989. Experience with a new self-retaining intraurethral catheter in patients with urinary retention. J. Urol. 142:92–94

Nissenkorn, I., Richter, S. 1990. A self-retaining intra-urethral device. Br. J. Urol. 65:197–200

Nordling, J., Holm, H.H., Klarskov, P., Nielson, K.K., Andersen, J.T. 1989. Intraprostatic spiral: new device for insertion with patient under local anaesthetic and with ultrasonic guidance with three months of follow-up. J. Urol. 142:756–758

Sarramon, J.P., Joffre, F., Rischmann, P., et al. 1989. Prosthese endourethrale Wallstent dans les stenoses recidivantes de l'urethre. Ann. Urol. 23:383–387

Shaw, P.J.R., Milroy, E.J.G., Eldin, A. 1990. Permanent external sphincter stents in spinal injured patients. Br. J. Urol. 66:297–302

Sigwart, U., Puel, J., Mirkovitch, V., et al. 1987. Intravascular stents to prevent occlusion and restenosis after transluminal angioplasty. N. Engl. J. Med. 316:701–706

Vincente, J., Salvador, J., Chechile, G. 1989. Spiral urethral prosthesis as an alternative to surgery in high risk patients with BPH. J. Urol. 142:1504–1506

Williams, G., Jager, R., McLoughlin, L., et al. 1989. Use of stents for treating obstruction of urinary outflow in patients unfit for surgery. Br. Med. J. 298:1429

Chapter 10

Prostatic Hyperthermia

T.J. Christmas

Introduction

The concept of hyperthermia as a medical treatment dates as far back as 400 BC when early medical practitioners such as Hippocrates noted the beneficial effect of hot steam baths. This non-specific treatment persisted through Roman times to the Victorian era when spa towns, some of which offered natural hot water spring therapy, were popular venues for the sick and infirm. The possible beneficial effects of hyperthermia as a treatment for tumours was first recognised in 1866 when complete resolution of a sarcoma was reported after an attack of hyperpyrexia due to erysipelas (Busch, 1866). It is now recognised that malignant cells are more susceptible to hyperthermia than normal cells, particularly at a temperature of 40–45 °C. In vitro and in vivo experiments have shown that neoplastic cells may be selectively destroyed by heat whilst normal cells survive in identical conditions (Giovanella et al. 1976). Heat alters cellular metabolism and neoplastic cells are particularly sensitive to such changes. Histological changes after hyperthermia include swelling and fragmentation of the cytoplasm, rupture of the plasma membrane and ultimately complete cellular necrosis may ensue. Normal cells are more efficient at reconstituting themselves after heat damage than neoplastic cells (Giovanella et al. 1976). Another reason for the selective hyperthermic damage of neoplastic cells as compared to normal cells is their relatively poor blood supply. Tumour cells are less able to increase their blood supply in response to heating and hence have an impaired cooling system rendering them more susceptible to the damaging effects of hyperthermia (Storm et al. 1979).

The degree of thermal damage depends upon the temperature and exposure time. Temperatures below 39 °C will not induce any injury and temperatures above 46 °C irretrievably damage all cells. Temperatures between 40 °C and 45 °C may be applied to destroy neoplastic cells and the duration of treatment should be doubled for each reduction of 1 °C in temperature to achieve equivalent therapeutic effect (Sterzer, 1980).

A combination of hyperthermia and radiotherapy has been advocated since the two treatments produce a mutually enhancing synergistic effect upon tumours (Yerushalmi, 1976). Hyperthermia apparently inhibits the repair of radiation-induced DNA damage and therefore decreases the dose of radiation required to achieve cell death. A similar additive effect has been reported with combined hyperthermia and chemotherapy (Hazan et al. 1984).

Hyperthermia may be administered to the whole body or locally to specific organs. A variety of heat sources have been used for hyperthermic therapy including hot water, local hot fluid instillation, infrared waves, ultrasound and microwaves.

Local Prostatic Hyperthermia

The first study of prostatic hyperthermia was in an animal model in which the prostate was treated by localised deep microwave hyperthermia administered transrectally with safe and efficacious results (Yerushalmi et al. 1983). Therefore, this treatment was commenced in human cases of both prostatic carcinoma and benign prostatic hyperplasia (BPH).

Transrectal Microwave Hyperthermia

Transrectal administration of microwave hyperthermia was first directed at the human prostate as a treatment for carcinoma of the prostate. The prostate was heated to 43 °C using a 2.45 GHz transrectal microwave probe while adjacent tissues were cooled to 32 °C. The results were encouraging with a reduction in the tumour mass as well as obstructive symptoms after this treatment (Yerushalmi et al. 1982; Servadio and Leib, 1984). The same apparatus was later used to evaluate the effect of transrectally applied microwaves in BPH. A total of 29 cases of histologically proven BPH were studied, 11 of whom had an in-dwelling urethral catheter for retention of urine. Each case was treated transrectally with the same equipment, as described above. Transrectal microwave hyperthermia was applied on an outpatient basis without sedation once every fortnight. Each treatment lasted for 1 hour and the mean number of treatments required was 11.7 (range 4–18). The temperature within the substance of the prostate was measured 10–15 minutes after commencing treatment and was shown to be within the range 42–43 °C. There was symptomatic improvement in voiding symptoms in all 18 cases without a catheter in situ and 8 of the 11 catheterised cases were able to void after treatment. The treatment was tolerated well and was free of side effects (Yerushalmi et al. 1985). However, the symptoms of outflow obstruction due to BPH are notoriously prone to a placebo effect (Chapple et al. 1990) and since there was no control group in this study or objective urodynamic evidence, in the form of flow rate estimation or cystometry, it is not possible objectively to conclude from the data presented that microwave therapy is beneficial as a treatment for BPH. Furthermore, the study reported a decrease in the size of the prostate after microwave therapy but only digital examination was used to assess the prostate volume and this is an inaccurate and non-reproducible technique that has now been surpassed by transrectal ultrasonography (TRUS).

The equipment used for transrectal microwave therapy was later modified incorporating a cooling system to prevent thermal damage to the rectal wall, a 100 watt/915 MHz microwave generator with a probe to specifically direct the waves, a probe to monitor the temperature within the prostatic urethra and a computer to control and coordinate treatment and monitor the effects. The temperature within the prostatic urethra was maintained at 42.5 ± 1 °C for 60 minutes. TRUS showed no diminution in the size of the prostate after treatment. Two patients developed small prostatorectal fistulae after treatment but both resolved with conservative management (Servadio et al. 1986). The Prostathermer (TM) Model 99-D (Biodan Medical Systems) incorporating a 915 MHz microwave generator, a cooling system, a temperature probe and a controlling computer was used to treat 6 men with BPH leading to intermittent retention of urine. In 5 of the 6 cases spontaneous voiding was achieved after treatment, the only failure had a large prostate of 5 cm diameter. The duration of treatment, divided into sessions of 60 minutes, lasted a total of between 298 and 690 minutes administered at between 5 and 10 sessions. The maximum flow rate improved in 5 of the 6 cases and the mean increase was 11.2 ml/sec. The post-micturition residual volume decreased after treatment in all but one case. Although digital examination suggested a diminution of the prostate TRUS showed no change in the dimensions of the prostate after treatment (Lindner et al. 1987). It is difficult to understand how the maximum flow rate can rise from 5 to 32 ml/sec (a 640% increase) after microwave therapy, as described in one case, with no apparent change in the dimensions of the prostate on TRUS when even prostatectomy may not achieve such a dramatic improvement in the maximum flow rate (Turner-Warwick et al. 1973). A more recent review of the treatment of BPH with the Prostathermer (TM) in a total of 37 cases, with a minimum of 6 months follow-up, has shown persistent relief of symptoms and successful trial without urethral catheter in 15 of the 23 treated cases with retention of urine (Servadio, 1989).

The most objective study of transrectal microwave therapy using the Prostathermer (TM) Model 99-D, reported to date has examined voiding parameters before and 4 weeks after treatment in 30 cases of BPH. The changes in urinary symptoms did not reach statistical significance. The objective results were also poor with an improvement in the mean maximum flow rate of only 1.1 ml/sec, which was not statistically significant. The increase in flow rate did however just reach statistical significance when corrected for the initial bladder volume according to the nomogram defined by Siroky and associates (Siroky et al. 1979). The post-micturition residual volume and volume of the prostate assessed by TRUS were both unchanged by treatment with the Prostathermer. There was an overall improvement in only 2 of the 28 evaluable cases which represents a success rate of only 7.1% (Strohmaier et al. 1990a) which is lower than the temporary spontaneous improvement rate for untreated BPH (Birkhoff, 1983).

Transrectal hyperthermia appears to be a safe procedure relatively free of side effects. A review of 435 cases of BPH treated by transrectal microwave using the Prostathermer has shown that there are few side effects: haematuria occurred in 1.4%, urinary tract infection in 1.6%, epididymitis in 0.4% and rectal pain in 0.9% (Lindner et al. 1990b). However, some doubt has been cast upon the efficacy of transrectal hyperthermia in the short term but an objective analysis of the long-term results of this treatment is awaited. It is interesting to note that the serum levels of prostate specific antigen (PSA) do not increase after transrectal hyperthermia of the prostate (Lindner et al. 1990) whilst inflammation of the prostate in prostatitis leads to a rise in serum PSA and even relatively minor trauma such as core biopsy may increase serum PSA levels over 50-fold and even digital massage of the prostate will increase the serum PSA level 1.5- to 2-fold within 1 minute (Stamey et al. 1987). This suggests that treatment with the Prostathermer has little or no effect upon prostatic epithelial cells, which represent a major portion of the volume of the gland in BPH, and would explain why the short-term efficacy of treatment is so poor (Strohmaier et al. 1990).

Transurethral Microwave Hyperthermia

Although only two major local complications within the rectal wall have been reported in humans after transrectal administration of microwave hyperthermia to the prostate, there is a potential risk of local rectal damage that makes transurethral therapy advantageous. Also it makes sense to approximate the treatment module as closely as possible to the site of obstruction in BPH, namely the prostatic urethra.

A transurethral applicator incorporating conventional microwave devices was recently developed. The system developed by BSD Medical Corporation consists of a microprocessor-controlled microwave generator, a 300 watt 630 or 915 MHz amplifier, 12 or 14F transurethral balloon catheter applicators with two or three reusable radiating antennae. During treatment the urethral temperature is monitored and the temperature within the substance of the prostate regulated at between 44 and 47.5 °C (Astrahan et al. 1989). In a series of 21 cases the treatment was tolerated well and was not associated with significant long-term side effects. The mean number of treatment sessions was 8.4 with a mean treatment time of 56 minutes. There were statistically significant decreases in the nocturnal urinary frequency, the volume of the prostate on TRUS (a mean of 9.7 to 7.9 ml), and the post-micturition residual volume and an increase in the mean maximum flow rate from 11.0 to 15.9 ml/sec (Sapozink et al. 1990). Pressure/flow cystometric studies were not performed and the median follow-up period was only 12.5 months. Again no control group was included in the study. A later trial using the same equipment in 15 patients with symptomatic BPH assessed prior to treatment by symptom scores, estimation of the prostatic volume using TRUS, measurement of the maximum flow rate and post-micturition residual. There was a statistically significant diminution in the prostatic volume, although the mean change in volume was only small (from 29 to 26 ml). The mean post-micturition volume was decreased from 269 ml before treatment to 50 ml after treatment. There was also a significant increase in the mean maximum flow rate of more than 6 ml/sec. Although 93% had dysuria and urinary frequency post-treatment and 40% of cases noticed perineal pain during treatment, side effects were otherwise minimal. Flexible urethroscopy 3 months after treatment showed no macroscopic evidence of urothelial injury within the urethra. Histological analysis of the prostate after treatment showed oedema, haemorrhage and coagulation necrosis of smooth muscle in the very early stages. One week after treatment there was evidence of complete haemorrhagic necrosis and vascular thrombosis in the periluminal tissues with surrounding granulation tissue. At 28 days after treatment collagenisation was evident and thrombosed vessels showed luminal obliteration with hyalinised walls (Baert et al. 1990).

Another transurethral microwave applicator has been developed by a group from Lyon, France. The antenna is mounted on a 20F flexible catheter and also includes a cooling device to reduce thermal effects upon the urethral mucosa (Fig. 10.1). This equipment has been shown to heat the prostate to 44 °C at a distance of 15 mm from the urethra whilst the temperature of the rectal mucosa does not rise above 41 °C during treatment. Transurethral microwave hyperthermia using this apparatus was applied prior to cystoprostatectomy and histological sections of the prostate showed evidence of thermal damage at a distance of 5 to 15 mm from the urethra with apparent preservation of the urethral mucosa (Fig. 10.2). Histological examination of the treated tissue revealed breakdown of acinar glandular cells and coagulation necrosis of smooth muscle. A clear demarcation was evident between the treated and untreated prostate (Fig. 10.3) (Devonec et al. 1990a,b). This machine, the Prostatron, manufactured by Technomed International, is now available commercially (Fig. 10.4) and the manufacturers have renamed the technique using this apparatus as transurethral microwave thermotherapy (TUMT). A clinical trial in 34 patients with outflow obstruction due to BPH evaluated before and 8 weeks after treatment with the Prostatron has shown a mean increase in the maximum flow rate of 5.1 ml/sec. However, there was little change in the mean post-micturition residual (83 to 79 ml) or mean prostate length on TRUS (83 to 79 mm). Of the 13 catheterised patients with acute retention of urine 6 (46%) were voiding normally 3 months later. The only complication encountered was retention of urine in 1 case. (Carter et al. 1990).

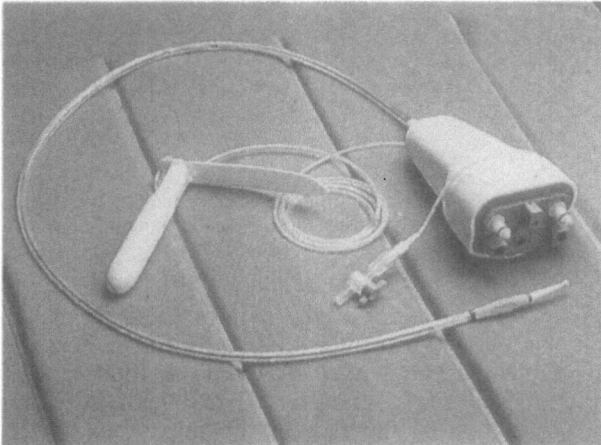

Fig. 10.1. Delivery system for transurethral prostate hyperthermia with rectal temperature sensor.

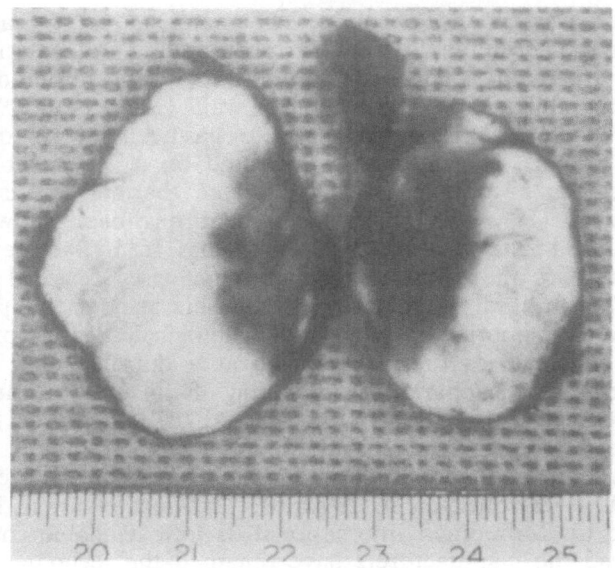

Fig. 10.2.   The effect of transurethral hyperthermia upon the prostate.

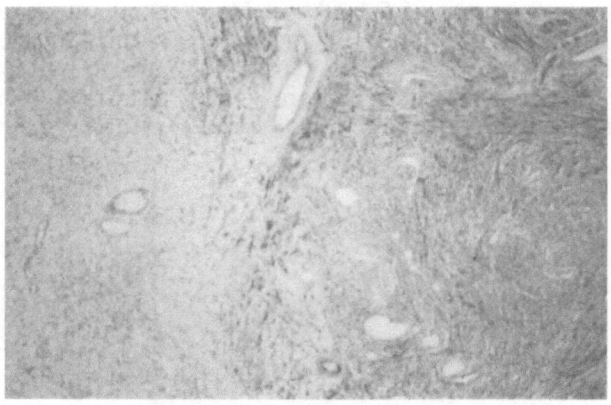

Fig. 10.3.   Histological section demonstrating the clear demarcation between benign prostatic hyperplasia that has been treated by transurethral hyperthermia and untreated tissue.

The results of the first study of transurethral microwave thermotherapy (TUMT) that has been performed including a sham treatment arm have recently been published (Ogden et al. 1993). A total of 40 patients were evaluated with follow-up for 3 months. There was a 70% improvement in the symptom score, a 53% increase in the maximum flow rate and 92% decrease in the post-micturition residual urine volume in the TUMT-treated group but no significant changes in these parameters in the sham group. The main complication in the TUMT-treated group was a 22% incidence of acute

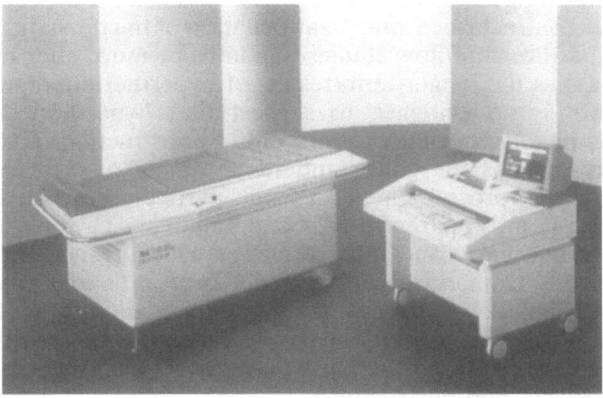

Fig. 10.4. Commercially available transurethral hyperthermia unit: the Prostatron[R].

retention of urine. This study is the first published work to have documented the efficacy of microwave treatment of BPH in a controlled trial.

Conclusion

The action of hyperthermia upon the prostate is to induce necrosis of cells and thrombosis of blood vessels. This is followed by an inflammatory cell infiltrate and ultimately collagenisation. Since the obstructive portion of the prostate is immediately adjacent to the prostatic urethra hyperthermic therapy administered transurethrally seems more likely to be effective than treatment with transrectal probes. The results reviewed here support the concept of greater efficacy of transurethral hyperthermia. The occurrence of recto-urethral fistulae after hyperthermia administered transrectally is a relative contraindication for the transrectal technique.

Although there is clear evidence of improvement in prostatic outflow obstruction the magnitude of the improvement does not appear to be great and is similar to that achieved with α-adrenoceptor blockade. Symptomatic improvement without a placebo group to compare and small increases in the maximum flow rate should be interpreted with caution when not accompanied by more objective data, in particular pressure/flow studies in which the outflow resistance is accurately quantified. Ogden and co-workers have demonstrated that TUMT significantly improves symptoms in BPH as opposed to sham treatment, and it is interesting that the irritative symptoms are particularly improved. Decrease in the volume of the prostate as estimated by TRUS does not necessarily imply a reduction in obstruction to the prostatic urethra particularly since glandular and smooth muscle elements of the prostate are apparently replaced by poorly compliant fibrotic tissue after hyperthermia. The study by Ogden et al. (1993) has shown a mild improvement in the flow rate at 3 months; however, there is a theoretical possibility that collagenisation of the prostatic tissue after hyperthermia could lead to fibrotic contracture leading to attenuation of the prostatic urethra after a longer period. Pressure/flow studies 6 months or more after treatment are indicated to assess the longer-term results of hyperthermia therapy.

So far there is no evidence to suggest that hyperthermia therapy is capable of completely relieving prostatic outflow obstruction and transurethral prostatectomy remains the gold standard treatment of choice in achieving this goal. However, prostatic hyperthermia, particularly when administered transurethrally, is an apparently safe and relatively cheap treatment that may in time prove more and more effective with advances in technology. The possible role of microwave therapy for prostatitis and prostate cancer needs to be examined. At present, further studies are indicated to evaluate the long-term efficacy of prostatic hyperthermia but it seems likely that this treatment will have a future role, particularly in younger men and those with small prostates and mild obstruction.

Acknowledgements   I am grateful to Technomed International for supplying the illustrations in this chapter and to Mr R.S. Kirby for his advice and comments.

References

Astrahan, M.A., Sapozink, M.D., Cohen, D., et al. 1989. Microwave applicator for transurethral hyperthermia of benign prostatic hyperplasia. Int. J. Hypertherm. 5:283–286

Baert, L., Ameye, F., Willemen, P., et al. 1990. Transurethral microwave hyperthermia for benign prostatic hyperplasia: preliminary clinical and pathological results. J. Urol. 144:1383–1387

Birkhoff, J.D. 1983. In: Benign prostatic hypertrophy. Hinman, F., Boyarsky, S., eds. Berlin, Heidelberg, New York, Springer, pp 5–21

Busch, W. 1866. Über den Einfluss welchen heftigere Erysipeln zuweilen auf organisiente Neubildungen ausuben. Verhandl. Naturh. Preuss. Rhein. Westphal. 23:28–30

Carter, S., Patel, A., Perrin, P., Devonec, M., Ramsay, J. 1990. Objective clinical results of transurethral microwave thermotherapy for benign prostatic obstruction. Proceedings of the World Congress on Endourology and ESWL, Washington

Chapple, C.R., Christmas, T.J., Milroy, E.J.G. 1990. Reduction in prostatic bladder outflow obstruction after long-term treatment with the 1 blocker prazosin. Urol. Int. 45:47–55

Devonec, M., Cathaud, M., Carter, S., Berger, N., Perrin, P. 1990a. Transurethral microwave application: temperature sensation and thermokinetics of the human prostate. J. Urol. 143:414A

Devonec, M., Cathaud, M., Carter, S. St., Berger, N., Guillaud, M., Perrin, P. 1990b. The effects of transurethral microwave thermotherapy (TUMT) in patients with benign prostatic hypertrophy. Eur. Urol. 18(suppl. 1):265

Giovanella, B.C., Stehlin, J.S., Morgan, A.C. 1976. Selective lethal effect of supranormal temperatures on human neoplastic cells. Cancer Res. 36:3944–3962

Hazan, G., Lurie, H., Yerushalmi, A. 1984. Sensitization of combined *cis*-platinum and cyclophosphamide by local hyperthermia in mice bearing the Lewis lung carcinoma. Oncology 41:68–75

Lindner, A., Golomb, J., Siegel, Y., Lev, A. 1987. Local hyperthermia of the prostate gland for the treatment of benign prostatic hypertrophy and urinary retention. Br. J. Urol. 60:567–571

Lindner, A., Siegel, Y.I., Korczak, D. 1990a. Serum prostate specific antigen levels during hyperthermia treatment of benign prostatic hyperplasia. J. Urol. 144:1388–1389

Lindner, A., Siegel, Y.I., Saranga, R., Korzcak, D., Matzin, H., Braf, Z. 1990b. Complications in hyperthermia treatment of benign prostatic hyperplasia. J. Urol. 144:1390–1392

Ogden, C.W., Reddy, P., Johnson, H., Ramsay, J.W.A., Carter, S. St. C. 1993. Sham versus transurethral microwave thermotherapy in patients with symptoms of benign prostatic bladder outflow obstruction. Lancet 341:14–17

Sapozink, M.D., Boyd, S.D., Astrahan, M.A., Jozsef, G., Petrovich, Z. 1990. Transurethral hyperthermia for benign prostatic hyperplasia: preliminary clinical results. J. Urol. 143:944–950

Servadio, C., Leib, Z. 1984. Hyperthermia in the treatment of prostate cancer. Prostate 5:205–211

Servadio, C., Leib, Z., Lev, A. 1986. Further observations on the use of local hyperthermia for the treatment of diseases of the prostate in man. Eur. Urol. 12:38–40

Servadio, C. 1989. Local hyperthermia for the treatment of prostatic disease. In: The prostate. Fitzpatrick, J.F., Krane, R.J., eds. Edinburgh, Churchill Livingstone

Siroky, M.B., Olsson, C.A., Krane, R.J. (1979) The flow rate nomogram. I. Development. J. Urol. 122:665–668

Stamey, T.A., Yang, N., Hay, A.R., McNeal, J.E., Freiha, F.S., Redwine, E. 1987. Prostate-specific antigen as a serum marker for adenocarcinoma of the prostate. N. Engl. J. Med. 317:909–916

Sterzer, F. 1980. Microwave apparatus for the treatment of cancer by hyperthermia. Microwave J. 23:39–44

Storm, F., Harrison, W.H., Elliot, R., Morton, D. 1979. Normal tissue and solid tumour effects of hyperthermia in animal models and clinical trials. Cancer Res. 39:2245–2249

Strohmaier, W.L., Bichler, K-H., Flüchter, S.H., Wilbert, D.M. 1990. Local microwave hyperthermia of benign prostatic hyperplasia. J. Urol. 144:913–917

Turner-Warwick, R.T., Whiteside, C.G., Arnold, E.P., et al. 1973. A urodynamic view of prostatic obstruction and the results of prostatectomy. Br. J. Urol. 45:631–645

Yerushalmi, A. 1976. Treatment of a solid tumour by local hyperthermia and ionising radiation: dependence on temperature and dose. Eur. J. Cancer 12:807–810

Yerushalmi, A., Servadio, C., Leib, Z., Fishelovitz, Y., Rakowsky, A., Stein, J.A. 1982. Local hyperthermia for treatment of carcinoma of the prostate: a preliminary report. Prostate 6:623–630

Yerushalmi, A., Shpirer, Z., Hod, I., Gottesfeld, F., Bass, D.D. 1983. Normal tissue response to localized deep microwave hyperthermia in the rabbit's prostate: a preclinical study. Int. J. Radiat. Oncol. Biol. Physics 9:77–81

Yerushalmi, A., Fishelowitz, Y., Singer, D., et al. 1985. Localized deep microwave hyperthermia in the treatment of poor operative risk patients with benign prostatic hyperplasia. J. Urol. 133:873–876

Chapter 11

Balloon Dilatation of the Prostate

J. Brantley Thrasher and K.J. Kreder

Introduction

Benign prostatic hyperplasia (BPH) is a common urologic problem in adult males. More than 80% of males over 50 years of age will be afflicted by the condition (Casteneda et al. 1987) and approximately 25% of patients in this age group will eventually require a prostatectomy (Birkhoff, 1983). An estimated 500 000 prostatectomies are performed in the United States annually, with 34 000 performed in the United Kingdom in 1985 (McLoughlin and Williams, 1990b). The majority of these patients undergo a transurethral resection of the prostate (TURP) with minimal morbidity and an associated mortality as low as 0.2% (Mebust, 1988). In spite of the proven safety and efficacy of this procedure, the relatively high cost and invasive nature of the operation have led many investigators to search for alternatives to transurethral prostatectomy. Currently, therapeutic options for the treatment of symptomatic BPH include medical management (Lepor, 1989), transurethral incision (Orandi, 1985), local hyperthermia, (Lindner et al. 1987), prostatic stents, (McLoughlin and Williams, 1990a; Chapple et al. 1990) and balloon dilatation (Reddy et al. 1988; Reddy, 1990; Dowd and Smith, 1990; Goldenberg et al. 1990; Klein and Lemming, 1989; Gill et al. 1989; Daughtry et al. 1990; Castaneda et al. 1989; McLoughlin and Williams 1990b). Transurethral balloon dilatation of the prostate (TUBDP) has been the subject of a great deal of interest and controversy in the recent literature. Herein, we present a review of the technique of balloon dilatation of the prostate, including our experience with the technique, its complications and those patients who benefit most from the procedure.

History of Prostate Dilatation

The concept of dilating the prostatic urethra to treat symptomatic BPH has been in existence for centuries. However, it was not until the mid-nineteenth century that effective instruments were developed for mechanical dilatation of the prostate. Guthrie in 1836, Civiale in 1841 and Mercier in 1850 pioneered prostatic dilatation using metal dilators to relieve urethral obstruction caused by BPH. In 1910, Hollingsworth described the use of a small suprapubic cystotomy and the index finger to stretch the bladder neck and disrupt the anterior and posterior prostatic commissures (Hollingsworth, 1910). This simple technique relieved obstructive symptoms and was associated with lower morbidity and mortality than an open prostatectomy. Franck reported similarly good results using this technique in 1938. In 1956, Werner Deisting and Otto Franck developed a metal dilator which was a modification of the instrument used by Mercier to disrupt transurethrally the anterior and posterior commissures and thus treat symptomatic BPH. Deisting reported excellent results in 324 patients with symptomatic BPH, treated with the metal dilator and followed for up to 8 years (Dersting, 1956).

Deisting's technique of transurethral dilatation gained popularity in Europe while transurethral resection of the prostate was gaining popularity in this country. Aalkjaer, in 1962, performed a comparison of transurethral or open prostatectomy to transurethral dilatation on 256 patients. He concluded that transurethral resection and open prostatectomy were more efficacious and were associated with fewer complications than transurethral dilatation of the prostate (Aalkjaer, 1962). As the optics and design of the transurethral endo-scopic instruments improved, interest in dilatation of the prostate waned.

Credit should be given to H. Joachim Burhenne for the resurgence of interest in dilatation of the prostate (Burhenne et al. 1984). He applied advances in balloon technology and knowledge gained from dilatation of other organ systems (Burhenne, 1975) to the prostatic urethra. Burhenne's first experimental work utilising humans involved 10 cadavers in which a 24F angio-graphic balloon catheter was used under fluoroscopic control. Post-procedure urethrograms following balloon dilatation demonstrated significant dilation of the prostatic urethra (Burhenne et al. 1984). Recent advances in pressure monitoring devices, larger balloons and more sophisticated positioning tech-niques have made balloon dilatation of the prostate a viable alternative to prostatectomy. Recently, investigators such as Castaneda et al. (1987) Reddy, (Reddy et al. 1988; Reddy, 1990) Dowd and Smith (1990) and Goldenberg et al. (1990) have used these technical advances objectively to research balloon dilatation of the prostate and provide information as to patient selection, mechanism of action, complications and evaluation of results.

Techniques

Regardless of the balloon dilatation technique chosen, the prostatic urethra must be adequately anaesthetised prior to dilatation to avoid the intense desire to void encountered with stretching of the prostatic capsule. Reddy and associates originally described the use of oral narcotics prior to the procedure with the addition of intravenous diazepam intra-operatively as needed (Reddy et al. 1988). Recently, however, they have advocated the use of a paraprostatic block at the junction of the prostate and seminal vesicle using 15 ml of 1% lidocaine solution to avoid the need for pre- or intraprocedural analgesics or sedatives (Reddy, 1990). Other investigators use intra-urethral 2% lidocaine with additional intravenous diazepam (Klein and Lemming, 1989) or intravenous analgesics and diazepams alone (Gill et al. 1989). It is our preference to use short-acting spinal anaesthesia as advocated by Dowd (Dowd and Smith, 1990) and Goldenberg (Goldenberg et al. 1990) to ensure absolute patient comfort and immobility during the procedure. It has been our subjective opinion that the immobility encountered with the use of spinal anaesthesia in the immediate post-operative period may decrease the amount of bleeding associated with the procedure. Further studies will be needed to investigate whether the type of anaesthesia administered has any bearing on the quantity of bleeding associated with TUBDP.

Although many studies do not address the issue of perioperative and post-operative antibiotic coverage, it is our practice to treat all patients undergoing TUBDP with perioperative antibiotics. While some authors have used intravenous aminoglycosides alone or in conjunction with ampicillin (Goldenberg et al. 1990; Daughtry et al. 1990), we prefer to administer 1 g of cefazolin intravenously 1 hour prior to surgery and then every 8 hours until the urethral catheter is removed. Using this regimen, we have had no problems with bacturia, fever, chills, or septicaemia.

Since the inception of balloon dilatation of the prostate, there have been three methods described for positioning the dilating balloon in the prostatic urethra. These three methods use cystoscopic, fluoroscopic, and digital guidance. A fourth method, transrectal sonographic monitoring, has been reported anecdotally and awaits further studies (Fornage and Toubas, 1989). Regardless of the type of placement procedure used, all patients are placed in the low lithotomy position for the procedure and sterilely prepped.

An example of a fluoroscopically guided dilating balloon catheter is the Medi-tech urethroplasty balloon (Medi-tech, Watertown, Mass.). When using this balloon dilating system, an 18 or 20F Councill-tip catheter is passed into the pendulous urethra and a retrograde urethrogram is performed to determine the position of the external sphincter. The position of the external sphincter is then marked by inserting a needle into the overlying drapes. The Councill-tip catheter is advanced into the bladder and a 0.038 inch guidewire is passed into the the bladder through the catheter. The Councill-tip catheter is then replaced with the dilating balloon catheter using the guidewire to manoeuvre it into proper position. Two radiopaque markers at the distal and proximal extent of the balloon (approximately 4 cm apart) are positioned so that the distal marker on the catheter does not extend into the region of the external sphincter. The balloon catheter is connected through a pressure gauge to a hand-held inflating syringe. The balloon is inflated with one-half strength contrast to a diameter of 25 mm (75F) and a pressure of 3 atmospheres at full inflation. During balloon inflation, all balloons have a tendency to migrate into the bladder, and therefore traction on the catheter is required to maintain proper balloon position within the prostatic urethra. Intermittent fluoroscopic monitoring during balloon dilatation confirms proper location of the dilating balloon and ensures that the external sphincter is not being dilated. As the prostatic capsule stretches, additional contrast is injected in order to maintain the pressure of 3 atmospheres. After dilation for 10–15 minutes, the balloon is deflated and the dilating balloon catheter is removed from the urethra. A retrograde urethrogram is performed to document the effect of dilation on the prostatic urethra. An 18F Councill-tip catheter is then passed over the guidewire into the bladder, and any blood clots evacuated. Catheter drainage is maintained until the urine is free of clots and relatively clear (24 to 48 hours).

A digitally positioned balloon (Microvasive Division of Boston Scientific Corporation) (Fig. 11.1) uses a positioning nodule which is located 8 mm proximal to the apical margin of the dilating balloon. This nodule can be used to position the balloon although alternative methods for positioning such as fluoroscopy and cystoscopy can still be used. The apical margin of the balloon has a radiopaque marker and the balloon is small enough that cystoscopy is possible with a small instrument (usually a flexible cystoscope). To use this dilating balloon catheter a flexible-tip 0.038 inch guidewire is inserted into the bladder through a cystoscope and the cystoscope removed. The penis is placed on stretch and the dilating catheter is passed over the guidewire up to the traction ring. With a palpating finger in the rectum, the dilating catheter is withdrawn from the bladder until the positioning nodule is felt at the apex of the prostate (Fig. 11.2). With continued palpation to ensure good positioning, an associate inflates the balloon to 45–50 ml by manual injection of one-half strength radiocontrast. The balloon is subsequently attached to the 10 ml LeVeen inflator in line with the Microvasive pressure gauge and inflated to 4 atmospheres (90F) and the stopcocks closed. Balloon pressure is maintained by injecting more contrast since the balloon pressure will decrease as the prostatic capsule stretches. The dilating balloon is maintained in position for 10 to 15 minutes; the contrast is removed from the balloon, and the balloon catheter is gently retracted over the guidewire. An indwelling urethral catheter is then placed into the bladder and the bladder is irrigated until all clots have been removed. This catheter is left in place until the urine is clear (usually 24–48 hours). Dowd and associates advocate the use of a suprapubic tube instead of a urethral catheter to allow the patients to be discharged on the same day as the procedure and begin voiding trials (Dowd and Smith, 1990).

The ASI (Advanced Surgical Intervention Inc., San Clemente, California) uroplasty catheter (Fig. 11.3) is a cystoscopically positioned catheter used by Goldenberg and associates (1990) and currently undergoing investigation at our institution in a prospective randomised trial comparing its use to TURP. (Donatucci et al. 1992) As an initial step in the use of this balloon catheter, the length of the prostatic urethra is measured using the ASI calibration catheter placed through a 21F cystoscope. The calibration catheter balloon is inflated with 10 ml sterile saline and positioned against the bladder neck without traction. The distance from the bladder neck to the external sphincter is determined by counting the 1 cm markings on the catheter. The calibration balloon is deflated; the bladder is filled with sterile fluid and the catheter removed. The appropriate length dilating balloon catheter is chosen corresponding to the distance from the bladder neck to the external sphincter. The 26F sheath with obturator is then passed into the bladder and the obturator removed. The dilating catheter is then placed into the sheath until the first blue mark (labelled FOLEY) is reached. This places the distal tip of the catheter beyond the end of the sheath within the bladder. The Foley balloon is then inflated with 15 ml of sterile fluid and pulled snug against the bladder neck. The third lumen of the catheter is attached to the irrigating solution and the sheath

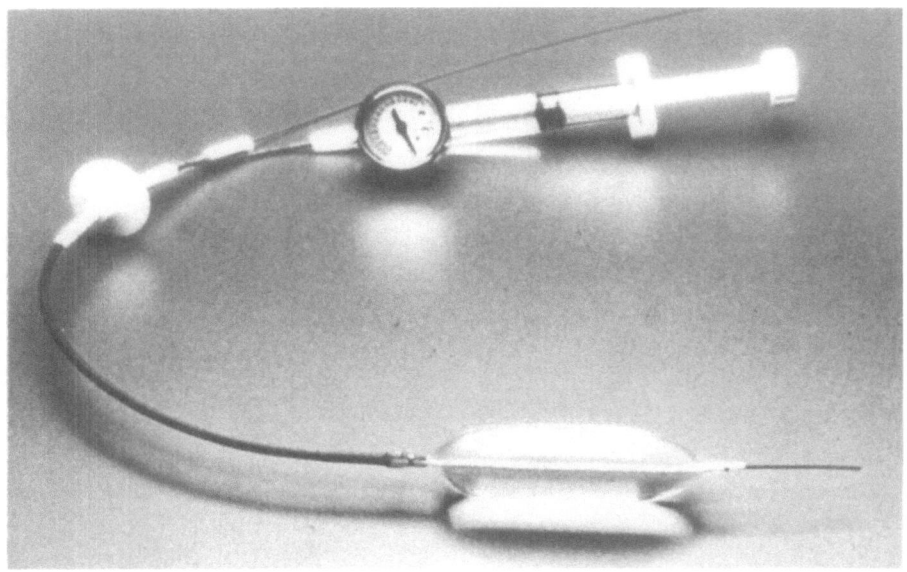

Fig. 11.1. Microvasive prostatic balloon dilatation system.

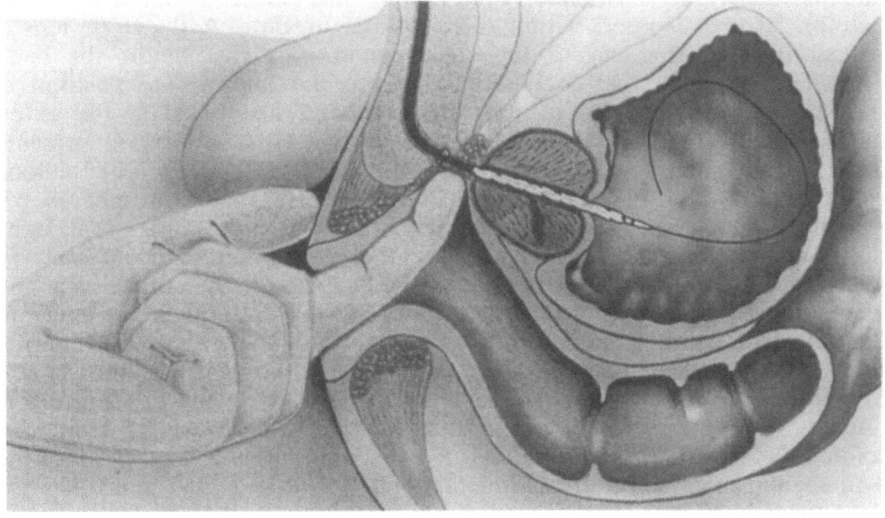

Fig. 11.2. Proper balloon position confirmed by transrectal palpation.

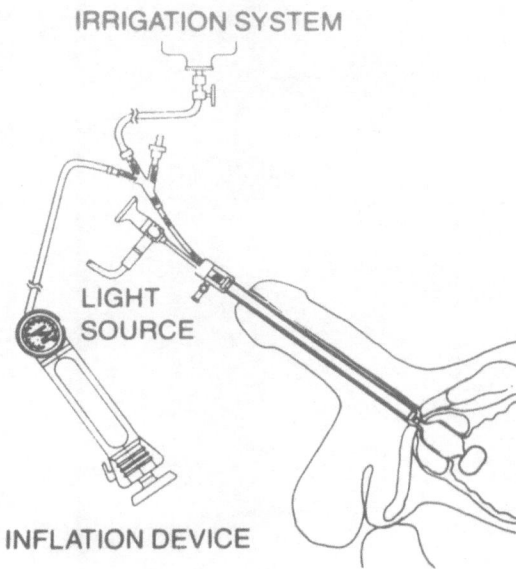

Fig. 11.3.   The Advanced Surgical Intervention Inc. uroplasty catheter.

is retracted back over the catheter until the second mark on the catheter labelled DILATE is reached (Fig. 11.4). This indicates that the dilating balloon is now exposed within the prostatic urethra. A 0 or 30° lens is placed through the end of the sheath in a port just below the catheter. The lens can then be used to ensure the appropriate position of the sheath by identifying a white marker band just distal to the external sphincter (Fig. 11.5). The inflation device with an integral pressure gauge is attached to the catheter port marked DILATE. The balloon is inflated to its full diameter of 25 mm (75F) at 3 atmospheres (45 pounds per square inch) pressure (Fig. 11.6). During the initial inflation, traction must be applied to the catheter in order to counteract the tendency of the balloon to migrate into the bladder. Dilatation is maintained for 10 minutes, during which time intermittent cystoscopy confirms that the balloon remains in position. At the end of the 10-minute period both balloons are deflated and the catheter is withdrawn into the sheath. The entire device is removed as a single unit to avoid distal urethral trauma. A repeat cystoscopy is performed specifically looking for anterior commissurotomies or mucosal tears. A 22F Foley catheter is placed into the bladder and maintained until after the urine is without clots and relatively clear (usually 48 hours).

Reddy and associates have recently described the use of a balloon dilating catheter manufactured by American Medical Systems (1101 Bren Road East, Minnetonka, MN. 55343–9058) called the Optilume catheter (Reddy, 1990). This catheter can be positioned in any one of the three ways previously mentioned. It has radiopaque markers on the catheter for fluoroscopic positioning and is small enough for rigid cystoscopy alongside the catheter.

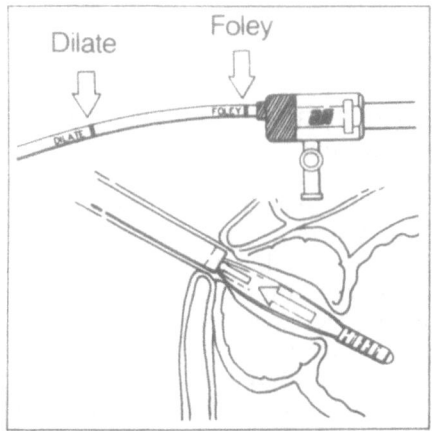

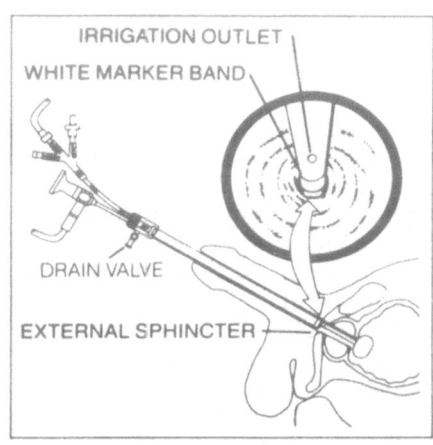

Fig. 11.4. The Advanced Surgical Intervention Inc. dilating balloon with marks for positioning.

Fig. 11.5. Appropriate positioning ensured by visual identification of the white marker band distal to the external sphincter.

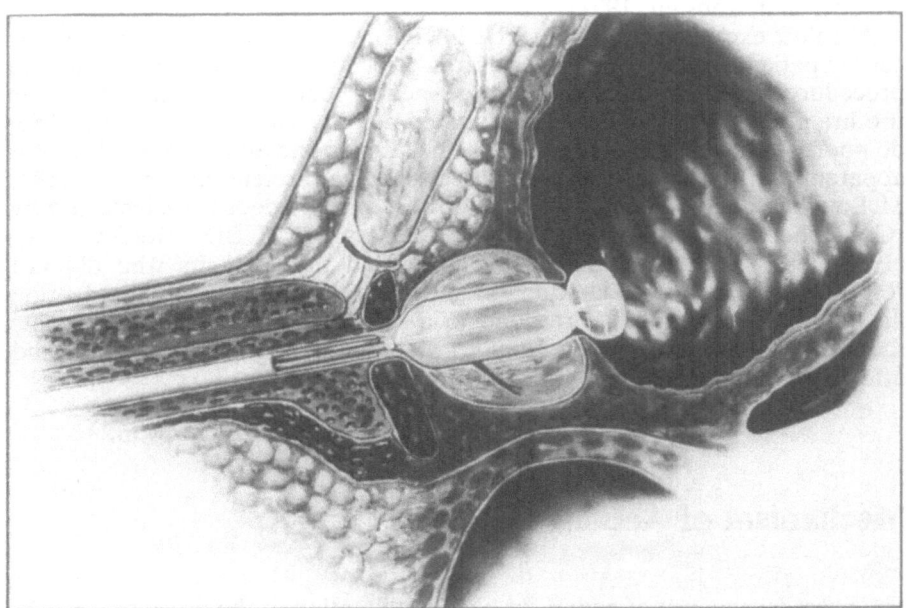

Fig. 11.6. The Advanced Surgical Intervention Inc. balloon inflated in the prostatic urethra.

It also has a locator which allows for digital placement and a fixation balloon which allows stabilisation of the dilating balloon. The fixating balloon is a smaller balloon positioned just distal to the external sphincter thus preventing migration of the dilating balloon into the bladder during inflation.

Patient Selection

Our selection criteria for patients undergoing TUBDP is similar to that used for patients undergoing TURP. The patients initially undergo a complete history including the completion of a symptom score sheet (Fig. 11.7), and a physical examination including a digital rectal examination. Pre-operative laboratory tests include haematology, liver function, prostate-specific antigen, prostatic acid phosphatase and urine culture. All patients also undergo cystoscopy and uroflowmetry prior to consideration for the procedure.

Those patients with obstructive symptoms (decreased force and calibre of the urine stream, hesitancy and dribbling), decreased flow rates and cystoscopic evidence of prostatic enlargement are considered for the procedure. Those patients with evidence of carcinoma or a positive urine culture require further treatment and evaluation prior to TUBDP. If the patient has predominantly irritative symptoms (frequency, urgency and nocturia), an overt or suspected neurologic lesion, is under age 55, or has failed previous TURP or TUBDP, further work-up with urodynamic assessment should be performed (Kreder and Websten, 1992).

Absolute exclusion criteria for TUBDP have not been established; however, certain patients have been identified from prior studies that do poorly with the procedure. Those patients with a large median lobe component, a prostatic urethra greater than 8 cm or an estimated prostate size of greater than 75 g do poorly following TUBDP (Reddy, 1990; Dowd and Smith, 1990). It is also apparent that those patients who present in urinary retention (Gillerd, 1989; McLoughlin and Williams, 1990b) and those with bladder neck hypertrophy (Goldenberg et al. 1990) are poor candidates for TUBDP. Reddy et al. (1988) and Dowd and Smith (1990) reported that patients who did not respond with the first dilatation (as judged by symptom scores and urine flow studies) also failed to respond to a second dilatation. These patients should probably be excluded from consideration for repeat dilatation and offered TURP instead.

Mechanism of Action

The exact mechanism of action for balloon dilatation of the prostate is yet to be elucidated. Several proposed mechanisms include the following:

1. The gland is compressed and dehydrated with subsequent atrophy and enlargement of the urethral lumen
2. A permanent stretching of the prostatic capsule
3. The smooth muscle tone of the prostate is lost by the high-pressure dilatation
4. The α-adrenergic receptors of the bladder neck and proximal prostatic urethra are disrupted

PATIENT NAME: _____   EVALUATOR:_____

Enter the number which most accurately describes each of the following symptoms

STREAM:	How would you describe your urinary stream:	0 Normal 1 Variable 3 Weak 4 Dribbling	
VOIDING:	Have you had to strain or push over your bladder to urinate?	0 No Strain 2 Abdominal Strain	
HESITANCY:	Have you noticed you can't begin urination well?	0 No 3 Hesitancy	
INTERMITTENCY:	Does your stream stop and start 2 or more times while your urinate?	0 No 3 Yes	
BLADDER EMPTYING:	How would you describe your ability to empty all of the urine out your bladder? (Have you ever had your bladder catheterized?)	0 Don't Know or Complete 1 Variable 2 Incomplete 3 Single Retention 4 Repeated Retention	
INCONTINENCE:	Have you noticed dribbling or urinating after you thought you were finished?	0 No 2 Yes (include terminal dribbling)	
URGE:	Have you had the feeling you can't wait to urinate?	0 No 1 Mild 2 Moderate 3 Severe	
NOCTURIA:	How often do you have to interrupt your sleep to urinate?	0 0-1 1 2 2 3-4 3 >4	

DIURIA:	How often do you have to urinate during the day?	0 < once every 3 hours
		1 < once every 2 hours
		   and up to 3 hours
		2 once an hour
		   and up to every 2 hours
		3 once or more an hour	

TOTAL SYMPTOM SCORE			
POTENCY	No Problem _____ Impaired _____ Impotent_____		
RETROGRADE EJACULATION	Yes_____ No_____		
OVERALL	Do you feel that your symptoms have improved? Yes_____ No_____		

DATE:_____

Fig. 11.7.   Symptom score sheet used in patient selection.

5. Anterior and/or posterior commissurotomies are performed.

It is unlikely that glandular atrophy plays a major part in relieving bladder outlet obstruction, since histological evaluation of resected tissue in patients who have failed TUBDP and subsequently come to transurethral resection reveals no evidence of necrosis, haemorrhage or glandular atrophy (Reddy et al. 1988). Ultrasonography and magnetic resonance imaging performed by the same authors before and after dilatation showed intraprostatic but no periprostatic haemorrhage and an intact prostatic capsule.

While Reddy and associates do not believe that commissurotomies occur with TUBDP, it has been our experience, as well as the experience of other investigators (Goldenberg et al. 1990; Castaneda et al. 1989), that endoscopic evidence of an anterior commissurotomy portends a good prognosis in the subjective and objective relief of the patient's symptoms. This is not to imply that we believe this to be the sole mechanism of action for the procedure; however, we do feel that it may play an important role. We also believe, as Reddy (1990), that the stretching of the prostatic capsule is another very important mechanism of action of TUBDP.

It is therefore apparent, based on the results of previous studies, that stretching of the prostatic capsule and possibly anterior commissurotomy play a role in the mechanism of action in TUBDP. It is less likely that glandular atrophy contributes to the mechanism of action and further studies will be needed to identify the contribution of disruption of the innervation of the prostatic urethra.

Results

The results of balloon dilatation trials to date have been difficult to compare, because the studies vary widely in the length of follow-up and in the parameters used to evaluate success. Table 11.1 reviews the results to date of six of the largest series in the literature.

Goldenberg et al. (1990) performed a very thorough evaluation of 42 men with symptom scores, endoscopy and urodynamic studies prior to TUBDP. The authors evaluated peak and corrected peak flow rates as well as post-void residuals and symptom scores. They note that the 14 patients in their study with primary bladder neck obstruction fared much worse than those with BPH. They also found an improvement of symptom scores after TUBDP in 70% of patients at 1 month but this decreased to 59% by 12 months after the procedure. They reported a similar gradual decrease in peak flow and corrected peak flow rates over a 1 year follow-up of the patients.

Gill et al. (1989) evaluated a total of 48 men with urodynamically proven bladder outflow obstruction and found that 89% remained obstructed by urodynamic criteria in spite of an almost 50% improvement in symptoms. Nineteen patients with urinary retention were also evaluated and only 3 were able to void spontaneously post-procedure. However, the authors speculate that their poor results found with patients in urinary retention may be due to dilatation with balloons 25 mm and smaller. They conclude that larger balloons

Table 11.1. A summary of previous clinical trials reporting on the use of balloon dilatation for prostatic bladder outflow obstruction

Reference	Number of patients	Symptom improvement	Flow rate improvement	Longest follow-up
Goldenberg et al. 1990	42	23/28 6 months	24/28	12 months
Dowd and Smith 1990	50	36/50	~23/50	41 months
Reddy 1990	62	70% 6 months 58% 12 months	–	24 months
Gill et al. 1989	67	<50%	–	11 months
Daughtry et al. 1990	55	46/55	30/41	26 months
Donatucci et al. 1992	21	16/21	7/21	12 months

should probably be used to obtain better results and that patients in urinary retention are poor candidates for TUBDP. Daughtry and associates (1990) noted that 40% of their study population (22 patients) were in retention prior to TUBDP. Of these patients 4 required repeat dilatation after initial failure and 5 went on to undergo TURP. This represents a significant improvement over the results obtained with patients presenting in urinary retention in Gill and associates' study. However, Daughtry and associates used larger calibre balloons and still demonstrated a relatively poor result with patients presenting in retention.

Reddy and associates (1988) initially used a 75F balloon for dilatation but have recently reported their experience with a balloon which expands to 90F. They report excellent results using the 90F balloon with 70% of the patients noting symptomatic improvement at 6 months post-procedure but a significant drop to 58% of the patients reporting improvement in symptoms at 1 year. They also noted that of the 14 patients that eventually came to TURP, 13 had median lobe enlargement. There is no information, however, on the number of patients who underwent repeat TUBDP. Dowd and Smith (1990) reported that no patient in their study benefited from repeat dilatation if the initial procedure failed.

A randomised study comparing balloon dilatation of the prostate to TURP compares two well-matched groups with 21 patients in the TUBDP group and 20 in the TURP group (Donatucci et al. 1992). Both groups demonstrated a statistically significant decrease in symptom score from pre-operative levels (TURP 12.5 to 5.14, ($p < 0.01$); TUBDP 14.15 to 7.14 ($p < 0.01$)). There was no significant difference between groups in post-operative symptom score. The TURP group demonstrated a significantly improved peak urinary flow (13.64 to 27.64 ml/sec, $p < 0.05$); as did the TUBDP group (11.24 to 15.57 ml/sec, $p < 0.05$). This study is still ongoing with the longest follow-up to date being 12 months. Initial results however, support

TUBDP as a safe and effective procedure when compared to the gold standard of TURP.

In summary, the results of the initial clinical trials of TUBDP have demonstrated that it is a safe procedure. When compared to TURP, patients experience similar subjective and objective improvement. However, these results tend to be short-lived with a significant number of patients reporting recurrence of symptoms after 1 year.

Complications

The complications of TUBDP include bleeding, infection, retrograde ejaculation, incontinence and pain. Fortunately, these complications are infrequent and short-lived. The most common post-operative complication is bleeding. Virtually all patients experience some haematuria in the immediate post-operative period but prolonged haemorrhage is extremely uncommon. Haematuria usually clears within 24 hours and there has been no need for transfusions in any of the large series reported (Reddy et al. 1988; Reddy 1990; Dowd and Smith, 1990; Goldenberg et al. 1990; Klein and Lemming, 1989; Gill et al. 1989; Daughtry et al. 1990; Donatucci et al. 1992; Castaneda et al. 1989; McLoughlin and Williams, 1990b.

Complications such as urinary tract infections are also uncommon. Goldenberg and associates reported two documented urinary tract infections after treating a total of 42 patients (Goldenberg at el. 1990). Gill and associates reported a much higher incidence of infection with 9 of the 48 men suffering uncomplicated urinary tract infections which responded to oral antibiotics. However, 4 of these patients had a chronic indwelling Foley catheter pre-operatively. It is also noted that in this study, patients received piperacillin 2 g intravenously pre-operatively without further antibiotic coverage post-operatively (Gill et al. 1989). In many large studies urinary tract infections are distinctly uncommon with Dowd and Smith (1990) and Reddy (1990) reporting none in a total of 112 patients treated.

Although retrograde ejaculation and incontinence have been noted quite frequently with TURP, they are rarely, if ever, encountered following TUBDP. Other complications such as bladder spasms and post-operative pain do occur, but are easily treated with analgesics and anticholinergics post-operatively. One major disadvantage of TUBDP, while not truly a complication, is the failure to detect occult malignancies, estimated to occur in 6% to 27% of the patients undergoing TURP (Agatstein et al. 1987; Pritchett et al. 1988).

Summary

In summary, transurethral balloon dilatation of the prostate is an exciting and innovative alternative to prostatectomy. It has proven to be both safe and effective with minimal morbidity. Studies to date have noted that patients with large prostate glands, significant median lobe hyperplasia, urinary retention or previous TUBDP failures do poorly following this procedure. The technique is a relatively easy one to master. Contemporary studies, however, have shown us that in spite of the excellent results reported with early experience using TUBDP, long-term follow-up has proven to be less optimistic. Further studies and longer follow-up will eventually define the place for this procedure in the urologist's armamentarium.

References

Aalkjaer, V. 1962. Transurethral resection versus dilatation treatment in hypertrophy of the prostate: a comparison of the effects of the methods. Urol. Int. 14:119–124

Agatstein, E.H., Hernandez, F.J., Layfield, L.J., Smith, R.B., deKernion, J.B. 1987. Use of fine needle aspiration for detection of stage A prostatic carcinoma before transurethral resection of the prostate: a clinical trial. J. Urol. 138:551–553

Birkhoff, J.J. 1983. Natural history of benign prostatic hypertrophy. In: Benign prostatic hypertrophy. Hinman, F. Jr., ed. New York, Springer, chapter 7

Burhenne, H.J. 1975. Dilatation of biliary tract strictures: a new roentgenologic technique. Radiol. Clin. (Basel) 44:153–159

Burhenne, H.J., Chisholm, R.J., Grenville, N.J. 1984. Prostatic hyperplasia: radiologic intervention. Radiology 152:655–657

Castaneda, F., Reddy, P., Wasserman, N., et al. 1987. Benign prostatic hypertrophy: retrograde transurethral dilation of the prostatic urethra in humans. Radiology 163:649–653

Castaneda, F., Isorna, S., Hulbert, J.C., et. al. 1989. The importance of separation of prostatic lobes in relief of prostatic obstruction by balloon catheter urethroplasty: studies in dogs and humans. A.J.R. 153:1301–1304

Chapple, C.R., Milroy, E.J., Rickards, D. 1990. Permanently implanted urethral stent for prostatic obstruction in the unfit patient. Preliminary report. Br. J. Urol. 66:58–65.

Civiale, J. 1983. Traite pratique des maladies des organes. Genito-Urinaire, Paris, 1841 (as cited in: Benign prostatic hypertrophy. Hinman, F. Jr., ed. New York, Springer, chapter 5)

Daughtry, J.D., Rodan, B.A., Bean, W.J. 1990. Balloon dilation of prostatic urethra. Urology 36:203–209

Deisting, W. 1956. Transurethral dilatation of the prostate: a new method in the treatment of prostatic hypertrophy. Urol. Int. 2:158–171

Donatucci, C.F., Donahue, R.E., Crawford, E.D., (1992) A randomized, community-based study of balloon dilatation of the prostate versus transurethral resection. Unpublished data.

Dowd, J.B., Smith, J.J., III 1990. Balloon dilatation of the prostate. Urol. Clin. North Am. 17:671–677

Fornage, B.D., Toubas, O. 1989. Transrectal sonographic monitoring of balloon dilatation of the prostatic urethra. J. Ultrasound Med. 8:53–55

Franck, O. 1938. Die Sprengung des Prostataringes. Munch. Med. Wochenschr. 85:777–782

Gill, K.P., Machan, L.S., Allison, D.J., Williams, G. 1989. Bladder outflow tract obstruction and urinary retention from benign prostatic hypertrophy treated by balloon dilatation. Br. J. Urol. 64:618–622

Goldenberg, S.L., Perez-Marrero, R.A., Lee, L.M., Emerson, L. 1990. Endoscopic balloon dilation of the prostate: early experience. J. Urol. 144:83–88

Guthrie, G.J. 1983. On the anatomy and diseases of the urinary organs. London, 1836 (as cited in: Benign prostatic hypertrophy. Hinman, F. Jr., ed. New York, Springer, chapter 5)

Hollingsworth, E. 1910. Dilatation of the prostatic urethra for the relief of the symptoms of prostatic enlargement. Ann. Surg. 51:597–608

Klein, L.A., Lemming, B. 1989. Balloon dilatation for prostatic obstruction. Urology 33:198–201

Kreder, K.J., Webster, G.D. 1992 Urodynamic assessment of bladder outlet obstruction. In: Controversies and advances in the diagnosis and treatment of BPH: Problems in urology. Lepor, H., ed. Philadelphia. Lippincott, in press

Lepor, H. 1989 Non-operative management of benign prostatic hyperplasia. J. Urol. 141:1283–1289

Lindner, A., Golomb, J., Siegel, Y., et. al. 1987. Local hyperthermia of the prostate gland for the treatment of benign prostatic hypertrophy and urinary retention: a preliminary report. Br. J. Urol. 60:567–571

McLoughlin, J., Williams, G. 1990a. Alternatives to prostatectomy. Br. J. Urol. 65:313–316

McLoughlin, J., Williams, G. 1990b. Prostatic stents and balloon dilatation. Br. J. Hosp. Med. 43:422–426

Mebust, W.K. 1988. Surgical management of benign prostatic obstruction. Urology 32 (suppl):12–15

Mercier, F. 1983. Recherches sur les valvules du col de la vessie. Paris, 1850 (as cited in: Benign prostatic hypertrophy. Hinman, F. Jr., ed. New York, Springer, chapter 5)

Orandi, A. 1985. Transurethral incision of prostate (TUIP):646 cases in 15 years – a chronological appraisal. Br. J. Urol. 57:703–707

Pritchett, T.R., Moreno, J., Warner, N.E., et al. 1988. Unsuspected prostatic adenocarcinoma in patients who have undergone radical cystoprostatectomy for transitional cell carcinoma of the bladder. J. Urol. 139:1214–1216.

Reddy, P.K., Wasserman, N., Castaneda, F., and Castaneda-Zuniga, W.R. 1988. Balloon dilatation of the prostate for treatment of benign hyperplasia. Urol. Clin. North Am. 15:529–535

Reddy, P.K. 1990. Role of balloon dilation in the treatment of benign prostatic hyperplasia. Prostate (suppl.) 3:39–48

Chapter 12

Is Pharmacotherapy a Satisfactory Alternative Treatment for Benign Prostatic Hyperplasia?

C.R. Chapple and I.R. Marshall

Surgical prostatectomy is the most commonly used treatment for benign prostatic hyperplasia (BPH) causing obstruction to the bladder outflow tract. Approximately 90% of patients will undergo a transurethral prostatectomy (Mebust, 1988) and this is the gold standard against which other therapies need to be judged. Prostatic surgery is associated with an improvement in patients' symptoms in the majority of cases; 75% at 3 years in the series reported by Bruskewitz (Bruskewitz et al. 1986) and 90% at 5 years in Meyhoff's experience (Meyhoff, 1987), with reoperation rates of the order of 2.8%–8% at 5 years (Bergman et al. 1955; Chilton et al. 1978; Meyhoff, 1987). The largest review of the results of prostatectomy so far reported (54, 077 patients) noted a reoperation rate of 8.9%–9.7% at 5 years, rising to 12%–15.5% at 8 years following transurethral prostatectomy (Roos et al. 1989). It is of particular note that the equivalent rates following open prostatectomy were 1.1%–3.4% at 5 years and 1.8%–4.5% at 8 years. This finding coupled with the significant mortality associated with surgery (Roos et al. 1989), in particular via the transurethral route, recognition of the slow clinical progression of benign prostatic obstruction (Craigen et al. 1969; Ball et al. 1981) and recently increased public awareness of alternative treatment options have increased interest in the use of pharmacotherapy as a treatment for benign prostatic hyperplasia.

Before considering any therapy which may be less effective than the existing first-choice treatment for benign prostatic hyperplasia (BPH), namely surgery, it is important to consider the natural history of the condition, and to exclude as far as possible other pathology affecting the prostate, in particular malignancy.

The natural course of untreated prostatic obstruction is very variable (Craigen et al. 1969; Castro et al. 1971) with slow progression of patients' symptomatology on conservative management alone (Ball et al. 1981;). It is therefore justifiable to attempt treatment with alternative therapies. On the other hand it must be remembered that the improvements seen after any short-term therapy may not therefore be a consequence of the treatment but may rather reflect natural fluctuations of the disease process itself (Table 12.1).

All patients should be properly investigated prior to the instigation of one of the newer treatment alternatives, in particular pharmacotherapy; not only so that a satisfactory appraisal of their efficacy can be obtained, but also so that prostatic malignancy and other complications of prostatic obstruction or other coexisting disease such as bladder cancer are not missed. Nevertheless, despite comprehensive investigation using contemporary techniques, the absence of the tissue diagnosis automatically obtained following prostatectomy is associated with the likelihood of missing up to one fifth of patients with focal carcinoma, (Chisholm, 1989).

Benign prostatic hyperplasia is an important cause of bladder outflow obstruction. Both a *static* factor due to the mechanical compression exerted by the increased bulk of prostate in BPH and fluctuating – so called *dynamic* influences – resulting from alterations in the neural control of prostatic muscle control are important. Certainly, benign prostatic enlargement of the prostate comprises both hypertrophy and in particular hyperplasia of prostatic stromal and glandular compartments. Indeed, contrary to popular belief morphometric quantification of this tissue has suggested that hyperplasia of the stromal compartment is the predominant feature (Bartsch et al. 1979). Although these authors did not carry out a separate analysis of the smooth muscle, it is likely that this would demonstrate a relative increase in the muscular component as contrasted to normal prostate.

Pharmacotherapy can potentially be effective by *reducing* prostatic size acting via a hormonal mechanism of action or *relaxing* prostatic smooth muscle by blockade of sympathetic adrenergic nerves. The assessment of such therapy must be carried out using double-blind placebo-controlled studies not only because of the random fluctuations in symptoms which occur in patients with symptomatic BPH, but also because of the significant placebo effects noted in controlled trials reported to date (Table 12.2).

Table 12.1. Natural history of untreated BPH based on four studies: 282 patients followed up for 2.6–5 years (after Isaacs, 1990)

% Response based on					
Subjective criteria			Objective criteria		
Worse	Better	No change	Worse	Better	No change
45 ± 7	38 ± 4	16 ± 9	63	22	16

Table 12.2. The placebo effect of drugs on BPH? Review of 12 studies: 260 patients followed up for 0.6–6 months (after Isaacs, 1990)

% Response based on					
Subjective criteria			Objective criteria		
Worse	Better	No change	Worse	Better	No change
12 ± 2	42 ± 5	46 ± 6	19 ± 7	24 ± 6	58 ± 11

Hormonal Therapy

Whilst the precise mechanisms underlying the development of BPH are poorly understood it seems clear that hormonal factors are important in its pathogenesis. John Hunter was the first clearly to document the relationship between the testes and prostatic growth, when in 1786 he noted that castration of animals produced a reduction in prostatic size and function. The earliest hormonal therapy used in man was the treatment of BPH by surgical castration (Cabot, 1896; White, 1895). In a study of 111 cases treated by castration, White noted a marked reduction in prostatic size. Of 61 patients who had undergone castration who were reported by Cabot the following year, urinary retention disappeared in 27 and the majority of patients were markedly improved. Moore (1944) reported the most comprehensive study in support of this relationship between the testes and the pathogenesis of BPH. In this study, absent testicular function (castration or hypopituitarism) prior to the age of 40 years prevented the occurrence of BPH or prostate cancer in men who lived into the BPH age group (over 55 years). Further evidence in support of these observations is provided by study of the Russian Skoptzys sect which undergoes ritual castration for men at the age of 35 years and who appeared to be spared the development of BPH (Zuckerman, 1936).

Although there are no significant differences in androgen levels in age-matched men with and without BPH (Bartsch et al. 1979), it seems likely that androgens provide a hormonal milieu that is essential to the development of BPH. A number of theories exist as to the mechanism of development of BPH (Geller, 1989), further consideration of which is beyond the scope of this chapter.

Despite the efficacy of castration the advent of endoscopic resection of the prostate resulted in a diminution of interest. However, Geller and associates were amongst the first in this field with a study of the progestational agent megesterol acetate in an uncontrolled study reported in 1965 (Geller et al. 1965). Subsequently a number of drugs have been used competitively to antagonise the trophic effects of androgens on the prostate, using drugs acting at various levels on the neuroendocrine axis (Figure 12.1). A representative selection of these studies is summarised in Table 12.3.

It is evident from this data that hormonal therapy is effective in double-blind trials but noticeably less so than surgery. It is becoming increasingly clear that certain subgroups of patients are more likely to respond to hormonal blockade than others. It may be that the reason for this lies with the underlying prostatic histology in particular the relative proportions of epithelial and stromal components. Indeed, the observation by Huggins and Stevens (1940) when reviewed in retrospect provides some interesting insight into the potential limitations of anti-androgen therapy. In three patients whose BPH was treated by castration, significant epithelial atrophy did not occur until 90 days after hormonal withdrawal and there was little change in the

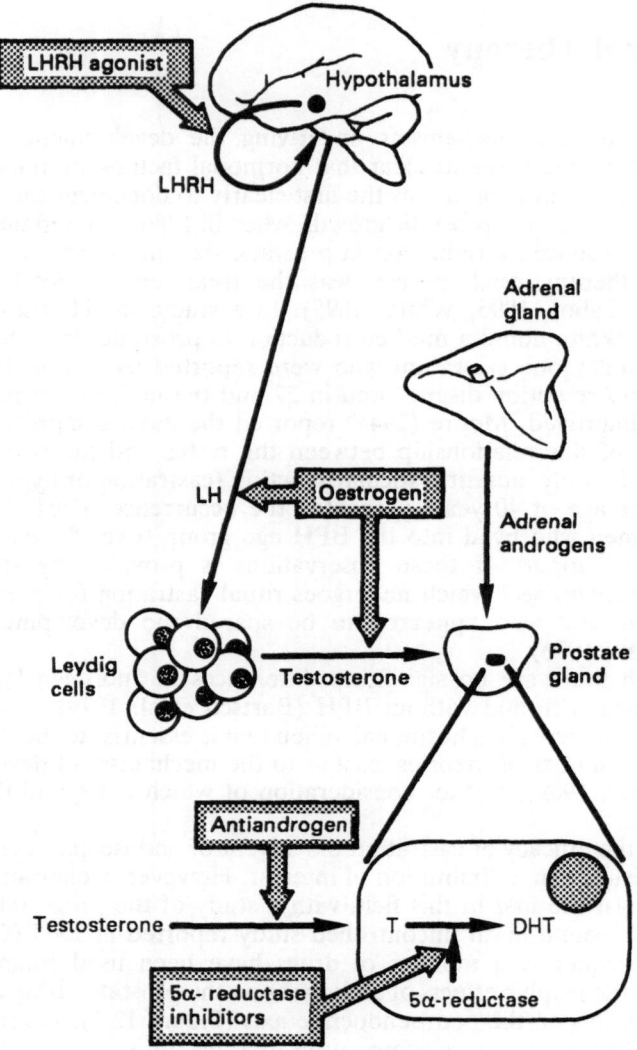

Fig. 12.1. Schematic diagram indicating the mechanism of action of the various groups of hormonal agents which are currently available.

stroma. Recent evidence has been put forward which suggests that serum prostatic specific antigen (PSA) may be helpful in predicting response to hormonal therapy (Matzkin et al. 1991; Levine et al. 1989). Serum PSA appears to reflect the ratio between epithelial and stromal components within the prostate; although PSA is positively correlated with prostatic volume, PSA is also correlated with the degree of prostatic epithelial hyperplasia. The patients who respond best to this therapy are those with a higher serum PSA and a smaller prostatic volume.

Table 12.3 A selection of representative clinical studies evaluating androgen deprivation for BPH (after Lepor, 1989)

Reference	Drug	Randomised placebo-controlled	Patient no.	Weeks of study	Change in prostate size	Change in urinary flow rate	Improved symptom score	Conclusion
Scott and Wade 1969	Cyproterone acetate	No	13	Variable	Not measured	Increased	Not measured	Effective
Caine et al. 1975	Flutamide	Yes	30	12	Not measured	Significant increase	Not measured	Effective
Geller et al. 1979	Megesterol acetate	Yes	61	20	Not measured	Significant increase	Not measured	Effective
Donkervoort et al. 1975	Megesterol acetate	No	36	16	Not measured	Increase	Yes	Inconclusive
Meiraz et al. 1977	17-hydroxy progesterone	No	39	14	No significant change	Not measured	No significant change	Ineffective
Peters and Walsh, 1987	Nafarelin acetate	No	8	27	24% decrease in size	Increase in some patients	Improved in 6/9 patients	Inconclusive
Matzkin et al. 1991	Triptorelin	No	17 10	24 48	27% decrease in size	Increase in some patients	Improved in 10/17 patients	Limited role

A major disadvantage of all these therapies has been the high incidence of unwanted side effects many of which can be attributed to a reduction in systemic circulating androgens (loss of libido, impotence). The development of specific androgen blockade within the prostate by inhibition of the enzyme 5α-reductase, thereby preventing the conversion of testosterone to the active derivative dihydrotestosterone (DHT), was potentially a major advance. This would provide a prostate specific hormonal effect without reducing circulating extra-prostatic androgen which results in unwanted side effects consequent upon androgen withdrawal. The initial clinical studies have provided disappointing results with improvements in mean urinary flow rate of only 1–2 ml/sec, despite significant reductions in prostatic size and quantitative symptom scoring (Stoner, 1991; Kirby et al. 1991). Really this is not surprising since the results would not be expected to be superior to those to be obtained following castration. From the preliminary results which are available, there do appear to be significant inter-subject variations in response within the studies similar to those noted with previous studies of hormonal therapy for BPH, no doubt for the same reasons.

While there are advantages for this specific therapy acting solely on production of DHT there is the disadvantage that 5α-reductase inhibition does not prevent the peripheral conversion of testosterone to oestrogen carried out by the enzyme aromatase. Oestrogen may be important in addition to DHT in the genesis of BPH, by an action predominantly on the stromal component of the prostate (Geller, 1989). The only aromatase inhibitor which has so far been investigated (testolactone) is a relatively weak antagonist; it has been investigated in an uncontrolled fashion, but was found to improve symptoms in 7 of 13 patients (Tunn et al. 1985) and in half of the treated patients decreased prostatic size by 15%–26% (Schweikert and Tunn, 1987). This is an area which warrants further investigation, especially in combination with inhibition of 5α-reductase.

Adrenergic Blockade

Learmonth (1931) reported that stimulation of the pre-sacral nerve in man contracted the prostatic musculature. Total neural blockage using spinal anaesthesia produces a 47% reduction in urethral closure pressure (Furuya et al 1982) and α blockade similarly results in a decrease in urethral closure pressure (Donker et al. 1972). Dynamic changes such as these in recent years have highlighted the potential clinical importance of pharmacological blockade of the motor sympathetic adrenergic nerve supply to the prostate. The consequences of blockade will vary according to the level of sympathetic stimulation acting on the prostate gland (Furuya et al. 1982).

Experimental Studies

Functional Muscle Strip Studies

Functional isometric muscle strip experiments have suggested that in both the normal and hyperplastic prostate there is a functional predominance of α_1-adrenoceptors. The evidence in support of this comes from studies using agonists and antagonists.

Noradrenaline and phenylephrine (3×10^{-7} to 3×10^{-5} M) produce concentration-dependent contractions of adenomatous, peripheral and normal prostate tissue preparations. The maximum effect obtained with phenylephrine (α_1 agonist) is about 75% of that found with noradrenaline (α_1/α_2 agonist) (Hedlund et al. 1985; Figure 12.2). In contrast agonists selective for α_2-adrenoceptors are either ineffective (e.g. UK 14,304; Fig. 12.2) or only exert effects at high concentrations at which they act via the α_1-adrenoceptor (e.g. clonidine; Hedlund et al. 1985).

Studies with α-adrenoceptor antagonists in strips of prostate have always been carried out using noradrenaline as the agonist. The highly selective

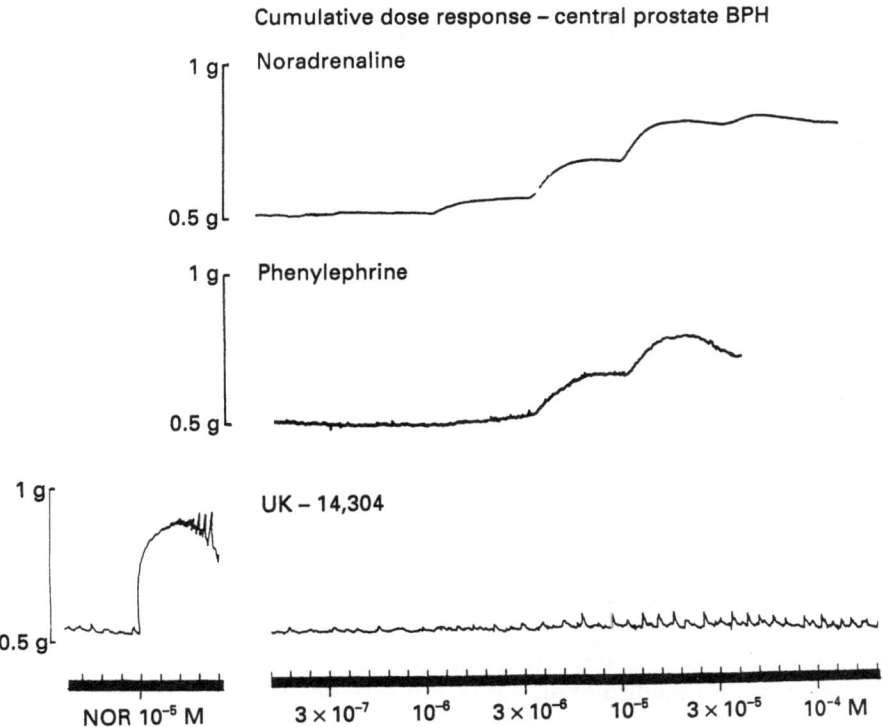

Fig. 12.2. Cumulative dose response curve to noradrenaline, phenylephrine and UK 14,304. (x axis, drug concentration in moles; y axis, tension in muscle strip preparations in grams).

α_1-adrenoceptor antagonist prazosin competitively antagonised contractions to exogenous noradrenaline (Fig. 12.3; Hieble et al. 1985) with a pA_2 value of 9.1 and a slope of the Schild plot not significantly different from 1.0 (Fig. 12.4). The conclusion that α_1-adrenoceptors are involved is supported by the relative ineffectiveness of rauwolscine which is selective for α_2-adrenoceptors. This compound antagonised noradrenaline contractions only around 10^{-6} M or higher (Hieble et al. 1985; Hedlund et al. 1985), concentrations at which rauwolscine is no longer selective but also has affinity for α_1-adrenoceptors.

Field stimulation of the nerve terminals in isolated prostatic strips evoked frequency-dependent contractions (nerve-mediated as they are inhibited by tetrodotoxin, (TTX) (Fig. 12.5) which were abolished by prazosin and phentolamine but not by rauwolscine or scopolamine (Hedlund et al. 1985) or atropine (Fig. 12.5). Thus these contractions appear to be due to the release of transmitter, probably noradrenaline, onto α_1-adrenoceptors and this response is not mediated via α_2-adrenoceptors or muscarinic receptors. The latter is consistent with the lack of contraction to either exogenous acetylcholine or carbachol (Hedlund et al. 1985). Measurement of the release of ^{3}H-noradrenaline by field stimulation was inhibited by clonidine and potentiated by rauwolscine (Hedlund et al. 1985) showing that the pre-synaptic α_2-adrenoceptor mechanism which can regulate noradrenaline release was functional.

These functional studies suggest that contraction of the prostate is mediated via adrenergic nerves and post-junctional α_1-adrenoceptors. Therefore antagonism of these receptors may relax prostatic smooth muscle in vivo if there is activity in the sympathetic nerves. The same α_1-adrenoceptors also mediate contractions to exogenous noradrenaline. These observations provide the rationale for the use of α_1-adrenoceptor antagonists in the treatment of BPH. The demonstration of the pre-synaptic α-adrenoceptors, through which the release of noradrenaline can be regulated, suggests that non-selective α-adrenoceptor antagonists will be less effective in treating BPH. This is because, through α_2-adrenoceptor blockade, they will increase the release of noradrenaline from sympathetic nerves and this extra amount of agonist may offset the post-junctional antagonism at the α_1-adrenoceptors.

Radioligand Binding Studies: Homogenates

Ligand binding techniques have only recently been applied to the investigation of human prostatic α_1- and α_2-adrenoceptors. These studies have raised an as yet unexplained paradox; one study demonstrating an excess of α_2 over α_1 receptors in adenomatous prostate (Hedlund et al. 1985) and another suggesting equivalent densities for both groups of α receptors (Lepor and Shapiro, 1984; Shapiro and Lepor, 1986) despite the demonstrable functional predominance of α_1 receptors (see above). It has been suggested that α_2 receptors may have an important role in mediating contraction of canine prostatic muscle (Shapiro et al. 1987), but care needs to be exercised in the extrapolation from animal models to man.

The results of saturation analyses carried out in our unit on tissue from adenomatous central prostate (7 patients), peripheral prostate (8 patients),

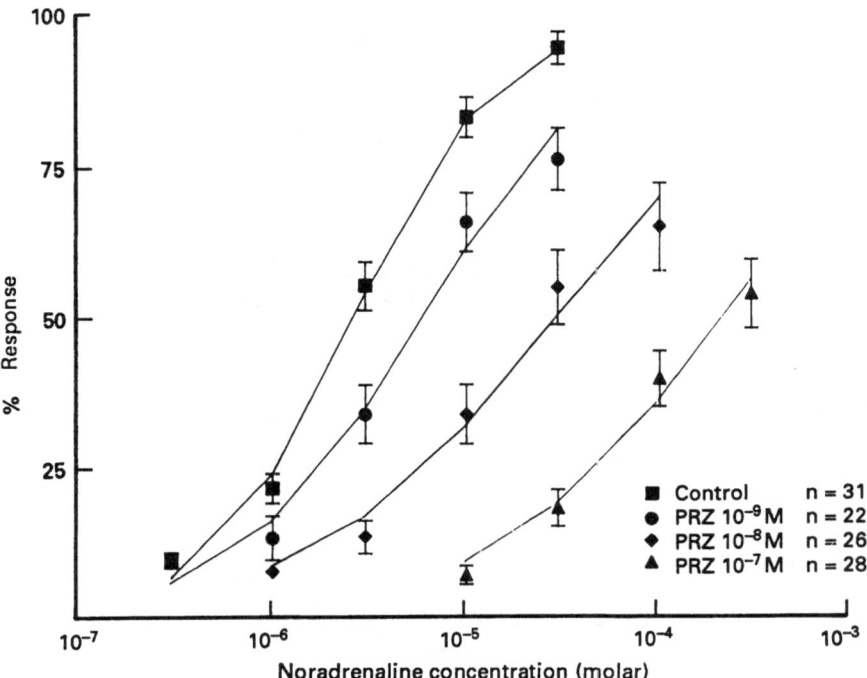

Fig. 12.3. Fitted dose response curves, contractile response to noradrenaline contrasting the response in the presence of differing concentrations of prazosin (PZR) (10^{-9}M–10^{-7}M).

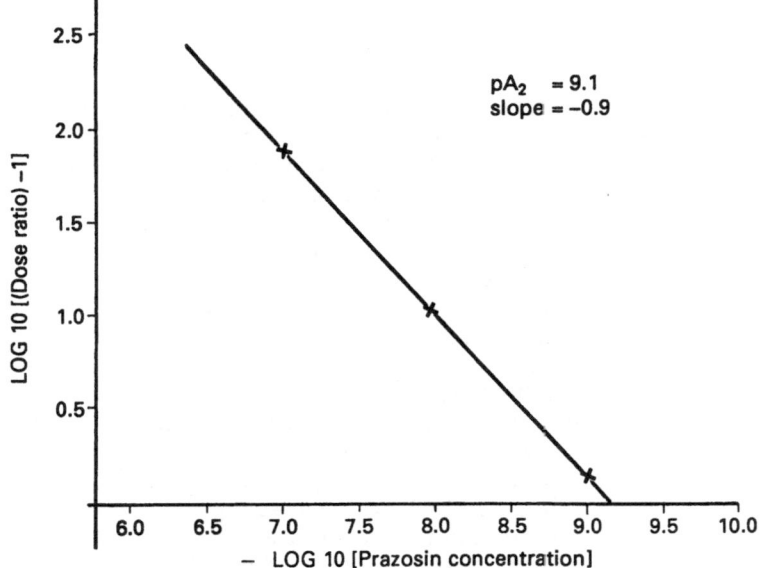

Fig. 12.4. Schild plot for prazosin in central prostate.

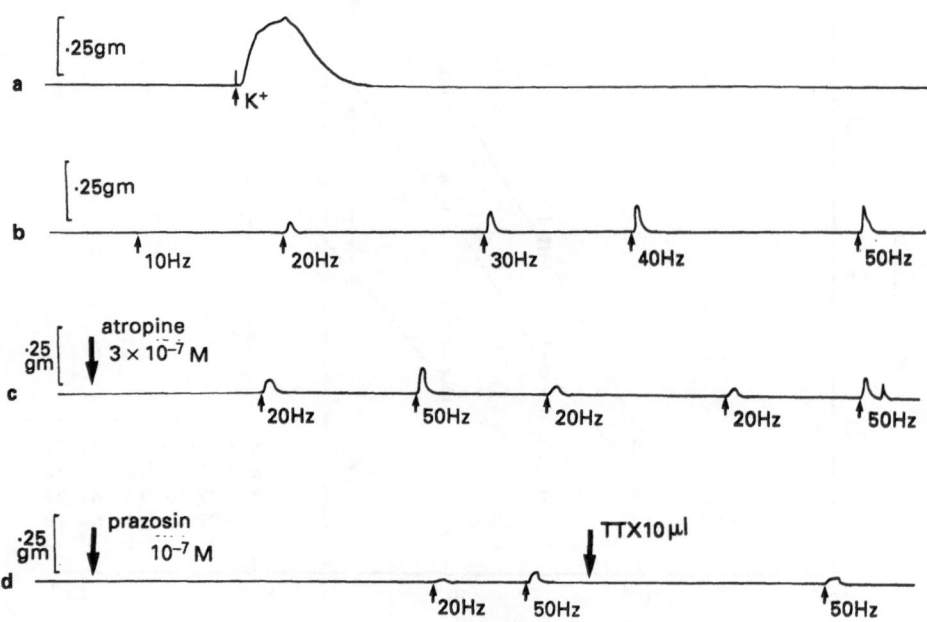

Fig. 12.5. **a** Response to maximal stimulation with K⁺. **b** Response to nerve stimulation.
c Effect of pre-incubation with atropine 3×10^{-7}M on the response to nerve stimulation.
d A comparison of pre-incubation with prazosin 10^{-7}M and TTX on the response to
nerve-mediated stimulation.

and normal control prostate (3 patients) are summarised in Table 12.4 and
Fig. 12.6 (Chapple et al. 1989). The binding of ³H-prazosin and ³H-UK 14,304
was saturable and in each case a single class of binding sites was identified,
as confirmed by a linear Scatchard analysis plot. The equilibrium dissociation
constants (K_D) ranged between 0.32 and 0.52 nM for α_1 receptors and 1.8 and
3.10 nM for α_2 receptors (³H rauwolscine gave similar results). In some tissues
it was not possible to measure α_2 binding sites but α_1 receptors were always
present in all of the tissues examined. All tissues contained a much higher
density of α_1-adrenoceptors than α_2, therefore the detection of α_1 receptors
was taken as a marker of tissue viability and the results for α_2 receptors were
analysed. In contrast, if both α_1 and α_2 receptors were absent, then the
results were not included in the analysis, as it was assumed that the tissue
was damaged. The adrenergic receptor concentration (B_{MAX}) was calculated
in fmoles/mg protein. The range of values measured was 61.1–79.4 fmoles/mg
protein for α_1 binding sites and 12.1–36.1 fmoles/mg protein for α_2 binding
sites. Fig. 12.6 contains representative Scatchard analysis curves for peripheral
prostate, but similar patterns were also obtained with both central and normal prostate. This is demonstrated by the correlation coefficients for the
representative curves; control prostate ³H-prazosin $r=-0.96$, ³H-UK 14,304

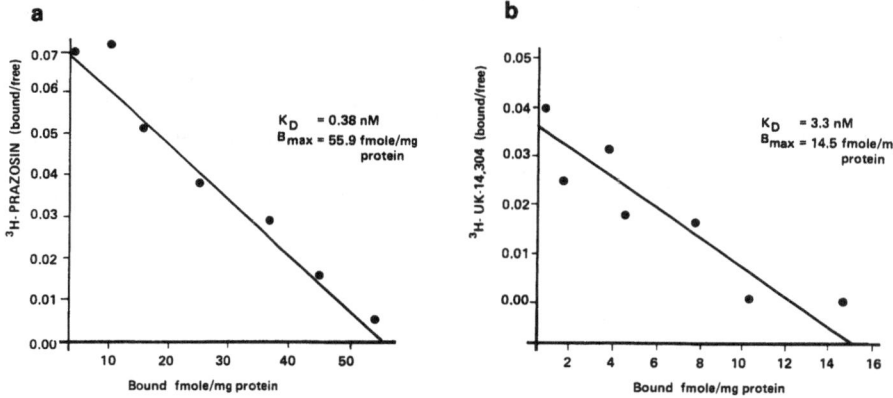

Fig. 12.6. Representative Scatchard plots for **a** ^{3}H-prazosin and **b** ^{3}H-UK 14,304 binding to homogenates from seven adenomatous prostatic tissues. Plots represent one experiment performed in triplicate and repeated seven times on membranes obtained from different patients in each experiment. Equilibrium dissociation constant (K^D), receptor concentration (Bmax) and linear correlation coefficient (LCC) values were determined from the Scatchard plots presented.

Table 12.4 Summary of mean values ± standard error of mean for α-adrenoceptor ligand binding studies (separate experiments performed in triplicate)

Sample	[3]H Prazosin α^1		[3]H UK14,304 α^2	
	K_D (nM)	B_{max} (fmoles/mg)	K_D (nM)	B_{max} (fmoles/mg)
Prostate (BPH) (central) $n = 7$	0.51 ±0.07	65.9 ±5.2	2.34 ±0.26	36.1 ±6.2
Prostate (BPH) (peripheral) $n = 8$	0.32 ±0.03	79.4 ±11.1	3.1 ±1.0	18.4 ±3.1
Prostate (control) $n = 2$	0.52	61.1	1.8	12.1

$r=-0.94$; peripheral prostate ^{3}H-prazosin $r=-0.97$, ^{3}H-UK 14,304 $r=-0.89$; central prostate ^{3}H-prazosin $r=-0.98$, ^{3}H-UK 14,304 $r=-0.92$. The ratio of α_1 to α_2 receptors was approximately 2 : 1 in adenomatous central prostate, and 4 : 1 in peripheral non-adenomatous tissue. Statistical comparison of these data using the Mann-Whitney U statistic confirmed a significant difference between α_1 and α_2 receptor binding sites in the peripheral prostate ($p < 0.005$). Conversely the apparent difference between α_1 and α_2 receptors for central prostate failed to reach significance ($p > 0.05$).

Radioligand Binding Studies: Slide-Mounted Tissue Sections

The autoradiographic images obtained from the three different radioligands used to identify $\alpha_{1\&2}$-adrenoceptor and muscarinic receptor binding sites contrasted the localisation of the three binding sites (Fig. 12.7). The majority of ^{3}H-prazosin binding identified was confined to the stroma. In comparison, a sparse grain distribution was seen with ^{3}H-rauwolscine in the same region, but extensive labelling was seen on the numerous blood vessels present in these tissue sections. Muscarinic cholinoceptors, identified using ^{3}H-QNB, were principally located on glandular epithelium, as reported in previous studies (Hedlund et al. 1985; Lepor and Kuhar, 1984). In addition to

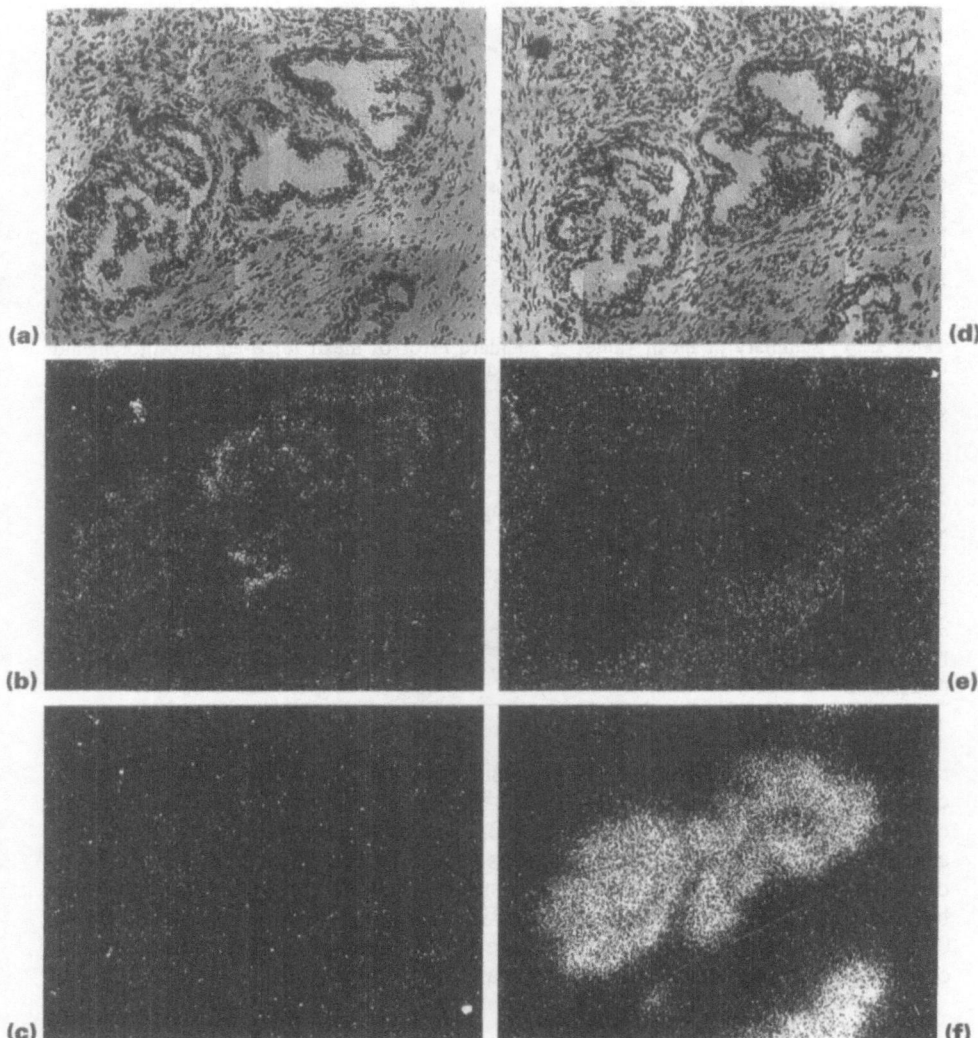

Fig. 12.7. Consecutive serial sections of human prostate (magnification × 60) are shown here. These include the following: **a,d** stained with toluidine blue to demonstrate the anatomy; **b** demonstrating the distribution of α_2-adrenoceptors; **c** control; **e** demonstrating the distribution of α_1-adrenoceptors; **f** demonstrating the distribution of muscarinic cholinoceptors.

extensive blood vessel labelling, a population of α_2-adrenoceptors was seen in close proximity to the base of some of the ^{3}H-QNB-labelled glandular epithelial cells.

The mean specific binding value (% grain occupancy/unit area) in the stroma of each prostate specimen was calculated for both adrenoceptor radioligands used (Table 12.5). The mean specific binding values for the α_1- and α_2-adrenoceptors were 4.5 ± 0.39 and 1.6 ± 0.37 respectively, and the average ratio of $\alpha_1 : \alpha_2$ binding sites in the prostatic stroma was 3.9 ± 0.75. The differences between these two groups were very highly significant (Mann-Whitney, $p < 0.0001$).

Muscarinic cholinergic receptors have been found exclusively on glandular epithelium in this and other reports. Both adrenergic and cholinergic nerve axons have been detected subepithelially in the human prostate (Vaalasti and Hervonen, 1980a), and cholinoceptor stimulation, resulting from sympathetic activity in the canine prostate, causes an increase in the amount of secretion expelled into the urethra (Bruschini et al. 1978). In this study, occasional high α_2 receptor densities were found in close proximity to these epithelial cells bearing muscarinic receptors, in the region of the basal lamina. This arrangement is a well-recognised feature in the autonomic nervous system. For example, α_2-adrenoceptors have been reported on cholinergic nerve terminals in the guinea-pig ileum (Drew, 1978). It is interesting to speculate that in the prostate gland there could be adrenoceptor modulation of acetylcholine release.

Receptor autoradiography has two substantial advantages over biochemical (homogenate) studies, in that it combines specific anatomical resolution with high sensitivity. The availability of slide-mounted intact histological sections allowed densitometric computer-assisted quantification of the α-adrenoceptor binding within prostatic stromal tissue. This degree of specificity is not achieved in homogenate studies although the latter allow more precise measurement of

Table 12.5. Quantification of autoradiographically demonstrable adrenoceptor sites

Specimen number	Specific receptor binding[a]		Approximate ratio Alpha−1 / Alpha−2
	Alpha-1	Alpha-2	
1	5.9	1.1	5:1
2	2.2	1.5	3:2
3	3.9	1.6	5:2
4	3.4	0.8	9:2
5	5.0	1.0	5:1
6	5.6	4.5	5:4
7	4.2	0.6	7:1
8	4.7	2.6	2:1
9	6.2	0.8	8:1
10	3.6	1.8	5:2
Mean	4.5	1.6	3.9
± SEM	± 0.39	± 0.37	± 0.75

[a] % grain occupancy/unit area

the density of receptors and ligand affinity. While a discrepancy exists in the literature regarding adrenoceptor density in human prostatic tissue (Hedlund et al. 1985; Shapiro and Lepor, 1986), the present study using ligand binding and autoradiography clearly shows an α_1-adrenoceptor predominance over α_2-adrenoceptors in the prostatic stroma. These results are consistent with the pharmacological data.

Conclusions

The results of the in vitro pharmacological isometric studies reported here confirm that there is a functional predominance of α_1-adrenoceptors in human prostatic muscle. The α_2-adrenoceptors, however, are associated with blood vessels. The results of radioligand studies confirm the trend of an increase in α_2 binding sites towards parity in adenomatous tissue reported by previous studies, but demonstrate an overall predominance of $\alpha_1 : \alpha_2$ receptors of approximately 3 : 1 which is in accordance with the results of the functional studies. A potential source of error would be if there were significant differences in innervation and histological structure between different areas of the same gland. We have carefully investigated this possibility by examining tissue from a number of different areas within prostatic adenomata removed at the time of open operation and, although there was significant regional variation, this appeared to be occurring randomly with no clearly identifiable regional trends.

These studies have shown that the principal motor control of the prostate is adrenergic via an action on α_1-adrenoceptors, which are localised predominantly within the stromal compartment of the prostate (Chapple et al. 1989; James et al. 1989). These results provide a scientific basis for the use of α_1-adrenoceptor antagonists in the provision of symptomatic relief to selected patients with benign prostatic hyperplasia.

Clinical Studies

The initial clinical application of adrenergic blockade to the lower urinary tract utilised the combined $\alpha_{1\&2}$-adrenergic antagonist phenoxybenzamine, and this produced encouraging improvements in urinary flow and clinical symptoms in most clinical studies (Caine et al. 1976, 1978; Boreham et al. 1977; Abrams et al. 1981, 1982; Gerstenberg et al. 1980), with few exceptions (Brooks et al. 1983). The incidence of side effects in 30% of patients on treatment with phenoxybenzamine (Caine et al. 1976), combined with evidence of mutagenicity in bacterial and mouse-cell cultures (Anonymous, 1983) has, despite its clearly documented efficacy, precluded its more widespread acceptance in the treatment of benign prostatic obstruction. These adverse effects have been attributed to the blockade of pre-synaptic α_2- adrenoceptors which is thought to interfere with the normal negative feedback control of noradrenaline release at the presynaptic adrenergic nerve terminal, resulting in high circulating noradrenaline levels.

With recognition of the importance of the α_1 receptor in mediating sympathetic action in the normal and adenomatous prostate, attention has turned to the therapeutic use of selective α_1 antagonists such as prazosin (Shapiro et al. 1981), with the intention of reducing unwanted side effects. Prazosin was introduced as an anti-hypertensive agent in 1977 (Cambridge et al. 1977) and was subsequently reported to produce urinary incontinence (Thien et al. 1978; Straughan, 1978). This incidental observation contributed to recognition of the potential role of selective α_1-adrenoceptor blockade as therapy in the lower urinary tract.

The majority of the existing short-term studies have demonstrated that selective α_1-adrenergic blockade can be effective with few adverse side effects. All of the contemporary α blockers appear to be very similar in terms of pharmacological and clinical efficacy and safety, producing up to a 50% increase in urinary flow rate with a significant improvement in patients' symptoms (Tables 12.6, 12.7). They are a useful addition to the therapy of patients on a waiting list for surgery, where it is contraindicated for medical reasons and those who don't want surgery. Nevertheless, it must be remembered that optimal pharmacological blockade of α receptors by producing a relaxation of prostatic smooth muscle is unlikely to produce more than 50% of that to be expected from a surgical prostatectomy (Lepor et al. 1990).

Table 12.6.   Efficacy of α-adrenoceptor antagonists in improving the urinary flow rate

Drug and author (no. of patients no. of weeks' treatment)	Mean increase in maximum flow rate (ml/sec)	Mean increase in mean flow rate (ml/sec)
Phenoxybenzamine		
Caine et al. 1978 (50,2)	6.2 (88%)	3.2 (82%)
Abrams et al. 1982 (41,4)	3.1 (43%)	–
Brooks et al. 1983 (28,4)	0.9 (14%)	–
Prazosin		
Hedlund et al. 1983 (20,4)	2.0 (41%)	1.1 (42%)
Martorana et al. 1984 (18,2)	6.9 (96%)	2.2 (48%)
Kirby et al. 1987 (55,4)	4.8 (59%)	–
Hedlund and Andersson 1988 (8,4)	2.0 (28%)	1.1 (29%)
Chapple et al. 1990 (58,12)	3.2 (34%)	–
Le Duc et al. 1990 (39,4)	5.35 (54%)	–
Alfuzosin		
Ramsay et al. 1985 (31,12)	0	–
Jardin et al. 1991 (518,26)	1.4 (11.5%)	0.9 (14%)
Indoramin		
Iacovou and Dunn, 1987 (30,8)	10 (118%)	–
Chow et al. 1990 (139,8)	4.9 (59%)	–
Stott and Abrams, 1991 (40,4)	2.6 (39%)	–
Terazosin		
Fabricius et al. 1990 (57,24)	4.2 (54%)	2.7 (55%)
Lepor et al. 1990 (39,8)	3.6 (42%)	1.9 (48%)
YM 617 & 12617		
Kawabe and Niijimah, 1987 (77,2)	3.0 (43%)	2.3 (85%)
Kawabe et al. 1990 (270,4)	3.6 (35%)	2.0 (41%)

Table 12.7. Efficacy of α-adrenoceptor antagonists in improving symptoms

Drug and author (no. of patients, no. of weeks' treatment)	Obstructive symptoms	Irritative symptoms	Combined symptoms
Phenoxybenzamine			
Caine et al. 1978 (50,2)	–	–	Y
Abrams et al. 1982 (41,4)	–	–	Y
Brooks et al. 1983 (28,4)	–	–	N
Prazosin			
Hedlund et al. 1983 (20,4)	Y	N	Y
Martorana et al. 1984 (18,2)	–	–	Y
Kirby et al. 1987 (55,4)	Y	Y	Y
Hedlund and Andersson, 1988 (8,4)	–	–	–
Chapple et al. 1990 (58,12)	N	N	Y
Le Duc et al. 1990 (39,4)	–	N	Y
Alfuzosin			
Ramsay et al. 1985 (31,12)	–	Y	–
Jardin et al. 1991 (518,26)	Y	Y	Y
Indoramin			
Iacovou and Dunn, 1987 (30,8)	N	N	Y
Chow et al. 1990 (139,8)	–	–	Y
Stott and Abrams, 1991 (40,4)	N	Y	N
Terazosin			
Fabricius et al. 1990 (57,24)	Y	Y	Y
Lepor et al. 1990 (39,8)	Y	Y	Y
YM 617 & 12617			
Kawabe and Niijimah, 1987 (77,2)	Y	Y	Y
Kawabe et al. 1990 (270,4)	Y	Y	Y

N, No change as compared to placebo; Y, significantly improved as compared to placebo.

Criticism has been levelled at the current literature which reports the efficacy of selective α_1 blockade, since it is based on detailed study of short treatment periods (Wein, 1989), with little effect on urodynamic parameters other than the urinary flow rate. Certainly, it must be borne in mind, that the symptomatic consequences of secondary detrusor instability are the commonest cause of referral to the urologist and it is possible that longer periods of treatment are required to demonstrate a therapeutic effect.

A report of the results of the first double-blind long-term study reporting the use of prazosin confirmed the observations of prior workers that there was an increase in the mean maximum urinary flow rate on treatment. In addition, it provided the first evidence for a significant change in cystometric parameters, with a 19% reduction in maximum micturition pressure (Chapple et al. 1990). The only other published long-term studies report the use of the selective α_1 antagonist terazosin (Lepor et al. 1990; Lepora and Knapp-Maloney, 1991; Fabricius et al. 1990), indoramin (Iacovou and Dunn 1987; Chow et al. 1990) and alfuzosin (Ramsay et al. 1985; Jardin et al. 1991). With the exception of the work by Ramsay et al. which used videocystometrography at entry and exit from the 3-month study, the other authors studied patients with flow rates, post-voiding residuals and symptom scoring, but did not evaluate other urodynamic parameters. Indeed, in the study reported by Jardin et al. (1991), only 45% of the patients had had a urinary flow rate estimation and only 36% a post-voiding urinary residual prior to entry into the trial. The work reported by Ramsay et al. was the only one which failed to demonstrate any improvement in the urodynamic parameters of outflow obstruction. The other studies all demonstrated a significant increase in urinary flow rate which then decreased on continuing therapy by 1.3 ml/sec (29.5%), (Lepor et al. 1990); 0.6 ml/sec (14.4%), (Fabricius et al. 1990); and 1.8 ml/sec (67%), (Jardin et al. 1991) over a subsequent follow-up period of at least 13 weeks. In a subsequent open study of the longer-term use of terazosin there was an increase in maximum flow rate of 4.7 ml/sec at 6 weeks which reduced to 1.6 ml/sec at 72 weeks (Lepor and Knapp-Maloney 1991). These observations are compatible with the development of tolerance to the effects of this drug therapy. However, the findings reported here support the alternative hypothesis that there is a dynamic rebalancing of the relationship between pressure and flow during voiding, which results from α_1 blockade and that these effects on detrusor function take more than 1 month to occur. This would also explain why the increase in urinary flow rate was not as large as previously reported in an earlier 1-month study using a similar protocol (Kirby et al. 1987). Indeed, in support of this suggestion it is well recognised that the reduction in detrusor instability which occurs after prostatectomy may take up to 6 months. In view of the fixed time period of this study it is not possible to comment on whether the observed relationship between micturition pressure and flow was maintained at a longer follow-up period such as 6 months; but by inference from the terazosin studies which have data (not double-blind) of up to 18 months (Lepor and Knapp-Maloney 1991) this does seem likely.

Conclusions

The therapeutic effect of the α_1/α_2-adrenoceptor antagonist phenoxybenzamine has been reported to be superior to that achieved by selective α_1 blockade and one possible explanation being that this difference might be due to an additional action on α_2-adrenoceptors. Certainly, human prostatic α_2-adrenoceptors have been demonstrated using ligand binding studies (Hedlund et al. 1985; Chapple et al. 1989; Gup et al. 1990) to be present in an increased density in patients with symptomatic benign prostatic enlargement. However, it seems unlikely that they subserve a significant motor role, since selective slide-mounted autoradiography studies of the human prostate have demonstrated them to be primarily localised to blood vessels and the basement membrane of glandular acini rather than to the stromal compartment which is the site of prostatic smooth muscle (James et al. 1989). An alternative possibility is that if there is any benefit from α_2-adrenoceptor antagonism it is not exerted locally in the prostate but elsewhere.

These results suggest that selective α_1 blockade needs to be given for a period longer than 1 month to achieve maximum benefit. The increase in urinary flow rate is not as great as might be expected and this can be partly attributed to a reduction in voiding detrusor pressure. Optimal pharmacological blockade of α receptors by producing a relaxation of prostatic smooth muscle is unlikely to produce more than a 47% decrease in the total urethral closure pressure (Furuya et al. 1982), which is likely to be substantially less than that which could be obtained with surgical intervention.

The Future

Laboratory Studies

Selective α_1 blockade of prostatic adrenoceptors using the current non-specific α_1 antagonists is restricted by the systemic (predominantly cardiovascular) side effects which limit the maximum therapeutic dose. Recent animal studies have demonstrated the presence of α_1-adrenoceptor subtypes, α_{1A} and α_{1B}. Laboratory studies need to be directed at the search for more prostate-specific α_1 receptor subtypes, which would allow the development of therapy which might produce fewer systemic side effects. Preliminary work which we have conducted has investigated the existence and distribution of specific α_1-adrenoceptor subtypes within the human prostate as contrasted to a systemic blood vessel, the human inferior epigastric artery.

Strips of human prostatic tissue were obtained at the time of endoscopic prostatectomy and lengths of inferior epigastric artery obtained at the time of open surgery were subjected to in vitro pharmacological study in an organ bath. Dose-dependent responses were obtained to adrenoceptor stimulation by noradrenaline. These contractions were competitively antagonised by the α_1 antagonists doxazosin and prazosin at concentrations of 1×10^{-8} M– 1×10^{-6} M. In addition, the effects of the antagonists WB4101 (1×10^{-8} M–1×10^{-7} M) and SZL-49 (3×10^{-8} M – 1×10^{-7} M) which have some selectivity for α_{1A}-adrenoceptors and chlorethylclonidine (CEC, 1×10^{-5} M–1×10^{-4} M) which has selectivity for α_{1B}-adrenoceptors were investigated (Minneman 1988; Piascik et al. 1990). CEC and SZL-49 produce non-competitive antagonism since they bind covalently to receptors.

In the prostate, prazosin, doxazosin and WB4101 produced a shift to the right of the dose response curves to noradrenaline as expected from competitive antagonism at α_1-adrenoceptors. The relatively low affinity of WB4101 suggested there were α_{1B} receptors present. In agreement with this finding, CEC not only resulted in a similar shift to the right but also reduced the maximal contractile responses by up to 75% (Fig. 12.8). Conversely, the alkylating agent with some selectivity for α_{1A} receptors, SZL-49, was only effective at concentrations affecting both subtypes of α_1 receptor. Thus, SZL-49 3×10^{-8}M reduced the maximum contractile response to 65% $\pm$ 5% of the maximum response to noradrenaline 3×10^{-3} M and the corresponding value at a concentration of 1×10^{-7} M SZL-49 was 35% $\pm$ 2% (Fig. 12.9).

In contrast, whilst doxazosin and prazosin had a similar effect in both tissues, there was a difference in the responses to CEC, which was less effective, and SZL-49, which was more effective in the inferior epigastric artery than in the prostate. At a concentration of CEC 3×10^{-5} M the

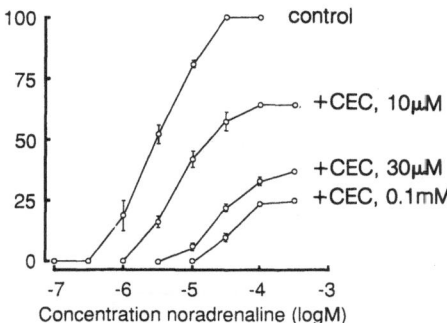

Fig. 12.8. Fitted dose response curves, contractile response of prostate to noradrenaline contrasting the response in the presence of differing concentrations of chlorethylclonidine (CEC) (10^{-5}M–10^{-4}M).

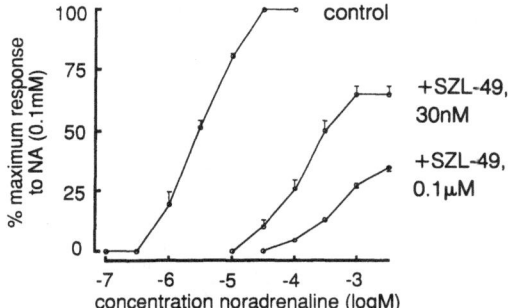

Fig. 12.9. Fitted dose response curves, contractile response of prostate to noradrenaline contrasting the response in the presence of differing concentrations of SZL-49 (3×10^{-8}M–10^{-7}M).

maximum contractile response was 93% ± 7% of the maximum obtained with 3×10^{-5} M noradrenaline and was reduced to a corresponding figure of 76% ± 12% at a concentration of 1×10^{-4} M CEC (Fig. 12.10). SZL-49 3×10^{-8} M reduced the maximum contractile response to 1×10^{-4} M noradrenaline to 41% ± 7% and at a concentration of 1×10^{-7} M further reduced it to 10% ± 6% (Fig. 12.11).

These findings provide evidence in support of different distributions of α_1-adrenoceptor subtypes within the human prostate and inferior epigastric artery. In the prostate it is likely that α_{1B}-adrenoceptors form the majority while α_{1A}-adrenoceptors predominate in the inferior epigastric artery. Existing α_1-adrenoceptor antagonists have been developed on the basis of their efficacy in the cardiovascular system. If the α_1 receptors in the systemic vasculature are similar to those in the inferior epigastric artery, the development of α_{1B}-specific antagonists could improve the therapeutic efficacy of these agents in relaxing prostatic smooth muscle while reducing systemic side effects.

Subsequent ongoing research work in our laboratory validated against receptor clones has identified that the responses in the human prostate

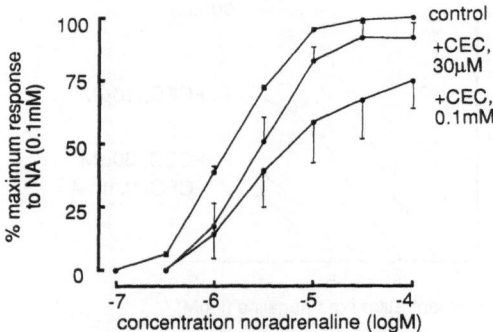

Fig. 12.10. Fitted dose response curves, contractile response of inferior epigastric artery to noradrenaline contrasting the response in the presence of differing concentrations of chlorethylclonidine (CEC) ($10^{-5}M–10^{-4}M$).

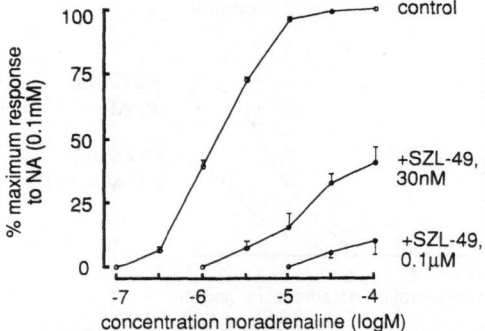

Fig. 12.11. Fitted dose response curves, contractile response of inferior epigastric artery to noradrenaline contrasting the response in the presence of differing concentrations of SZL-49 ($3 \times 10^{-8}M–10^{-7}M$).

previously attributed to the α_{1B} receptor subtype are in fact due to stimulation of the α_{1C}-adrenoceptor subtype. There is now clear evidence that the α_{1C}-adrenoceptor is the most important functional subtype in the human prostate.

Clinical Studies

Further clinical studies should utilise both comprehensive urodynamic assessment and the detailed analysis of changes in symptomatology and investigate the comparability of these two methods of assessing drug efficacy. Work needs to be directed at the investigation of drug combinations, for example, these should be directed at the investigation of the potential therapeutic efficacy of the concurrent use of selective α_1-adrenergic blockade to relax the stromal prostatic smooth muscle combined with prostate selective hormonal blockade (e.g. 5α-reductase inhibitors) to shrink the epithelium containing glandular tissue. Additional attention should be directed at parameters which could be used to identify the specific subgroups of patients likely to respond to pharmacotherapy.

References

Abrams, P.H., Shah, P.J.R., Stone, A.R., Choa, R.G. 1981. Bladder outflow obstruction treated with phenoxybenzamine. Prog. Clin. Biol. Res. 78:269–275

Abrams, P.H., Shah, P.J.R., Stone, A.R., Choa, R.G. 1982. Bladder outflow obstruction treated with phenoxybenzamine. Br. J. Urol. 54:527–530

Abrams, P.H. 1985. Detrusor instability and bladder outlet obstruction. Neurourol. Urodynamics 4:317–328

Anonymous. 1983. Phenoxybenzamine for symptoms of bladder neck obstruction. Drug. Ther. Bull. 21:15–16

Ball, A.J., Feneley, R.C.L., Abrams, P.H. 1981. The natural history of untreated prostatism. Br. J. Urol. 53:613–616

Bartsch, G., Muller, H.R., Oberholzer, M., Rohr, H.P. 1979. Light microscopic stereological analysis of the normal human prostate and of benign prostatic hyperplasia. J. Urol. 122:487

Boreham, P.F., Braithwaite, P., Milewski, P., Pearson, H. 1977. Alpha-adrenergic blockers in prostatism. Br. J. Surg. 4:756–757

Brooks, M.E., Sidi, A.A., Hanani, Y., Braf, Z.F. 1983. Ineffectiveness of phenoxybenzamine in treatment of benign prostatic hypertrophy. A controlled study. Urology 21:474–478

Bruschini, H., Schmidt, R.A., Tanagho, E.A. 1978. Neurologic control of the prostatic secretion in the dog. Invest. Urol. 15:288–290

Bruskewitcz, R.C., Larsen, E.H., Madsen, P.O., Dorflinger, T. 1986. Three-year follow-up of urinary symptoms after transurethral resection of the prostate. J. Urol. 136:613–615

Cabot, A.T. 1896. The question of castration for enlarged prostate. Ann Surg 24:265–309

Caine, M., Perlberg, S., Gordon, R. 1975. The treatment of benign prostatic hypertrophy with flutamide (SCH 13521): a placebo-controlled study. J. Urol. 114:564

Caine, M., Pfau, A., Perlberg, S. 1976. The use of alpha adrenoceptor blockers in benign prostatic obstruction. Br. J. Urol. 48:255–263

Caine, M., Perlberg, S., Meretyk, S. 1978. A placebo-controlled double-blind study of the effect of phenoxybenzamine in benign prostatic obstruction. Br. J. Urol. 50:551–554

Cambridge, D., Davey, M.J., Massingham, R. 1977. Prazosin, a selective antagonist of post-synaptic alpha-adrenoceptors. Br. J. Pharmacol. 59:514P–515P

Castro, J.E., Griffiths, H.J.L., Edwards, D.E. 1971. A double-blind, controlled, clinical trial of spirinolachtone for benign prostatic hyperplasia. Br. J. Surg. 58:485–489

Chapple, C.R., Aubry, M.L., James, S., et al. 1989. Characterisation of human prostatic adrenoceptors using pharmacology receptor binding and localisation. Br. J. Urol. 63:487–496

Chapple, C.R., Christmas, T.J., Milroy, E.J.G. 1990. A twelve-week placebo-controlled study of prazosin in the treatment of prostatic obstruction. Urol. Int. 45(suppl. 1):47–55

Chapple, C.R., Carter, P., Christmas, T.J., et al. 1991. A three-month, double-blind, placebo-controlled study of doxazosin as treatment for benign prostatic bladder outflow obstruction. Neurourol. Urodynamics 10:308–309

Chapple, C.R., Burt, R., Marshall, I. 1991. α_1-adrenoceptor subtypes in the human prostate and inferior epigastric artery. Neurourol. Urodynamics 10:306–308

Chapple, C.R., Stott, M., Abrams, P.H., Christmas, T.J., Milroy, E.J.G. 1992. A twelve-week, placebo-controlled study of prazosin in the treatment of prostatic obstruction due to benign prostatic hyperplasia. Br. J. Urol. (in press)

Chisholm, G.D. 1989. Benign prostatic hyperplasia: the best treatment. Br. Med. J. 299:215–216

Chow, W., Hahn, D., Sandhu, D., et al. 1990. Multicentre controlled trial of indoramin in the symptomatic relief of benign prostatic hypertrophy. Br. J. Urol. 65:36–38

Craigen, A.A, Hickling J.B., Saunders C.R.G., Carpenter R.G. 1969. Natural history of prostatic obstruction. J. R. Coll. Gen. Pract. 18:226–232

Donker, P.J., Ivanovici, F., Noach, E.L. 1972. Analyses of the urethral pressure profile by means of electromyography and the administration of drugs. Br. J. Urol. 44:180–193

Donkervoort, T., Zinner, N.R., Sterling, A.M., Donker, P.J., Van Ness, J., Ritter, R.C. 1975. Megesterol acetate in treatment of benign prostatic hyperplasia. Urology 6:580

Fabricius, P.G., Weizert, P., Dunzendorfer, U., MacHannaford, J., Maurath, C. 1990. Efficacy of once-a-day terazosin in benign prostatic hyperplasia: a randomised placebo controlled clinical trial. Prostate (suppl. 3):85–93

Furuya, S., Kumamoto, Y., Yokoyama, E., Tsukamoto, T., Izumi, T., Abiko, Y. 1982. Alpha-adrenergic activity and urethral pressure profilometry in prostatic zone in benign prostatic hypertrophy. J. Urol. 128:836–839

Garraway, W.M., Collins, G.N., Lee, R.J. 1991 High prevalence of benign prostatic hypertrophy in the community. Lancet 338: 469–471

Geller, J., Bora, R., Roberts, T., et al. 1965. Treatment of benign prostatic hypertrophy with hydroxyprogesterone caproate: effect on clinical symptoms, morphology and of endocrine function. JAMA 193:121

Geller, J., Nelson, C.G., Albert, J.D., Pratl, C. 1979 Effect of megesterol acetate on uroflow rates in patients with benign prostatic hypertrophy: double-blind study. Urology 14:467

Geller, J. 1989. Pathogenesis and medical treatment of benign prostatic hyperplasia. Prostate 2 (suppl.):95–104

Gerstenberg, T., Blaabjerg, J., Nielsen, M.L., Clausen, S. 1980. Phenoxybenzamine reduces bladder outlet obstruction in benign prostatic hyperplasia. A urodynamic investigation. Invest. Urol. 18:29–31

Glynn, R.J., Campion, E.W., Bouchard, G.R., Silbert, J.E., 1985. The development of benign prostatic hyperplasia among volunteers in the normative aging study. Am. J. Epidemiol. 121:78–82

Gup, D., Shapiro, E., Baumann, M. et al. 1990. Autonomic receptors in human prostate adenomas. J. Urol. 143:179–185

Hedlund, H., Andersson, K.E., Ek, A. 1983. Effects of prazosin in patients with benign prostatic obstruction. J. Urol. 130:275–278

Hedlund, H., Andersson, K.E. 1988. Effects of prazosin and carbachol in patients with benign prostatic obstruction. Scand. J. Urol. Nephrol. 22:19–22

Hedlund, H., Andersson, K.E., Larsson, B. 1985. Alpha-adrenoceptors and muscarinic receptors in the isolated human prostate. J. Urol. 134:1291–1298

Hieble, J.P., Caine, M., Zalaznik, E. 1985. In vitro characterization of the α-adrenoceptors in human prostate. Eur. J. Pharmacol. 107:111–117

Huggins, C., Stevens, R.A. 1940. The effect of castration on benign hypertrophy of the prostate in man. J. Urol. 43:705–714

Hunter, J. 1786. Observations on the glands situated between the rectum and the bladder called vesiculae seminales. In: Collected works. Vol. 14, Palmer, J.F., ed. London, Longman, p 31

Iacovou, J.W., Dunn, M. 1987. Indoramin: an effective new drug in the management of bladder outflow obstruction. Br. J. Urol. 60:526–528

Issacs, J.T. 1990. Importance of the natural history of benign prostatic hyperplasia in the evaluation of pharmacologic intervention. Prostate 3 (suppl.):1–7

James, S., Chapple, C.R., Phillips, M.I., Burnstock, G. 1989. Autoradiographic analysis of alpha-adrenoceptors and muscarinic cholinergic receptors in hyperplastic human prostate. J. Urol. 142:438–444

Jardin, A., Bensadoun, H., Delauche-Cavallier, M.C., Attali, P. 1991. Alfuzosin for treatment of benign prostatic hypertrophy 337:1457–1461

Kawabe, K., Niijima, T. 1987. Use of an α_1-blocker, YM-12617, in micturition difficulty. Urol. Int. 42:280–284

Kawabe, K., Ueno, A., Takimoto, Y., Aso, Y., Kato, H. 1990. Use of an α_1-blocker, YM617, in the treatment of benign prostatic hypertrophy. J. Urol. 144:908–912

Kirby, R.S., Coppinger, S.W.C., Corcoran, M.O., Chapple, C.R., Flannagan, M., Milroy, E.J.G. 1987. Prazosin in the treatment of prostatic obstruction: a placebo-controlled study. Br. J. Urol. 60:136–142

Kirby, R.S., Eardley, I., Bryan, J., et al. 1991. A urodynamic study of 5-α reductase inhibiters in the treatment of infra-vesical obstruction due to BPH. Neurourol. Urodynamics 10:300–301

Learmonth, J.R. 1931. A contribution to the neurophysiology of the urinary bladder in man. Brain 54:147–176

Le Duc, A., Cariou, G., Baron, J.C., et al. 1990. A multicenter, double-blind, placebo-controlled study of the efficacy of prazosin in the treatment of dysuria associated with benign prostatic hypertrophy. Urol. Int. 45(suppl. 1):56–62

Lepor, H. 1989. Non-operative management of benign prostatic hyperplasia. J. Urol. 141:1283–1289

Lepor, H., Knapp-Maloney, G., Sunshine, H. 1990. A dose titration study evaluating terazosin, a selective, once-a-day α_1-blocker for the treatment of symptomatic benign prostatic hyperplasia. J. Urol. 144:1393–1398

Lepor, H., Knapp-Maloney, G. 1991. Outcome assessment of terazosin for benign prostatic hyperplasia (BPH): 18-month follow-up. J. Urol. 145:263A

Lepor, H., Kuhar, M.J. 1984. Characterization and localization of the muscarinic cholinergic receptor in human prostatic tissue. J. Urol. 132:397–402

Lepor, H., Shapiro, E. 1984. Characterization of α-1 adrenergic receptors in human prostatic hyperplasia. J. Urol. 132:1226–1229

Levine, A.C., Kirschenbaum, A., Kaplan, P., Droller, M.J., Gabrilove J.L. 1989. Serum prostate-antigen levels in patients with benign prostatic hyperplasia treated with leuprolide. Urology 34:10

Martorana, G., Giberti, C., Damonte, P., et al. 1984. The effect of prazosin in benign prostatic hypertrophy: a placebo-controlled double-blind study. IRCS Med. Sci. 12:11–12

Matzkin, H., Chen, J., Lewysohn, O., Braf, Z. 1991. Treatment of benign prostatic hypertrophy by a long-acting gonadotropin-releasing hormone analogue: 1-year experience. J. Urol. 145:309–312

Mebust, W.K. 1988. Surgical management of benign prostatic obstruction. Urology 32:12

Meyhoff, H.H. 1987. Transurethral versus transvesical prostatectomy: clinical, urodynamic, renographic and economic aspects. A randomised study. Scand J Urol Nephrol (Suppl) 102:1

Meiraz, D., Margolin, Y., Lev-Ran, A., Lazebnik, J. 1977. Treatment of benign prostatic hyperplasia with hydroxyprogesterone-caproate: placebo-controlled study. Urology 9:144

Minneman, K.P. 1988. α_1-Adrenergic receptor sub-types, inositol phosphates and sources of cell calcium. Pharmacol. Rev. 40:87–119

Moore, R.A. 1944. Benign hypertrophy and carcinoma of the prostate: occurrence and experimental production in animals. Surgery 16:152–167

Noble, J.G., Chapple, C.R., Milroy, E.J.G. 1991. Long-term selective α_1-adrenoceptor blockade versus surgery in the treatment of benign prostatic hyperplasia. Neurourol. Urodynamics 10:296–298

Perlberg, S., Caine, M. 1982. Adrenergic response of bladder muscle in prostatic obstruction. Urology 20:524–527

Peters, C.A., Walsh, P.C. 1987. The effect of nafarelin acetate, a luteinizing hormone-releasing hormone agonist, on benign prostatic hyperplasia. N. Engl. J. Med. 317:599

Piascik, M.T., Butler, B.T., Pruitt, T.A., Kusiak, J.W. 1990. Agonist interaction with alkylation-sensitive and resistant α_1-adrenoceptor subtypes. J. Pharmacol. Exp. Ther. 204:982–991

Ramsay, J.W.A., Scott, G.I., Whitfield, H.N. 1985. A double-blind controlled trial of a new α^{-1} blocking drug in the treatment of bladder outflow obstruction. Br. J. Urol. 57:657–659

Roos, N.P., Wennberg, J.E, Malenka D.J., et al. 1989. Mortality and re-operation after open and transurethral resection of the prostate for benign prostatic hyperplasia. N. Engl. J. Med. 320:1120–1123

Schweikert, H.U., Tunn, U.W. 1987. Effects of the aromatase inhibitor testolactone on human benign prostatic hyperplasia. Steroids 50:191–199

Scott, W.W., Wade, J.C. 1969. Medical treatment of benign prostatic hyperplasia with cyproterone acetate. J. Urol. 101:89

Shapiro, E., Lepor, H. 1986. Alpha-2 adrenergic receptors in hyperplastic human prostate: identification and characterisation using (3H) Rauwolscine. J. Urol. 135:1038–1042

Shapiro, A., Mazouz, B., Caine, M. 1981. The α-adrenergic effect of prazosin on the human prostate. Urol. Res. 9:17–20

Shapiro, E., Tsitlik, J.E., Lepor, H. 1987. Alpha-2 adrenergic receptors in canine prostate: biochemical and functional correlation. J. Urol. 137:565–570

Stoner, E. (1991) Phase III studies evaluating 5α-reductase inhibitor and proscar. J. Urol. 145:57A

Stott, M.A., Abrams, P.H. 1991. Indoramin in the treatment of prostatic bladder outflow obstruction. Br. J. Urol. 67:499–501

Straughan, J.L. 1978. Urinary incontinence with prazosin. S. Afr. Med. J. 53:882

Thien, T., Delaere, K.P., Debruyne, F.M., et al. 1978. Urinary incontinence caused by prazosin. Br. Med. J. ii:622–623

Tunn, U.W., Kaivers, P., Schweikert, H.U. 1985. Conservative treatment for benign prostatic
    hyperplasia. In: Regulation of androgen action. Bruchovsky, N., Chapdeleine, A., Newmann,
    F. eds. West Berlin, Congressdruck R. Bruckner, pp 87–90
Vaalasti, A., Hervonen, A. 1980. Autonomic innervation of the human prostate. Invest.
    Urol. 17:293–297
Wein, A.J. 1989. Prazosin in the treatment of prostatic obstruction. Editorial review. J.
    Urol. 141:693–694
White, J.W. 1895. The results of double castration in hypertrophy of the prostate. Ann.
    Surg. 22:1–80
Zuckerman, S. 1936. The endocrine control of the prostate. Proc. R. Soc. Med. 29:1557–1568

Chapter 13

Bladder Neck Dyssynergia and Prostatitis

J.G. Noble

The term "bladder neck obstruction" is widely used in clinical practice to describe a variety of conditions which cause voiding dysfunction at the level of the outlet of the bladder. The term is non-specific and therefore is open to misinterpretation, often being used to describe a specific lesion affecting the bladder neck mechanism itself, lesions causing outflow obstruction at the level of the bladder neck (these include all forms of prostatic enlargement) or rarely nowadays the term is used to denote bladder outflow obstruction in general without any distinction between proximal and distal location. (Turner-Warwick, 1973) (Table 13.1).

The pathophysiology of outflow obstruction secondary to prostatic hypertrophy has been discussed previously (Chapter 4). This chapter reviews the conditions of "bladder neck dyssynergia" and "prostatitis".

Bladder Neck Dyssynergia

It has long been recognised that urinary outflow obstruction can occur in the absence of prostatic enlargement but is was not until 1836 that Guthrie described a specific condition of bladder neck obstruction. He suggested that the condition was secondary to inflammation at the bladder neck producing contraction and loss of elasticity. He also noted that it could

Table 13.1. Causes of male bladder neck obstruction

Bladder neck	Bladder neck dyssynergia
	Bladder neck hypertrophy (detrusor hypertrophy)
	Fibrosis/stenosis (iatrogenic)
	Foreign body (e.g. stones)
Prostate	Infection: acute/chronic prostatitis
	Neoplasia: BPH, carcinoma
Urethra	Congenital urethral valves
	Congenital urethral hypoplasia
	Urethral stricture

occur in an early period of life and was often associated with the formation of "bladder pouches". Subsequently Mercier (1933) in France commented that the underlying problem was due to lack of bladder tone and atrophy of the detrusor muscle rather than outflow obstruction and the term "prostatisme sans prostate" was popularised. In America, Keyes, Fuller and Chetwood (Chetwood, 1913) recognised an obstructive condition of the bladder neck and considered it due to contracture or stricture within the prostatic urethra. In 1913, Young reported 52 cases of whom 17 were under 50 years of age.

Marion reported four cases of bladder neck obstruction in 1933 noting that all had had symptoms since adolescence and considered that the condition was caused by hypertrophy of the bladder neck musculature. He was the first worker to suggest that the condition was congenital in origin and to this day bladder neck obstruction is commonly referred to as "Marion's disease". Badenoch delivered a Hunterian Lecture in 1948 on the subject of bladder neck obstruction and agreed with the findings of Marion that the condition was probably congenital in origin and due to muscle hypertrophy probably analogous to congenital pyloric stenosis and cardiospasm.

It was not until the establishment of synchronous cine/pressure/flow cystography in the late 1960s that the concept of a functional rather than mechanical cause of bladder neck obstruction was raised. Turner-Warwick (1973) described in detail the urodynamic features of the condition and along with Bates (1975) provided evidence that the bladder neck muscle actively tightens during voiding; so-called bladder neck dyssynergia (BND). Despite this evidence no suitable model for bladder neck dysfunction has been demonsrated in functional studies and the mechanism for active contraction/relaxation of bladder neck smooth muscle remains unclear (Hills, 1984; Walker, 1985, Klarskov, 1987).

Bladder Neck Function

Under normal circumstances the bladder neck acts as an important sphincter remaining closed at rest and not normally opened by straining. The exact anatomical arrangement of the bladder neck sphincter remains a matter for debate but the most modern and acceptable theory suggests a true smooth muscle sphincter which is different in morphology and innervation from the detrusor and which contracts in a reciprocal rather than similar fashion. (Abrams, 1981) In the male the bladder neck seems to act as a sphincter which contracts during ejaculation preventing the reflux of semen into the bladder. In the female the bladder neck muscle is less well developed and is probably functionally unimportant (Chapple, 1989).

The smooth muscle of the bladder neck contains many α-adrenergic receptors and contracts in response to noradrenaline (Walker, 1985; Torrens, 1975). The observation that patients with BND occasionally have anxious personality characteristics and associated features of increased sympathetic activity, e.g. sweating, flushing, has led to the theory that the underlying disorder may be associated with high levels of circulating sympathomimetics and/or increased numbers of adrenoceptors. Certainly current research in our own department confirms that there is a significant level of anxiety within these patients

(Fig. 13.1) and work is in progress to demonstrate or refute the theory of autonomic overactivity (Methias, 1991, personal communication).

Clinical Features

The typical patient is male, aged between 20 and 60 years of age, who complains of symptoms of urinary outflow obstruction, i.e. hesitancy, poor urinary stream, terminal dribbling and incomplete bladder emptying. The age of presentation is considerably younger than that associated with prostatic pathology. However, many patients have a lifelong history of BND and therefore may not recognise these classical symptoms regarding their own stream as totally normal. Even on direct questioning these features may not become apparent. The commonest feature is the recognition that their urinary stream has never been "competitive" in comparison to others, i.e. voiding times in public, school games, etc. Some patients have visited psychiatric departments with an inability to void in the company of others in public lavatories; a symptom which can cause considerable stress and inconvenience. These symptoms should not regarded as functional until an organic cause has been excluded with urodynamic evaluation.

Occasionally patients present with urinary tract infections or symptoms attributable to "prostatitis". The differentiation of prostatitis and bladder neck dyssynergia is often extremely difficult on clinical grounds and indeed in 10% of patients with BND the conditions coexist. Approximately 50% of patients develop secondary detrusor instability such that irritative symptoms of frequency, urgency and nocturia may predominate.

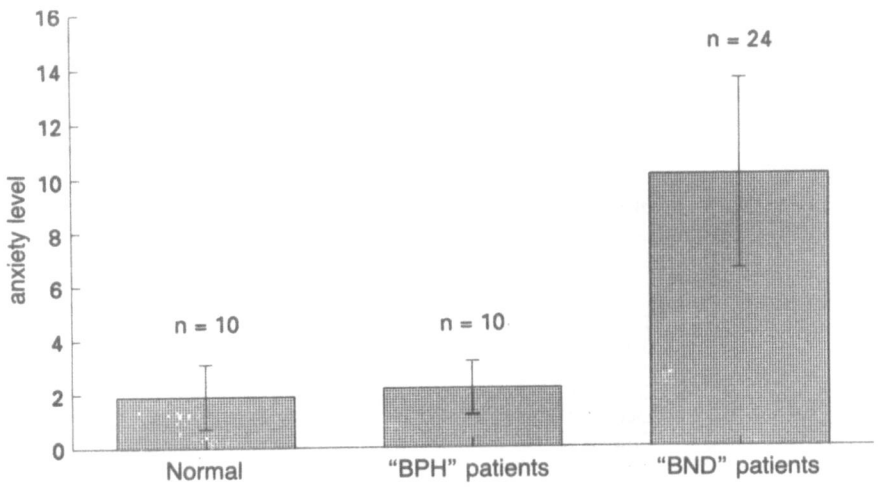

Fig. 13.1.   Chart comparing anxiety levels in age-matched groups of normal males, males with BPH, and males with BND

The combination of prostatic enlargement superimposed on subclinical BND is a common situation and should be suspected in patients who have relatively minor degrees of prostatic enlargement associated with a comparatively rapid onset of symptoms of outflow obstruction. In these conditions the lateral lobes of the prostate expand into the mid-prostatic urethra but fail to expand the bladder neck, and therefore a relatively small enlargement of the prostate gland augments the pre-existing outflow obstruction to a significant degree. This condition has been termed the "trapped prostate" and patients commonly respond well to treatment because resection of both the bladder neck and prostate relieves both recent prostatic obstruction and hitherto unrecognised life-long bladder neck obstruction. Post-operatively these patients with "double obstruction" often declare with delight that they have never voided so well.

Examination is usually entirely normal with the observation of a normal prostate gland on digital examination. Occasionally the bladder may be palpable in older patients who have detrusor decompensation has occurred secondary to long-term outflow obstruction.

Investigation

Patients presenting with the clinical features described require careful assessment to evaluate possible urological pathology (Table 13.2). These symptoms should never be ignored on the basis that the patient appears neurotic and is "too young" to have developed prostatic disease.

The importance of uroflowmetry in the diagnosis of BND cannot be over-emphasised as the great majority of patients will demonstrate an impaired voiding pattern even if they have failed to recognise the fact themselves. Uroflowmetry must be carried out in an private, non-stressful environment; the classical exercise of watching them void merely may inhibit micturition altogether. The voiding pattern alone is a helpful but non-specific indicator of the underlying pathology and should not, therefore be over-interpreted. However, certain patterns are highly suggestive of a particular lesion (Fig. 13.2). In cases where there is a strong suspicion of prostatitis it is essential to record the flow rate to avoid overlooking a treatable element of obstruction. However, it is prudent to check flow rates in between attacks of inflammation which may themselves create a mild outflow obstruction.

Table 13.2. Differential diagnosis of bladder neck dyssynergia

Detrusor-sphincter dyssynergia
Detrusor failure
Primary detrusor instability
Bladder neoplasia
Bladder neck stenosis/fibrosis
Urethral stricture
Psychogenic voiding dysfunction

Upper tract function is not normally compromised but should be assessed as part of a general investigation of the urinary system. Traditionally the intravenous urodynamogram has been used to confirm upper tract normality (this information is of vital importance if conservative treatment is planned); however, in our practice, we increasingly rely on ultrasonography as a reliable, safe and better tolerated investigation (Webb, 1990).

Cystourethroscopy is a mandatory investigation whose primary importance is to exclude other pathology, e.g. bladder neoplasia, and certainly conservative treatment should never be recommended unless endoscopy is normal. There are no endoscopic appearances by which a dyssynergic bladder neck can be unequivocally identified or excluded. So-called bladder neck hypertrophy is often described at endoscopy but does not necessarily constitute BND. Global hypertrophy of the detrusor and bladder neck musculature secondary to outflow obstruction, e.g. urethral stricture, does not result in a dyssynergic bladder neck mechanism. Thus the behaviour of the bladder neck cannot be assessed accurately by endoscopic evaluation as it does not permit observation of bladder neck opening and closing during micturition (Turner-Warwick, 1973).

With the development and refinement of urodynamic studies in the late 1960s more accurate assessment of lower urinary tract function became avaliable. The details of urodynamics are discussed in Chapter 1. Videocystometrography (VCMG) has the great advantage over simple inflow and outflow cystometry of demonstrating not only the presence of outflow obstruction (i.e. high pressure/low flow rate voiding) but also the actual site of obstruction whether it be at the bladder neck, prostate or distal sphincter. During the filling phase of the investigation approximately 50% of patients will demonstrate detrusor instability and many will have an increased cystometric bladder capacity probably related to detrusor decompensation reflecting the chronicity of the obstruction. Bladder trabeculation and diverticulae are also

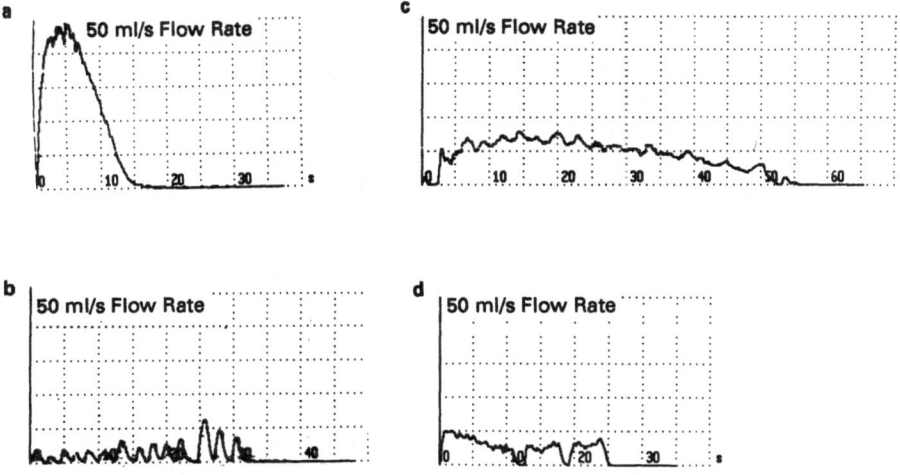

Fig. 13.2. Voiding flow patterns: **a** normal pattern; **b** detrusor failure with evidence of abdominal straining; **c** bladder neck dyssynergia; **d** stricture.

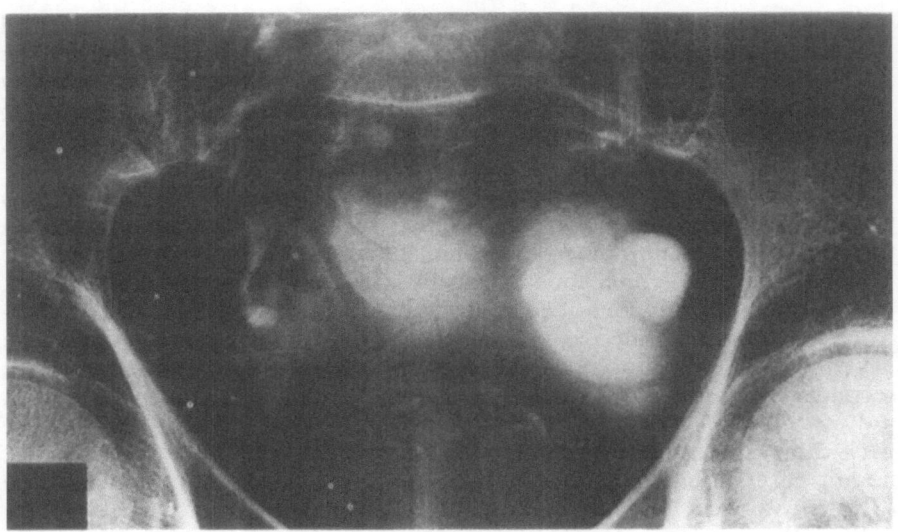

Fig. 13.3. Cystogram of a patient with BND showing extensive bladder trabeculation and diverticula.

often pronounced and are well demonstrated on VCMG (Fig. 13.3). As soon as micturition commences the recording of high pressure/low flow indicates the presence of outflow obstruction and the patient is then asked to interrupt his urinary flow; the so-called stop test. This is achieved by voluntary contraction of the distal sphincter mechanism and under normal circumstances urine/contrast is "milked" back into the bladder through the bladder neck which then closes. If the patient has BND then the bladder neck can not only be seen to cause outflow obstruction during voiding, but also prevents normal milk-back. Contrast is then seen to be "trapped" within the prostatic urethra (Fig. 13.4), this appearance being known as a positive Whiteside sign (Turner-Warwick and Whiteside, 1969). This appearance confirms the bladder neck as the site of the obstruction and excludes prostatic obstruction by virtue of a readily distensible prostatic urethra.

Urethral pressure profilometry adds little to the diagnosis of BND as recordings are made during filling and not voiding and it has been suggested that the resting pressure within the bladder neck regions remain normal in patients with BND (Bates, 1975).

Transrectal ultrasound (TRUS) is increasingly being used in evaluating lower urinary tract anatomy and we have recently studied the appearances of the bladder neck region in patients with BND. To date 53 male patients aged 24–67 years (mean = 41 ± 4.4), with the clinical and urodynamic features of BND, have undergone TRUS using a 7 MHz Aloka linear array probe. The findings have been compared with TRUS appearances in 170 male patients aged 21–85 years (mean = 54 ± 5.2) who underwent urodynamic assessment without evidence of BND; prostate obstruction $n = 95$, normal VCMG $n = 55$. In 23/54 of the patients with BND studied, biopsies of the bladder neck have been taken with an

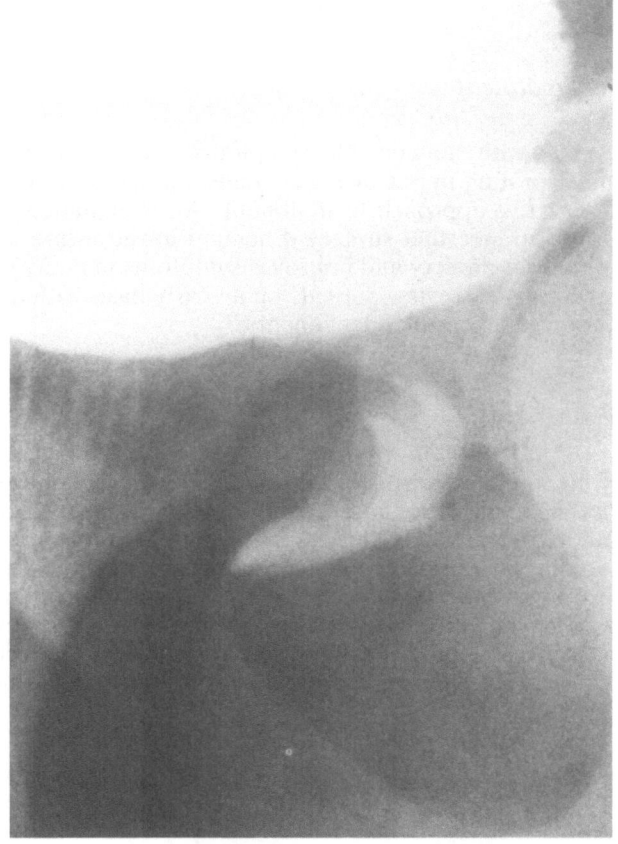

Fig. 13.4. "Stop test" during voiding phase of videocystometrography showing classical Whiteside trapping.

18G "trucut needle" via the transperineal route under ultrasound control (Fig. 13.5). These biopsy specimens have been assessed both histologically and functionally. In all of the patients studied with BND an ovoid, echo-poor area was seen in the bladder neck region which was absent in the other patient groups (Fig. 13.6). The position of the urethra was identified by a reference catheter inserted prior to VCMG and showed the area to be predominantly anterior to the urethra. Areas of intraduct prostatic calcification have also been identified suggesting intraprostatic reflux which may provide an explanation for the coexistence of prostatitis in approximately 10% of patients with BND (Turner-Warwick, 1979). The diameter of this area varied between 10 and 26 mm (mean = 17 ± 4.5mm). These specific features of BND have not been previously reported and potentially provide an effective, safe, well tolerated and cheap method of diagnosing BND without the use of specialised urodynamic investigation (Rickards, 1991).

Treatment

Conservative Treatment

In young patients with manageable symptoms and in whom there is no evidence of deteriorating upper or lower tract function then it is reasonable to offer a conservative approach to treatment. An explanation of the condition along with assurance that surgery if needed in the future is simple and curative often relieves anxiety and improves symptoms in many patients. It is usually only necessary to review patients on a yearly basis with an ultrasound cystodynamogram to assess bladder function.

Medical Treatment

As previously mentioned it seems that bladder neck smooth muscle contracts primarily under the influence of noradrenaline acting on α_1-adrenoceptors and theoretically therefore blocking this response may help to relax the bladder neck during voiding. The selective α_1-adrenoceptor antagonist prazosin has been shown to have some beneficial effects in the treatment of BND and certainly causes fewer cardiovascular side effects than the non-specific α antagonist phenoxybenzamine (Hedlund, 1989). However the results of long-term therapy are less convincing and at present therapy should be limited to

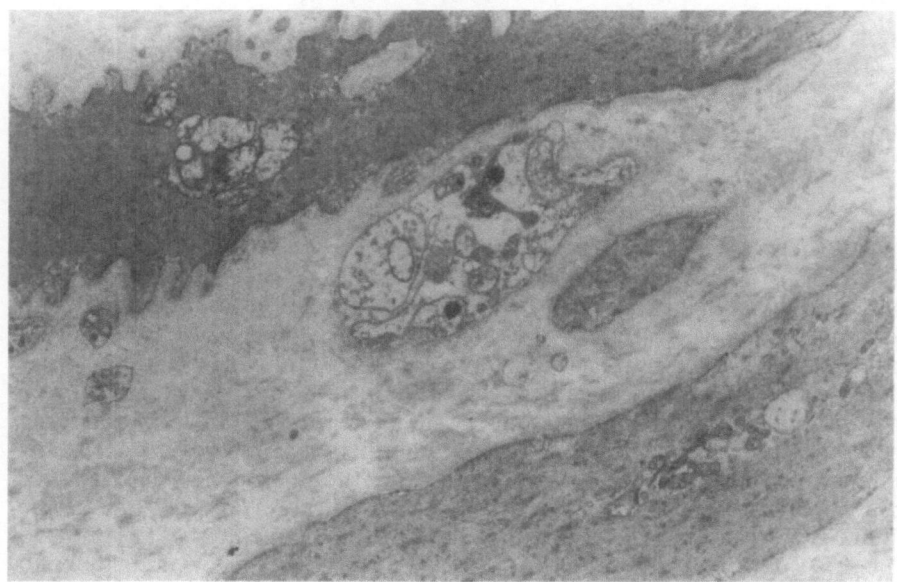

Fig. 13.5. Histological examination of bladder neck smooth muscle.

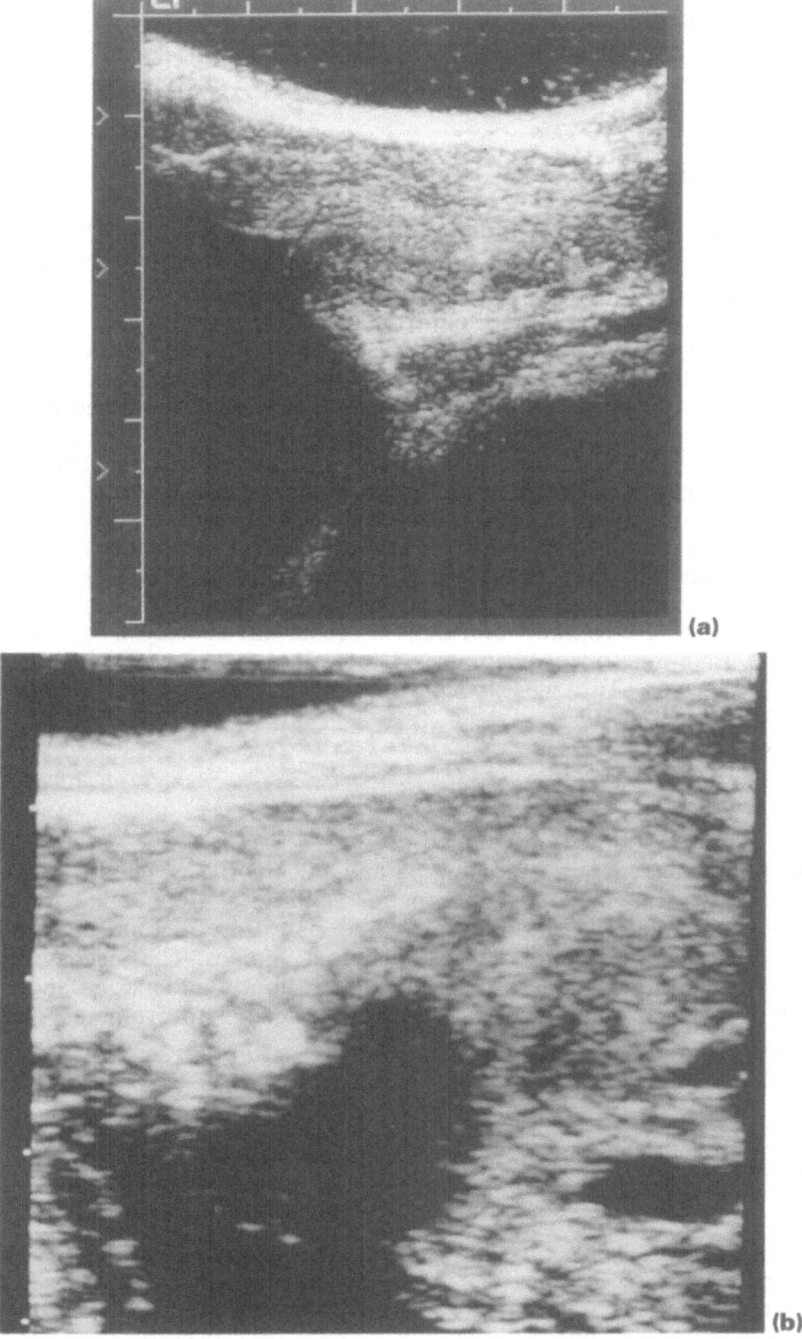

Fig. 13.6. Transrectal ultrasound appearances of the bladder neck: **a** normal, **b** bladder neck dyssynergia.

those patients planning a family, in whom surgery is contraindicated because of the risk of retrograde ejaculation and subsequent infertility. Undoubtedly more research is needed into the mechanism of bladder neck contraction and relaxation with the aim of developing more effective pharmacotherapy.

Surgical Treatment

The definitive treatment for BND is endoscopic incision of the full thickness of the bladder neck (BNI) in one or more positions with a Collins knife electrode (Turner-Warwick, 1973). The 5 or 7 o'clock incision is preferable as these avoid the veins within the prostatic capsule and thus avoid excessive bleeding. The cut is made from just distal to the ureteric orifice towards the verumontanum down to perivesical fat and the bladder neck is seen to spring open as the cut is deepened. Haemostasis should be carried out with the bladder empty so that larger bleeding vessels may not escape detection. Post-operative recovery is usually rapid with the catheter being removed after 24–48 hours and the patient returning home shortly afterwards.

The results of surgery are generally excellent and provided the incision is sufficiently deep the urinary flow rate is nearly always improved. Associated symptoms and especially those where coexistent prostatitis is evident are less commonly improved and patients should be made aware of this fact pre-operatively. Retrograde ejaculation occurs in 14%–16% of patients following BNI and once again it is imperative to warn patients of this effect in all cases (Turner-Warwick, 1973; Moisey et al. 1983; Delaere et al. 1983; Jonas et al. 1979)

Summary

Bladder neck dyssynergia is a common and still poorly recognised cause of outflow obstruction in young male patients. Surgical treatment with BNI is simple and effective but does carry the risk of retrograde ejaculation which is of special relevance to those planning families. The mechanism of normal and abnormal bladder neck function is poorly understood and thus further anatomical and functional research is needed to evaluate possible pharmacotherapeutic treatment.

Prostatitis

In recent years the pathophysiology and pathogenesis of various forms of prostatitis have become clearer. However, the aetiology of non-bacterial prostatitis and of the non-inflamed painful prostate remains poorly understood. The classification of the various forms of prostatitis has recently been revised (Drach et al. 1978) and depends upon objective features in the expressed prostatic secretion (EPS; Table 13.3).

Pathogenesis

The prostate is most commonly infected by an ascending pathway from the urethra. Support for this theory is based upon the fact that organisms found in the introitus and vagina of the sexual partners of patients with prostatitis have also been isolated and are from EPS specimens. These organisms may be asymptomatic within the urethra or may be the cause of urethritis as demonstrated by the association of prostatitis with gonococcal urethritis in 30% of cases (Thin, 1974). The progression of infection from the urethra to the prostate seems to be associated with turbulent flow within the prostatic urethra and it has been shown that spasm within the external sphincter, for whatever cause, may lead to prostatitis. The gland itself is infected via the prostatic ducts; the most vulnerable being those from the peripheral zone where the mode of entry into the urethra is non-valvular, i.e. perpendicular to or obliquely against the direction of flow. This has been confirmed in studies showing that the peripheral zone is most commonly affected in prostatitis whereas the central zone, whose ducts open obliquely into the urethra in the direction of flow, is spared. Outflow obstruction caused by phenomena other than external sphincter "spasm" produces turbulence in a similar way and also predisposes to prostatitis, e.g. urethral stricture and, in cases of bladder neck dyssynergia, 10% of patients develop symptoms of prostatitis presumably secondary to high intraprostatic urethral pressures on interrupting the flow of urine at the end of micturition (see "Whiteside sign" above).

The rate of detecting bacteria in EPS is not high with figures varying between 48.5% and 30% depending on whether the inclusion of *Staphylococcus albus* is considered relevant. The pathogenicity of this organism in prostatitis is the subject of much debate. The high incidence of negative culture in cases of prostatitis raises the question of a viral aetiology and the presence of high levels of IgA and IgM in such patients, even during periods of symptomatic regression, supports this argument along with possible autoimmunity (Gray et al. 1974). The most common organisms isolated are listed in Table 13.4.

Prostatic calculi are frequently seen in association with prostatitis and may be classified as either intrinsic or extrinsic. The intrinsic stones are formed from prostatic secretion and may represent normal progression of the corpora amylacea which predominate in the central zone. Extrinsic calculi are formed from elements which are found in the urine and are probably associated with a degree of reflux into prostatic ducts. Both types of stone may act as a nidus for infection and thus predispose to recurrence and chronicity (Blacklock, 1985).

Table 13.3. Classification of prostatitis

Acute bacterial prostatitis
Chronic bacterial prostatitis
Non-bacterial prostatitis
Prostatodynia
Psychogenic voiding dysfunction

Clinical Features

Patients usually present with the symptoms of prostatitis in early adult life corresponding to the period of maximum sexual activity. Acute bacterial prostatitis presents with a short history of general malaise with or without a fever associated with dysuria and urinary frequency. Pain may be localised suprapubically or to the perineum and is variable in severity. Haematuria may supervene as the attack progresses. In chronic bacterial prostatitis the symptoms are less dramatic and usually the patient presents with a history of relapsing bouts of pain and urinary difficulties. Pain on ejaculation is not an uncommon feature. Non-bacterial prostatitis is similar in presentation to chronic bacterial prostatitis and prostatodynia is characterised by persistent "prostatic" pain associated with a wide variety of urinary symptoms. These patients are often tense, anxious individuals with multiple symptoms and complaints.

General examination may confirm that the patient is unwell with a tachycardia and pyrexia but is otherwise unhelpful. Digital palpation of the prostate will be exquisitely tender in acute exacerbations of the disease but is not otherwise unduly painful. The prostate may feel nodular in more chronic disease.

Investigations

The diagnosis of bacterial prostatitis is obtained on analysis of three samples as described by Meares and Stamey (1968). The first 10 ml of voided urine is collected along with a midstream sample. A prostatic massage specimen is then obtained and the first 10 ml of urine voided thereafter is collected. In prostatitis the leucocyte and bacterial counts are low in the first two specimens but significantly higher in the post-massage specimen. The pH of the prostatic fluid seems to be raised in cases of prostatitis and should be requested on each sample obtained as it may provide a useful indicator as to the activity of the disease at a particular time. In chronic forms of the disease the sexual partner of the patient should be interviewed and relevant swabs obtained as this may prove to be the source of reinfection.

TRUS is a relatively new investigation which allows visualisation of foci of inflammation within the gland and can aid planned surgical drainage by localising abscesses etc. (Fig. 13.7).

Table 13.4 Common pathogens isolated in prostatic fluid from patients with prostatitis

Staphylococcus albus?
Staphylococcus aureus
Coliforms and other faecal organisms
Chlamydia trachomatis
Ureaplasma urealyticum

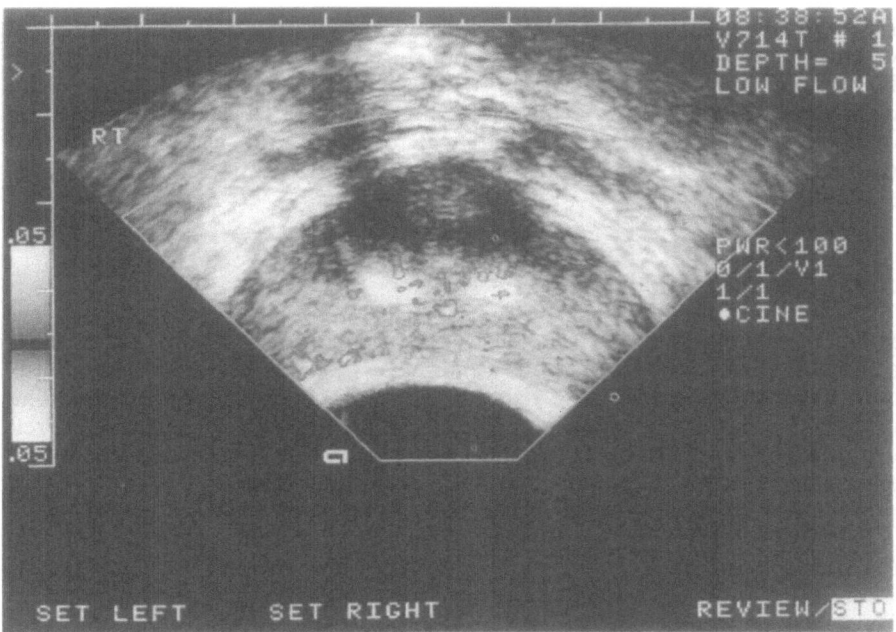

Fig. 13.7.   Transrectal ultrasound appearance of prostatitis.

All patients should undergo careful urological investigation to evaluate possible underlying pathology which may have predisposed to an attack of prostatitis, e.g. urethral stricture, bladder neck dyssynergia, etc.

Treatment

Acute Bacterial Prostatitis

Antibiotics form the mainstay of treatment along with simple analgesia and bed rest. Most of the common organisms are sensitive to trimethoprim and this drug is well distributed within the prostate gland after absorption. Treatment should be continued for at least 2 weeks and not stopped until there is good clinical evidence of regression of the inflammation. *Staphylococcus albus* infections are probably best treated with erythromycin until relevant sensitivities are obtained. The role of long-term antibiotic administration, e.g. Nitrofurantoin to prevent repeated attacks of prostatitis, has not been fully evaluated.

Chronic Bacterial Prostatitis

The choice of antibiotics in the treatment of chronic bacterial prostatitis should generally be influenced by the results of sensitivities of organisms grown from

EPS. Once again trimethoprim or various forms of tetracyclines are most often effective but they must be administered for at least 2 to 3 months to be sure of eradicating the infection. Chronic foci of infection may require drainage endoscopically and the use of TRUS facilitates accurate localisation of these lesions. Regular bacteriological review of EPS is required so that the identification of resistant organisms whilst on therapy can be made at an early stage.

Non-bacterial Prostatitis

It has been suggested that the cause of non-bacterial prostatitis stems from a viral infection with or without *Chlamydia trachomatis* and on this basis it is reasonable to treat these patients with anti-chlamydial antibiotics. The preferred drugs are doxycycline or monocycline and should be administered for at least 1 month to be of benefit. Once again close follow-up is needed to ensure eradication of the infection and/or superinfection.

Prostatodynia

These patients are generally extremely difficult to treat and certainly there is no justification for the injudicious use of long-term antibiotics, in the absence of evidence of a bacterial infection, in the hope that this will improve symptoms. The theory that there is a functional cause for the symptoms has been reinforced by the finding of elevated frontalis muscle electromyogram levels and pulse and respiration rates in some patients. This may be associated with voluntary or involuntary spasm of the urethral sphincter and account for prostatodynia symptomatology (Florante, 1980). On this basis both striated muscle relaxants, e.g. baclofen and α-adrenoceptor blockade have been used to treat this condition with success in some instances (Osborn et al. 1981).

With the advent of more effective culture techniques and antibiotics and a better understanding of the pathogenesis of the disease, complications arising from prostatitis are less commonly seen (Table 13.5).

Summary

Prostatitis is a common condition causing considerable morbidity in some cases. Careful and planned investigation will reveal the infecting agent in approximately 40% of cases allowing appropriate antibiotic therapy and relief of symptoms. Unfortunately in the majority of cases, symptoms return

Table 13.5. Complications of prostatitis

Prostatic abscess
Chronic bacterial prostatitis
Epididymo-orchitis
Pyelonephritis

at regular intervals and persist in some cases without culture of organisms from the prostate gland. These patients are notoriously difficult to treat but therapy with striated and smooth muscle relaxants may prove to be of benefit. Psychotherapy seems to be of help in those patients with prostatodynia where neurosis and anxiety are predominant features.

References

Abrams, P.H. 1981. Voiding disorders in the younger male patient. Urology 18:107–110

Badenoch, A.W. 1948. Congenital obstruction at the bladder neck. Ann. R. Coll. Surg. Engl. 4:295–307

Bates, C.P. 1975. The nature of the abnormality in bladder neck obstruction. Br. J. Urol. 47:651–656

Blacklock, N.J. 1985. Prostatitis. In: Textbook of genito-urinary surgery. Whitfield, Hendry, eds. 48:526–535

Buck, A.C. 1975. Disorders of micturition in bacterial prostatitis. Proc. R. Soc. Med. 68:508–511

Chapple, C.R. 1989. Asymptomatic bladder neck incompetence in nulliparous females. Br. J. Urol. 64:357–359

Chetwood, C.H. 1913. Contracture of the neck of the bladder. J.A.M.A. 60:265

Delaere, K.P.J., et al. 1983. Extended bladder neck incision for outflow obstruction in male patients. Br. J. Urol. 55:225–228

Drach G.W. 1974. Problems in the diagnosis of bacterial prostatitis: gram-negative, gram-positive and mixed infections. J. Urol. 111:630–636

Drach, G.W., et al. 1978. Classification of benign diseases associated with prostatic pain; prostatitis or prostatodynia? J. Urol. 120:266

Florante, J. 1980. Baclofen in the treatment of detrusor-sphincter dyssynergia in spinal cord injury patients. J. Urol. 124:82–84

Gray, S.P., et al. 1974. Distribution of immunoglobulins G, A and M in the prostatic fluid of patients with prostatitis. Clin. Chim. Acta 57:163–169

Guthrie, G.J. 1836. On the anatomy and disease of the urinary and sexual organs. London, Churchill, p 60

Hedlund, H. 1989. Effects of prazosin in men with symptoms of bladder neck obstruction and a non-hyperplastic prostate. Scand. J. Urol. Nephrol. 23:251–254

Hills, J. 1984. A novel non-adrenergic, non-cholinergic nerve-mediated relaxation of the pig bladder neck: an examination of possible neurotransmitter candidates. Eur. J. Pharmacol. 99:287–293

Jonas, U., et al. 1979. Indications and value of bladder neck incision. Urol. Int. 34:395–397

Klarskov, P. 1987. Non-cholinergic, non-adrenergic nerve mediated relaxation of pig and human detrusor muscle in vitro. Br. J. Urol. 59:414–419

Marion, G. 1933. Surgery of the neck of the bladder. Br. J. Urol. 5:351

McNeal, J. 1968. Regional morphology and pathology of the prostate. Am. J. Clin. Pathol. 49:347–357

Meares, E.M., Stamey, T.A. 1968. Bacteriologic localisation patterns in bacterial prostatitis and urethritis. Invest. Urol. 5:492–518

Mercier, L.A. 1933. In: History of urology. Baltimore, Williams and Wilkins, p 93

Moisey, C.U., et al. 1983. A subjective and urodynamic assessment of unilateral bladder neck incision for bladder neck obstruction. Br. J. Urol. 54:114–117

Osborn, D.E., et al. 1981. Prostatodynia: physiological characteristics and their rational management with muscle relaxants. Br. J. Urol. 53:621–623

Rickards, D. 1991. Bladder neck dyssynergia in the male: a new finding on transrectal ultrasonography. J. Urol. 145:369A

Thin, R.W.T. 1974. Prostatitis after urethritis in Singapore. Br. J. Vener. Dis. 50:370–372

Torrens M.J. 1975. Communication to the Vth Annual Meeting of the ICS, Glasgow

Turner-Warwick, R.T. Bladder outflow obstruction in the male. Urodynamics 19:184–203

Turner-Warwick, R.T., Whiteside, C.G. 1969. Investigation and management of bladder neck dysfunction. In: Modern trends in urology. Riches E., ed. London, Butterworth, pp 295–311

Turner-Warwick, R.T. 1973. A urodynamic view of the clinical problems associated with bladder neck dysfunction and its treatment by endoscopic incision and trans-trigonal posterior prostatectomy. Br. J. Urol. 45:44–59

Turner-Warwick, R.T. 1979. Observations on the function and dysfunction of the sphincter and detrusor mechanisms. Urol. Clin. North Am. 6:13–30

Walker, J. 1985. Responses of isolated smooth muscle from the human bladder neck. Proc. 15th Int. Continence Soc., pp 168–169

Webb, J.A.W. 1990. Ultrasonography in the diagnosis of renal obstruction. Br. Med. J. 301:944–946

Young, H.H. 1913. A new procedure (punch operation) for small prostatic bars and contracture of the prostatic orifice. J.A.M.A. 16:253–257

Subject Index